THE MEDICAL LIBRARY ASSOCIATION

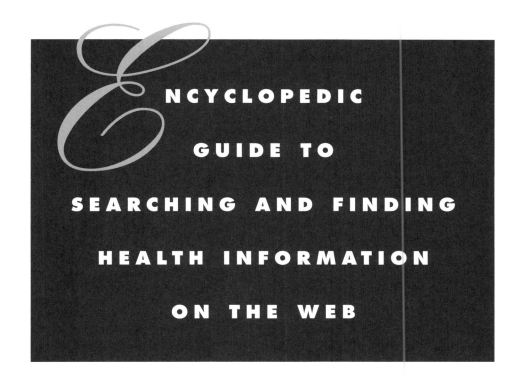

*E*NCYCLOPEDIC

GUIDE TO

SEARCHING AND FINDING

HEALTH INFORMATION

ON THE WEB

VOLUME 3:

HEALTH AND WELLNESS/
LIFE STAGES AND REPRODUCTION/
CUMULATIVE INDEX

Edited by

P. F. Anderson and Nancy J. Allee

Neal-Schuman Publishers, Inc.

New York   *London*

The Medical Library Association Encyclopedic Guide to Searching and Finding Health Information on the Web

Volume 1. Search Strategies/Quick Reference Guide
Volume 2. Diseases and Disorders/Mental Health and Mental Disorders
Volume 3. Health and Wellness/Life Stages and Reproduction/Cumulative Index

Published by Neal-Schuman Publishers, Inc.
100 William Street, Suite 2004
New York, NY 10038

The paper used in this publication meets the minimum requirements of American National Standard for Informational Sciences—Permanence of Paper for Printed Library Materials, ANSI Z39.48—1992

The very nature of information on the Internet means that we cannot guarantee that the information on a recommended site will remain the same, or that the site itself will continue to exist. Webmasters may change content; Web sites may change sites to which they link; ownership of a site may change; Web sites may be hijacked or stolen. We cannot control these circumstances, and cannot take responsibility for them.

This publication is designed to provide accurate and authoritative information on the subject matter covered. It is sold with the understanding that the authors, editors, and publishers are not engaged in rendering legal, medical, or other professional services. If medical or other expert assistance is required, the services of a competent professional person should be sought.

A cataloging record for this title is available from the Library of Congress (record number 2004042862).

Table of Contents

Comprehensive Overview of Volumes 1–3

VOLUME 1. SEARCH STRATEGIES/QUICK REFERENCE GUIDE

SEARCH STRATEGIES

CHAPTER 1. HEALTH INFORMATION ON THE WEB: WHAT'S GOOD AND WHAT'S GOOD FOR YOU

CHAPTER 2. STRATEGIC SEARCHING BY QUESTION
Questions and Question Types
Key Concepts and Example Questions
Using Health Concepts and Terms to
  Focus a Search
References

CHAPTER 3. STRATEGIC SEARCHING BY TERM
Identifying the Most Important Search-
  able Concepts in Your Question
Choosing Terms: Flexibility and
  Readability
Choosing Terms: Deciding What Type of
  Language You Should Use to Search

CHAPTER 4. STRATEGIC SEARCHING WITH SEARCH ENGINES
Background Information
Different Types of Search Engines
How Search Engines Work
General Search Engine Tips and Tricks
Reference

CHAPTER 5. RECOGNIZING THE LIMITA-TIONS OF SEARCH ENGINES
Things Search Engines Can and Cannot
  Do
404 Fun: Finding Missing Sites
More Things Search Engines Can't Find:
  The Invisible Web
Learning More about Search Engines
Reference

CHAPTER 6. CHOOSING A SEARCH ENGINE TO MATCH YOUR QUESTIONS
Selecting a Search Engine to Match Your
  Question
Search Engine and Strategy Favorites
Search Process

CHAPTER 7. STRATEGIC TALKING: WORK-ING WITH YOUR HEALTH CARE TEAM
Guidelines for Internet Communication
  for Health Care Providers
Shared Decision Making
Tips and Tools for Talking with Health
  Care Providers
Strategies for Using Information from the
Internet with Your Health Care
  Provider
Final Communication Tips for Internet-
Savvy Health Care Consumers
References

CHAPTER 8. COMPLETE STEP-BY-STEP SEARCH PROCEDURE
The Search Question
Initial Search Strategy: Recommended
  Keywords and Search Terms

CHAPTER 9. ANSWERING FREQUENTLY ASKED QUESTIONS: DIAGNOSIS
What Questions to Ask Your Doctor
Health in the News
Medical Procedures
Mammography
References

CHAPTER 10. ANSWERING FREQUENTLY ASKED QUESTIONS: TREATMENTS
Prescriptions and Drug Information
Herbal Information
Medical Devices
Remedies and Therapies

CHAPTER 11. BASIC HEALTH CONCEPTS: TERMS, IMAGES, AND STARTING POINTS
Health Terminology and Definitions
Medical Subject Headings, Disease,
  and Procedure Codes
Anatomical Locations, Terms, and Guides
Collections of Consumer Health
  Information

Other Recommended Tools and
Thoughts
Reference

CHAPTER 12. TOOLS AND SUPPORT
Personal Health Evaluation or
  Self-Diagnosis
Caregiving, Caregivers, and Supportive
  Care
Finding Health Care Facilities and
  Personnel
Insurance and Financial Resources
Where to Ask a Person Questions
Finding Supplies and Tools over the
  Internet
Finding Books, Magazines, Journals, and
  Libraries
Information about Health Professionals
Advance Directives and Related Legalities
Health Legislation
Medical Errors
Patient Advocacy and Rights

CHAPTER 13. STATISTICS AND STAN-DARDS, GUIDELINES AND GOVERNMENT RESOURCES
Government Resources: U.S.: Federal
Government Resources: U.S.: States and
  Local
Government Resources: International
Health Statistics
Health Guidelines and Standards of Care
References

QUICK REFERENCE GUIDE

1. Selected Health and Medical Terms
   according to Concept
2. Forms to Help You Search
3. General and Health Search Engines
4. Other Resources for Improving Your
   Searching Skills
5. State and Local Health Consultation
   and Information Services
6. Geographic, Language, and Location
   Codes
7. Favorite Overall Sources of Consumer
   Health Information

VOLUME 2. DISEASES AND DISORDERS/MENTAL HEALTH AND MENTAL DISORDERS

VOLUME 3. HEALTH AND WELLNESS/LIFE STAGES AND REPRODUCTION, AND CUMULATIVE INDEX

Preface

The number of Internet users has reached an all-time high—and grows larger every year. Both the number of searchers seeking health care information and the amount of information on the Web constantly increase. Consumers search for different types of health information in different ways. Studies show that women are more likely to search for information about their children's health and are more likely to worry about the reliability of information. Men are more likely to use the health information from the Web to ask follow-up questions of their physicians, to bookmark Web sites, and to search for sensitive health information. Teenagers search the Web for health information on topics such as weight issues, mental health, drugs and alcohol, and violence.

Librarians and other professionals who assist and direct searchers of health information on the Web are often asked to tackle the sometimes painful, often personal, and always very important questions of their clients. Just as all patrons want to find the best information available on the Web as quickly as possible, all librarians want to find the best answers for their clients.

HEALTH INFORMATION ON THE WEB

Librarians pay a great deal of attention to evaluating the quality of the health information available on the Web and identifying strategies for effective retrieval. Concurrently, lay people with health information needs have to sift through commercial Web sites as they seek trusted, reliable, unbiased information in answer to their health questions.

Before beginning a search, librarians and other professional researchers helping consumers have often had to decide *how* to search for health information on the Web. They could choose the undemanding searching of commercial sites, usually providing sufficient overviews and adequate results to general questions, but leaving the nagging sense that valuable information was overlooked. They might also choose the skilled, but more daunting, prospect of an individually designed search for specific information. The second search promises a superior exploration—but may seem fraught with risk. *The Medical Library Association Encyclopedic Guide to Searching and Finding Health Information on the Web* has been designed to help all individual consumers searching for personal information get the best possible answers available. It has also been created to help librarians—and all health information researchers on the Web—do an efficient, comprehensive job of an increasingly overwhelming task.

CHALLENGES

The main challenges to searching and finding health information on the Web are (1) knowing where to look and how to find the information and then (2) coping with the sheer volume of information that is available. *The MLA Encyclopedic Guide* is designed to tackle the undertaking in two basic ways. First, it teaches how to skillfully and thoughtfully search any health question in its entirety. Second, it provides an unparalleled reference tool of over 720 effective searches and strategies devised and tested by librarian–searching professionals, health care experts or practitioners, computer experts with health expertise, patient experts and advocates. Search topics cover 77 individual subjects in four broad subject areas, each a separate section of the *Guide*:

- "Diseases and Disorders"
- "Mental Health and Mental Disorders"
- "Health and Wellness"
- ."Life Stages and Reproduction"

GUIDE ORGANIZATION

These two purposes—learning how to search and providing a reference tool of actual searches—are mirrored in the organization of *The Medical Library Association Encyclopedic Guide to Searching and Finding Health Information on the Web.*

About Volume 1

Volume 1 is titled *Search Strategies/Quick Reference Guide,* and the first part of the volume is dedicated to explaining the essential background of effective searching of health information on the Internet. "Search Strategies" covers every aspect in theory and in practice. It begins with "Health Information on the Web: What's Good and What's Good for You," exploring the history, overview of current trends, and unique challenges of Web searching. Then it moves on to examine how to evaluate Internet health information and issues in using it, including criteria, confidentiality, standards, Web site accessibility, and many others.

Next "Search Strategies" progresses into a critical discussion of strategies and strategic searching that includes general tips, question types, and putting the pieces together. In particular:

- Strategic searching by question
- Strategic searching by term
- Strategic searching with search engines
- Limitations of search engines
- Choosing a search engine to match your questions
- Strategic talking: working with your health care team
- Complete step-by-step search procedure

This portion of the *Guide* contains general sources, tools, statistics, and standards. The "frequently asked questions" portion of this section gives ideas on how to find information on general health concerns—drug information, laboratory results, medical procedures, terminology, and more. The final section of volume 1, "The Quick Reference Guide," includes seven handy and useful guides to finding health information on the Web. Three of them are likely to be used most frequently:

- "Selected Health and Medical Terms according to Concept," a comprehensive listing of more 2,000 terms divided into eight broad areas: health, disease, core medical, medical specialties, common imaging tests, common laboratory and diagnostic terms, and surgical and non-surgical terms.
- Forms for quick-starting the process or helping people walk through the strategic thought process with their own questions
- The geographic, language, and location codes of over 220 countries and their related states and possessions.

About Volumes 2 and 3

Volume 2, *Diseases and Disorders/Mental Health and Mental Disorders,* examines specific diseases, illnesses, and conditions. The first half, "Diseases and Disorders," ranges from AIDS to arthritis, cancer to chronic fatigue syndrome, skin diseases to stroke and cerebrovascular diseases. It includes nearly 300 specific topics in 32 major areas. It features the top-reported causes of death and disability for all major populations in the United States, both by age group and ethnicity, as reported by the U.S. Census. To help address searching for those less common illnesses, it also includes a section on searching for information about rare diseases. The second half, "Mental Health and Mental Disorders," looks at more than 150 specific topics in 23 major areas. They cover key approaches to the topic, including causes, comorbidity, prevention, and risks; diagnosis; management, prognosis, recovery; therapies, therapists, and survival. Specific diseases range from addictions to anxiety, dementia to depression and eating and learning disorders, schizophrenia to suicide—and many other vital conditions.

Volume 3, *Health and Wellness/Life Stages and Reproduction*, shows how to use the strategic approach in a comprehensive series of real-life health situations. "Health and Wellness" includes more than 160 specific entries grouped under 11 general areas. The major groupings include wellness and lifestyle; safety; first aid; traffic accidents; multicultural health; alternative/complementary health sources; issues faced by the lesbian, gay, bisexual, and transgendered community; living with a chronic illness, living with a disability; pain and pain management; and hospice and end-of-life care. The second half of volume 2, "Life Stages and Reproduction," covers 114 specific entries grouped under 11 general areas. "Life Stages" examines newborns, children, adolescents, men, women, and seniors. "Reproduction" topics include birth defects, genetic diseases, pregnancy problems, prostate disorders, and sexual health issues.

Volume 3 also has the cumulative index for the entire *MLA Encyclopedic Guide*. The index will be particularly helpful when you are looking for a specific term and will direct you to the best places to begin your search. The page you are directed to will feature cross-references to more ideas or terms in other sections of the *Guide*. You will see that there are extensive "see references" to other pertinent material at the beginning of each separate entry.

Note: *The Medical Library Encyclopedic Association Guide to Searching and Finding Health Information on the Web* also features a companion Web site. An optional CD-ROM is also available. See page xxxi for further information on these elements.

The Arrangement of Volumes 2 and 3

Volumes 2 and 3, divided into more than 75 parts, cover a wide range of subjects from different perspectives, all with basically the same structure. Each part fully explores a given subject and features complete search strategies, actual searches of various discrete subtopics, and other important and helpful information.

The search strategies include the following subdivisions:

- "Special Searching Terms for This Topic"
  "What to Ask"
  "Where to Start"

- "Topic Profile" with four sections:
  "Who," Who is at risk?
  "What," What are the effects?
  "Where," Where in the body will the effects be seen?
  "When," When in life does it usually occur?

- "Abbreviations Used in This Section"

More than 600 "Procedures and Special Topics" sections feature recommended search terms and important sites. The recommended terms comprise a wide, authoritative vocabulary of medical terms and expressions producing comprehensive search results. "Important sites" are the dependable, respected sites that a researcher could consult directly or employ as part of an individualized search strategy.

The following list terms or important, helpful sites:

- "Hotlines"
- "FAQs"
- "Publications on the Internet"
- "Medical Specialty"
- "Professional Organizations"
- "Patient Support Organizations"
- "Best One-Stop Shops"

METHODOLOGY

The universe of health information needs is virtually infinite. To place realistic limitations, we employed the following methodology. We reviewed four primary sources to determine a topic's eligibility for inclusion in this section. Any topic that appeared in any of these sources at that time was included in the book, even if it is not widespread:

- statistics from the United States government for top-reported causes of death for all major populations reported;
- statistics from the United States government for top-reported causes of disability for all major populations reported;
- top-reported chronic, acute, and infectious disorders;
- FAQs reported by major health search engines and health information services.

This last category incorporated reported questions from healthfinder, HealthWeb, MedlinePlus, NetWellness, NOAH, and the United States Department of Health and Human Services. Using this methodology virtually ensured that all of the topics represented are common health issues and concerns.

Although we certainly tried to offer a broad range of subjects, *The MLA Encyclopedic Guide* could not be a comprehensive encyclopedia of every piece of health information on the Web. The first volume is a guide to searching, and the actual strategies and searches in the latter two volumes can be adapted to any health question. Also, although the diseases and special topics are common health issues and concerns, there is a section of searching rare diseases with samples that can be used to find information on any type of condition that is less common in the population as a whole.

A WORD ABOUT THE AUTHORS

Many people contributed to this reference source. In addition to the two main authors, more than 20 individual authors researched and created the individual sections. Most authors are librarians, but some authors are health care experts or practitioners, computer experts with health expertise, patient experts and advocates, or people with a blend of these skills. The range of authors was selected to embrace and illustrate the range of concepts and strategies available and to give a place for those different voices. Searching is an effort in which diversity truly brings strength, and many voices and many ideas are often better able to find a way to an answer.

Become an Expert Searcher

Whether you use *The Medical Library Association Encyclopedic Guide to Searching and Finding Health Information on the Web* as a librarian helping a patron research a topic or as an individual doing private research, we trust you will find the information arranged in a user-friendly, yet professional, manner. We aimed to provide the best of both worlds. The guide is designed to be an authoritative research tool as well as the intuitive searching strategy of a skilled professional. Doctors, nurses, health care professionals, and librarians (e.g., medical, public, academic, special) will find this work useful in a variety of ways. They may find it helpful in enhancing and enriching their own searching skills, but first and foremost we hope that they will find this a helpful reference in their dialogues with patients and patrons.

The Medical Library Association Encyclopedic Guide to Searching and Finding Health Information on the Web is dedicated to the idea that there is a wealth of helpful and life-saving health information available on the Internet—if you know the best way to find it. Too often seekers of this information—whether individual researchers or trained librarians—have only had the choice of consulting prepackaged information or searching without pointers from trained professionals in the field. Our guide has attempted to provide a comprehensive and cutting-edge assortment of information along with the best overall strategies to search. It is designed to bring together the best of health care information and the best of the Internet and—importantly—the best research methods. Health concerns demand nothing less.

Acknowledgements

Anyone who has ever asked us questions of the sort represented in this book has had a very special role in shaping our understanding of consumer health information needs, and we deeply appreciate the knowledge we gained from these interactions.

We want to extend our deep respect and gratitude to our colleagues who contributed chapters to the guide and to the staff of our respective libraries who assisted in a variety of ways in the completion of this book. A special note of appreciation goes to Deborah Lauseng and Helen Look for their project management roles: to Helen for establishing the initial process and procedures for submitting, reviewing, and revising chapters for the first manuscript and to Deborah for taking over this role and shepherding the book through the final manuscript.

We also thank the staff of Neal-Schuman Publishers for the roles they have played throughout the writing process. Thanks to Charles Harmon for the discussion that led to the original book concept, to Michael Kelley for his delightful and insightful personality and editing, and to Eileen Fitzsimons for her talented skills as copyeditor and as liaison between authors and publisher.

Many of our professional colleagues have also contributed in a variety of ways with much enthusiasm. This would include, at the minimum, those librarians and others at the University of Michigan (especially Barbara MacAdam); the marvelous librarians in the Consumer and Patient Health Information Special Interest Group (CAPHIS) of the Medical Library Association (MLA); and our friends and colleagues in HealthWeb, in the National Network of Libraries of Medicine (NNLM), and in the National Library of Medicine (NLM). We owe particular thanks to Janis Brown, Rosalind Dudden, Lynanne Feilen, and the members of the MLA Book Panel for their oversight and assistance.

Special thanks is due to those dedicated and generous souls who manage the various health-oriented search engines and information sites and who answered many of our questions about their sites, and offered suggestions and critiques of portions of our content in their areas of expertise.

Many of the above are also represented on the Medical Webmasters List from the Association of Online Cancer Resources (ACOR), whose members were uniformly generous with information and suggestions.

Patricia F. Anderson
Nancy J. Allee
Ann Arbor, 2004

A Special Note from Patricia F. Anderson

I would like to thank my early mentors:

- Manfred Kochen, who fought for the creation of what became the Web and who predicted its influence on personal and public decision making;
- Maurita Holland, who initiated and supported my explorations in decision making and information transfer;
- Gwen Cruzat, whose rigorous modeling of the health literature provided a context for further explorations and conceptual modeling in this area; and
- Faith VanToll Ross, who supported the integration of these inquiries into a real world setting and the expansion of these early interests to include interface design and quality evaluation.

David Brin graciously helped me find appropriate "sound bites" to synopsize his *Transparent Society* concepts as they related to this book. Warner Slack, M.D., was similarly generous regarding his book, *Cybermedicine*. Dr. Ahmad Risk, Dr. Col. Holly Doyne, Carolyn Petersen, and Alexandra Andrews were particularly generous with time and thought, asking many highly enlightening questions (both on and off of the Medical Webmasters List[MWM-L]), and reading and critiquing portions of the book. Dr. Risk, in particular, directed my attention to several relevant resources, which are cited in this work, and critiqued large portions of the work

Last, but far from least, my two children didn't get the kind of birthday celebrations or holidays or even regular dinners to which they had previously been accustomed during the years of writing the book. They deserve medals of honor (and enormous hugs) for their patience.

Readers and Discussants

The following health care professionals, librarians, educators, Web masters, informaticians, and patients or patient advocates generously volunteered time, information, resources, and particular expertise in discussing the concepts on which this book is based. They reviewed writing and subject content, offered technical tips and tricks, and provided other insights and support.

Ahmad Risk
Alana O'Neal
Aldo Leone
Alexandra Rivera-Rule
Alexandra Andrews
Allan Barclay
Rafael Becerra
Amid Ismail
Anna Schnitzer
Anne-Marie Glenny
Barbara MacAdam
Robert Bagramian
Brian Burt
Bryan Vogh
Carla Funk
Carol Shaw
Carolyn Petersen
Catherine Arnott Smith
Catherine Hayes
Cathy VanCamp
Chip Hart
Chris Shaffer
Christine Klausner
Darlene Nichols
David Baker
David Brin
Deb Lauseng
Dennis Lopatin
Elaine Lukasavitz
Eric Hellman
Erinn Faiks

Eve-Marie LeCroix
Fran Verter
Geri Durka-Pelok
Gillian Mayman
Gunther Eysenbach
Hassan Halawany
Heiko Spallek
Helen Look
Janet Clarkson
Janis Brown
Jim Hoyt
Joan Cadillac
Joan Durrance
John Paul Gobetti
Karen Ridley
Kari Gould
Katie Nesbitt
Khalifa Al-Khalifa
Kim and Marilyn Catalano
Kim Malo
Kristie Huige
Larry Jacobs
Lee A. Green
Lisa Tedesco
Lynanne Feilen
Lynn Johnson
Margeaux Martell
Marilyn S. Lantz
Marita Inglehart
Martin L. Knott
Matthew Bietz

Michael D'Alessandro
Michelle LeMay
Nancy Pulsipher
Nancy Yanes-Hoffman
Naomi Miller
Pat Redman
Patricia Munoz
Paul Hoffman
Paul Resnick
Rita Verheggen
Robert Feigal
Robert Waldstein
Robert Young
Ron Pytel
Rose Ann Anderson
Ruth Holst
Ruti Volk
Scott Pelok
Sharon Brooks
Steve Marine
Suresh Bhavnani
Susan Hipolite-Taichman
Terry Weymouth
Titus Schleyer
Tom Flemming
Tom Green
Virginia Hendricks
Warner Slack
Woosong Sung

How To Use the Guide

There are two basic ways (with thousands of variations) to search using the *Medical Library Association Encyclopedic Guide*.

- The "Search Strategies" in Volume 1 demonstrates *how* to thoroughly search the Internet for health-related questions.
- Volumes 2 and 3 focus on hundreds of individual health topics, providing specific search strategies outlining how a professional searcher would tackle each topic. A compilation of the most useful information available, in the form of recommended Web sites, is included.

HOW TO USE THE TABLE OF CONTENTS AND CUMULATIVE INDEX

The table of contents and the cumulative index provide two different tools for locating information contained in these three volumes.

The index provides a direct approach to specific medical terms, drugs, diagnoses, or treatments found in *The MLA Encyclopedic Guide*. Here you will find other terms to use on the Web, other index terms, and often cross-references to other relevant sections of the book.

The table of contents in volume 1, *Search Strategies,/MLA Guide Quick Reference*, is a straightforward list of chapters on learning the best strategies for searching a health question on the Internet, and quick reference tools that will assist in making the search successful. Since skills build step-by-step, it is best to read the chapters in order, though often you may prefer to skip around so that you can focus on a specific topic.

The table of contents in volume 2, *Diseases and Disorders/Mental Health and Mental Disorders*, covers specific medical or mental conditions and topics. The table of contents for volume 3, *Health and Wellness/Life Stages and Reproduction*, offers more general topics and situations relating to these broad areas of interest. The table of contents for these two volumes covers the entire scope of the material included. Where a broad topic area is presented (e.g., cancer), care has been given to provide a more detailed listing of the content to enable the user to locate a specific topic of interest (e.g., gallbladder cancer). The individual topics are arranged alphabetically within the main groupings. Please note that sometimes a topic may appear in more than one location—some mental conditions may have physical causes, and vise versa.

Sample Searches Using the Table of Contents

To search through volumes 2 and 3 using the table of contents, first pick the largest subject and then narrow the search. For example, a search for information about osteopororosis might be conducted as follows:

1. Turn to volume 2, "Diseases and Disorders."
2. Look up part XXIII, "Musculoskeletal Injuries and Disorders."
3. Note that entry 219, page 124, is Osteoporosis, one of 19 different musculoskeletal injuries and disorders examined in "Special Topics and Procedures."
4. Turn to page 124 to find a complete search for this particular topic featuring recommended search terms and important sites. Follow any cross-references to other pertinent sections of the *Guide*.

Note: There is a complete search strategy for "Musculoskeletal Injuries and Disorders" with special searching issues for this topic, a topic profile (including who, what, where, and when), and the abbreviations used in this section. This is followed by helpful information: publications on the Internet, hotlines, FAQs, medical specialties, professional organizations, patient support organizations and discussion groups, and "best one-stop shops."

A search for more general question about the health of older women might be conducted this way:

1. Turn to volume 3, *Life Stages/Reproduction*.
2. Look up part V, "Adults' Health Issues (Women)."
3. Note that entry 55, page 144, is Osteoporosis.
4. Turn to page 144 to see a complete search (by a different author) for Osteoporosis featuring recommended search terms and important sites. Again, follow cross-references to other pertinent sections of the Guide.

Note: There is a complete search strategy for "Adults' Health Issues (Women)" with special searching issues for this topic, including what to ask and where to start, additional search strategies, a topic profile (with who, what, where, and when) and the abbreviations used in this section. Following the 21 "Procedures and Special Topics" (subject-specific search strategies and recommended sites) is more helpful information about publications on the Internet, hotlines, FAQs, medical specialties, professional organizations, patient support organizations and discussion groups, and "best one-stop shops."

TIPS FOR SEARCHING AND FINDING INFORMATION

Volume 1 explains the thought processes and strategies used by searching experts in a way that will help readers learn to search the Web more effectively. Highlights of the strategy section include what the common questions are, how to ask good questions or searchable questions, how to tell if you have found good information, how to use information from the Web, and troubleshooting. The "Quick Reference Guide" shows how to find common types of information, as well as how to find answers to those general questions patients most frequently ask. This is an excellent place to learn more about health care in general.

To use volume 1 to search a specific health topic, move from section to section; play with the examples and search terms given by replacing them with your own questions, terms, and concerns. At helpful Web sites, make a note of other terms used to describe the same idea, and use those in a new search. Go back and forth between the book and the Web browser, and keep making notes of the terms or concepts that seemed to work best with your topic. Don't stop there—look through the final chapters of the "Quick Reference Guide" for ideas for different questions and ideas for other kinds of resources.

The various parts of volumes 2 and 3 demonstrate these ideas in practice, with many examples on different health topics. Please note that in these volumes, in addition to search strategies and recommended Web sites, each part contains valuable information, such as FAQs, hotlines, and professional and patient organizations. In addition, a companion Web site is available at http://www.neal-schuman.com/mlaguide/.

HOW TO USE EACH PART

In volumes 2 and 3, each part is uniform in the sense that it is built around the same basic structure. For example, each features:

- Special Searching Issues for This Topic
- Topic Profile—broken into "Who, What, Where, and When"
- Abbreviations Used in This Section
- Procedures and Special Topics

- Hotlines
- FAQs
- Publications on the Internet
- Medical Specialties
- Professional Organizations
- Patient Support Organizations/Discussion Groups
- Best One-Stop Shops

Within the "Procedures and Special Topics" individually numbered topic entries appear. Depending on the health topic, they range from a few to many topics (arthritis has 4, cancer has 38). For example, the "Procedures and Special Topics" in the AIDS and HIV part has 13 specific entries:

1. General
2. AIDS-Related Dementia
3. Clinical Trials
4. Complications and Common Manifestations
5. Diagnosis
6. Finding a Doctor
7. Finding Community
8. Finding Funding Support
9. Prevention
10. Privacy
11. Special Populations
12. Therapies and Treatments
13. Terminologies and Dictionaries

Each of these 13 individual entries features subject-specific information:

- Recommended Search Terms
- Important Sites

Using the Recommended Searches

To best make the most of the recommended searches, remember: *To find the right information, you need the right words. To find the right words, you must be flexible, willing to play, learn, and change.* For example, within each topic entry, topic authors explored what was available on the Internet much more broadly than the links that were selected. They also explored the range and variety of terminology or language used to describe some of the various significant concepts relating to that topic.

The "Recommended Search Terms" provide examples of useful terms and how to "play" with them. The sample searches try to avoid using special features unique to a specific search engine; instead, they feature examples that would work in most major search engines. Ideally, one could copy the recommended searches, exactly as they appear in the text, into the search box of any major search engine. The exception to this "straight copying" is if a strategy would be most effective if you supplied a more specific term from your own circumstances. For those cases, the authors have added instructions for customizing your search in square brackets like this:

- Health [with the name of your diagnosis]

If you see such a search string that includes square brackets, do not type it into the search box as shown, but provide the information that the text within the brackets requests.

Searching with the Plus and Minus

The plus and minus signs can use force a search engine to include, or exclude, a term. Some search engines only allow this from the advanced search page. In these cases, there will usually use a phrase such as "must include" or "must not include" with a search box where the term can be entered or selected. However, most search engines allow you to do this by placing a plus sign (+) or minus sign (-) in front of the word. Please note, there are no spaces between the plus or minus sign and the word.

The plus sign is most useful (1) when you would like to use phrase searching but are not certain of the best word order or (2) you are dissatisfied with your results after searching without phrase searching. The plus sign (+) adds focus to the search by telling the search engine that one of the words is more important than the others. With the breast cancer example, you might list the words breast cancer, but use the plus sign to say that cancer is very important to the results. This search would be shown in this book as follows.

- Breast +cancer

Using the Important Sites

The important sites are the most reliable ones you can expect when you use a comprehensive search strategy. These comprise an authoritative list of superior sites and a springboard to your own discoveries.

A NOTE ON URLs

Keep in mind that the main purpose of *The MLA Encyclopedic Guide* is to teach searching and finding information on the Internet, not to provide a list of Web sites. Although many of the "Important Sites" will remain stable, the nature of the Internet is constant growth and change. Even as the book went to press, documents were undoubtedly being moved, changed, or even deleted.

Suppose that under the "Important Sites" a specific URL does not work, or only the address of the organization home page is provided; how do you find the resource you are interested in? First, look at the name of the site carefully. In many cases, the name of the hosting organization (that is, the sponsor or publisher) is listed, followed by "the path" for locating the specific document or Web page. Each step of the path is separated by a colon (:), and these steps will help you locate the resource you are looking for.

Another way to locate a desired resource is to do a phrase search for the title of the resource. Also, adding the name of the author or publisher of the site or a shortened URL can be especially powerful. For example, suppose you have the following site name:

American Cancer Society (ACS): Ovarian Cancer: Detailed Guide

Here are some the different searches you can try:

- "ovarian cancer" "detailed guide"
- "ovarian cancer" "american cancer society"
- "ovarian cancer" ACS
- "ovarian cancer" "cancer.org"

Notice the strategy. The searches all include the main topic, "ovarian cancer," combined with the next step on the path ("detailed guide") or with a term or partial address leading directly to the specific page of the American Cancer Society. These same principles can be used to search for any resource with an incomplete URL.

Another way to do this is to type in the URL for the home page. Once there, follow these steps:

- Look for a list of links. If one of them has the same title or a similar title to that listed in the book, click on it to see if it is what you want.
- If there is no link that looks right, do some browsing. There ought to be a section of the site that would make sense as a place to hunt. Use the various levels of the title for clues.
- Check some obvious starting places, such as "patient information" or "publications."
- If the site has many levels of organization, try browsing by type of disease or body part.
- If there is a site map, be sure to consult it. It will help you with surfing to the correct page.
- Try searching for the page with the search engine on that site. To do this, you would simplify the search, usually using just the topic word or a few words from the title, instead of the Google-style search. Play around, you may need to use quotation marks.

Try to enhance these ideas with those listed in section of the "404 Fun: Finding Missing Sites" in volume 1. Also try to find a similar or new page on the site that has the information you want. There is no guarantee that the page is still there. And above all, be playful, curious, and inventive; try to find information that will help you to make thoughtful decisions about your health search.

HOW TO USE THE CD-ROM

A companion CD-ROM containing an HTML version of the complete text of all three volumes and featuring live links to almost 11,000 "Important Sites" is available from the publisher. This will enable you to quickly link back and forth from Web site to text as well as search the entire text by keyword.

Quick Guides to Searching for Health Information

BASIC

Don't rely on Google's "I Feel Lucky" button. Here are five tips for improving your searches.

1. Try the advanced search.
2. Use quotation marks (to group words as phrases).
3. Use different words (to describe the same idea).
4. Change the number of words in the search box: More words = fewer results; fewer words = more results.
5. Get rid of oddballs: Getting weird results? Pick a word from the oddball results, and add it to your search with a minus sign right before it (no spaces). This will "throw out" that idea from your search.

Always remember the bottom line: it's your health, ask more questions.

ADVANCED

F   Frame your search; phrase the question

R   Relevance (i.e., what is most important?)

I   Irrelevance (i.e., what is not searchable or not answerable?)

A   Alternates (i.e., find other terms for the most important concepts).

R   Review, revise, repeat

S   Select a search engine; search

E   Evaluate

C   Cite what was found

T   Tinker, or Try again

F = FRAME YOUR QUESTION

1. Put Your Question into Words

State your question. The question you ask determines the answers you will find.

2. Identify Question Qualities

Question Type	Simple	Complex		
Question Topic	Common	Rare	Technical	
Question Class	Etiology	Diagnosis	Therapy	Prognosis

3. Classify Questions

Etiology/Causation	Why/Who/When
Diagnosis	What/Where
Therapy/Prevention/Causation/Harm	What to Do/What Not to Do
Prognosis/Outcome	What Next/What to Expect

R = RELEVANCE

I = IRRELEVANCE

4. Select Key Concepts

	Are your concepts: Relevant? Searchable? Irrelevant? Answerable?

5. Rank Key Concepts by Importance

1. _____ 2. _____ 3. _____	Most questions have two to four important concepts, of which one is most important. Find that one most important concept before you start your search, and put it first when you search.

A = ALTERNATES

6. Find Other Terms for Most Important Concepts

1. _____ 2. _____ 3. _____	• Use a thesaurus. • The more technical or medical the term, the more technical results will be. • Be sure to check spelling and definitions of the most important concepts and terms.

R = REVIEW, REVISE, REPEAT

S = SELECT A SEARCH ENGINE (#7)

If the question is *simple* and *common*. . .	. . .then browse a major general health resource, or search in a health-specific search engine.
If the question is *complex* and *common*. . .	. . .then search two to three of the concepts as single words or phrases in a moderate to large general search engine. If this doesn't work, then vary the terms for the concepts.
If the question is *simple* and *rare* or *technical*. . .	. . .then use a two-part strategy. First, search the most specific or technical term in a large general search engine. Second, locate a specialized source on the topic, then repeat the search within the topic resource.
If the question is *complex* and *rare* or *technical*. . .	. . .then use a three-part strategy. Attempt both parts of the strategy for a rare/technical question of the simple type. Also search for an expert with whom you may need to consult.

S = SEARCH

8. Remember These General Search Tips
   - Use phrase searching (i.e., quotation marks).
   - To say a word must be included, prefix it with a plus sign (+).
   - To get rid of a word in the search results, do the search again, including that word prefixed by a minus sign (-).

9. Follow Sound Search Strategies

Always	• Be specific, be accurate. • Search by synonyms or aliases. • Search for related diseases or types of diseases.
Usually	• Spell out acronyms. • Search by phrase. • Search by most unique term.
Rarely	• Search by part of body affected. • Search by what's wrong.

10. Experiment If a Search Doesn't Work	11. Don't Give Up If the Site You Want Is Gone
• To refine a search, first change terms, not the search engine. • Use more specific terms if search retrieved too much. • Choose different terms if the information retrieved is off topic). • Try more general terms if search retrieved too little. • Change search engines if a few tries of new terms still does not work.	• Use the cache option in Google. • Backtrack up the hierarchy of directory levels. • Use the search engine at the main level of the Web site. • Use a general search engine to locate the page's title, publisher, or organization. • Try searching in the Internet Archive: <http://www.archive.org/>.

E = EVALUATE (#12)

Candor	They tell you the whole truth.
Honesty	They tell you nothing but the truth.
Quality	The information is accurate, up to date, and easy to understand.
Informed consent	They do not keep information about you without your permission.
Privacy	They protect any information you allow them to keep.
Professionalism	They tell you their limitations and ethical responsibilities.
Responsible partnering	They disclose influences and sources of information or funding; they choose all of these to foster trust.
Accountability	They say who they are, why they do this, and how to reach them.

C = CITE WHAT WAS FOUND

13. Discuss the Findings with Your Doctor

1. This is the information I found.
2. This is why I believe this to be a credible source of information.
   - OR: I would appreciate your judgment of this information.
   - OR: I have concerns about the quality of this information, and would appreciate a suggestion of a better source.
3. This information raised these questions or concerns. I would appreciate discussing them with you.
   - OR: Would you please recommend information to answer these questions or concerns?

T = TINKER OR TRY AGAIN

14. Know When to Stop

- If at first you don't succeed, try, try again.
- If at first you do succeed, try at least once more to see you find something better. Shop around. Second opinions count with health information, too.
- If you try and try again, and still don't succeed, decide how important this is for you, and then ask for help, take a break and try again later, or simply stop.

Health and Wellness

Part I: Wellness and Lifestyle

P. F. Anderson

Special Searching Issues for This Topic

Finding information on general health—how to maintain good health, and wellness—is one of the greatest search challenges encountered in the writing of this book. Using the most common health and wellness terms tends to retrieve almost exclusively commercial sites selling various over-the-counter home remedies or bogus and scam pseudo-information sites. This is true even when searching a group of health and wellness terms, such as "fitness diet health nutrition wellness." The word "healthy" seemed to retrieve more relevant information than other general health terms, and you will see this reflected in the search strings under specific topics. This may not last, as the preferred terminology used in Web site changes often over time.

For these reasons, the best strategies to locate this information are a little different than those through much of the rest of the book. First, for general health information, go to the Best One Stop Shops recommended in this chapter and elsewhere in the book. Second, search a specific health and wellness topic whenever possible. Third, try to focus your searches on non-commercial sites by adding one of the following search strings to the end of your topic search.

- ".gov"
- ".info"
- ".org"

Abbreviations Used in This Section

AAFP = American Academy of Family Physicians

AHRQ = Agency for Healthcare Research and Quality

BBC = British Broadcasting Corporation

CDC = Centers for Disease Control and Prevention

CFSAN = Center for Food Safety and Applied Nutrition

EPA = Environmental Protection Agency

FCIC = Federal Consumer Information Center

FDA = Food and Drug Administration

HON = Health on the Net Foundation

NCI = National Cancer Institute

NHS = National Health Service (United Kingdom)

NIDA = National Institute of Drug Abuse

NIMH = National Institute of Mental Health

NOAH = New York Online Access to Health

USDA = Department of Agriculture

Procedures and Special Topics

1. General

Recommended Search Terms

- Healthy
- "Well-being" health

Important Sites

American Self-Help Group Clearinghouse: <http://www.selfhelpgroups.org/>

Healthy People 2010: Leading Health Indicators: Resources for Action: <http://www.healthypeople.gov/LHI/EnglishFactSheet.htm>

Helpdoctor (UK): <http://www.helpdoctor.co.uk/>

National Health Information Center (NHIC): <http://www.health.gov/NHIC/>

Sympatico Health: Healthcentral.com: <http://health.sympatico.ca/>

U.S. Army: HOOAH4Health: <http://www.hooah4health.com/>

2. Beverages and Drinking Water

Recommended Search Terms

- Beverage safety ".gov" -alcohol
- "Health benefits" water
- "Health risks" water
- Healthy water

Important Sites

Chlorine Chemistry Council: Water Quality and Health: Drinking Water and Health Newsletter: <http://c3.org/news_center/ccc_periodicals/drinking_water/>

Environmental Protection Agency (EPA): Drinking Water and Health: What You Need to Know: <http://www.epa.gov/safewater/dwhealth.html>

Environmental Protection Agency (EPA): Kids' Stuff: Water for Kids: <http://www.epa.gov/water/kids.html>

Environmental Protection Agency (EPA): Water on Tap: A Consumer's Guide to the Nation's Drinking Water: <http://www.epa.gov/safewater/wot/wot.html>

International Medicine Center: Food and Beverage Safety: <http://www.traveldoc.com/info/foodsafety.asp>

MedlinePlus: Caffeine: <http://www.nlm.nih.gov/medline plus/caffeine.html>

MedlinePlus: Drinking Water: <http://www.nlm.nih.gov/medlineplus/drinkingwater.html>

Worksafe BC, Health and Safety Centre: Injury Prevention Resources for Tourism and Hospitality: Food and Beverage: <http://tourism.healthandsafetycentre.org/s/Prevention-FoodBeverage.asp>

HOTLINES

Food and Drug Administration (FDA): Center for Food Safety and Applied Nutrition (CFSAN):
1-888-SAFEFOOD/1-888-723-3366

Food and Drug Administration (FDA): Food Safety Information Service (FSIS):
1-800-535-4555; 1-800-256-7072 (TDD/TTY) or e-mail <mphotline.fsis@usda.gov>

University of Guelph (Canada): Food Safety Net:
1-866-50-FSNET/1-866-503-7638 or e-mail <fsnrsn@uoguelph.ca>

FAQs

Environmental Protection Agency (EPA): Ground Water and Drinking Water: Frequently Asked Questions: <http://www.epa.gov/OGWDW/faq/faq.html>

MEDICAL SPECIALTIES

Environmental health; Sanitation; Sanitary engineering

PROFESSIONAL ORGANIZATIONS

Chlorine Chemistry Council: <http://c3.org/>
Culinary Institute of America: <http://www.ciachef.edu/>

BEST ONE-STOP SHOP

U.S. Environmental Protection Agency (EPA): Office of Water: <http://www.epa.gov/ow/>

3. DIET AND NUTRITION

Recommended Search Terms

- Diet nutrition
- Dietary guidelines
- Dietary reference intakes
- Dietition guidelines
- Dietition recommendations
- Food nutrition
- Food pyramid
- Healthy diet
- Healthy nutrition
- Healthy weight

Important Sites

American Academy of Family Physicians (AAFP): Nutrition and Exercise: Healthy Balance for a Healthy Heart: <http://familydoctor.org/handouts/288.html>

American Dietetic Association: <http://www.eatright.org/>

American Medical Women's Association (AMWA):Exerpts from AMWA's Women's Complete Healthbook: Guidelines for a Healthy Diet: <http://www.amwa-doc.org/publications/WCHealthbook/dietamwa-ch03.html>

American Society for Clinical Nutrition: <http://www.faseb.org/asns/>

American Society for Nutritional Sciences (ASNS): <http://www.nutrition.org/>

British Broadcasting Corporation (BBC): Healthy Living: Nutrition: <http://www.bbc.co.uk/health/nutrition/>

British Nutrition Foundation: <http://www.nutrition.org.uk/>

Calorie Control Council (CCC): What's Your Body Mass Index?: <http://www.caloriecontrol.com/bmi.html>

Calorie Control Council (CCC): Healthy Weight Calculator: <http://www.caloriecontrol.com/ibw.html>

Center for Nutrition Policy Promotion: <http://www.usda.gov/cnpp/>

Food and Drug Administration (FDA): Center for Food Safety and Applied Nutrition. (CFSAN): <http://vm.cfsan.fda.gov/list.html>

Food and Drug Administration (FDA): Center for Food Safety and Applied Nutrition (CFSAN): Information about Losing Weight and Maintaining a Healthy Weight: <http://vm.cfsan.fda.gov/~dms/whwght.html>

Food and Drug Administration (FDA): "Daily Values" Encourage Healthy Diet: <http://www.fda.gov/fdac/special/foodlabel/dvs.html>

Food and Nutrition Information Center (FNIC): <http://www.nalusda.gov/fnic/>

Healthy Refrigerator: <http://www.healthyfridge.org/mainmenu.html>

Healthy Weight Forum: <http://www.healthyweightforum.org/>

MedlinePlus: Cholesterol: <http://www.nlm.nih.gov/medlineplus/cholesterol.html>

MedlinePlus: Nutrition: <http://www.nlm.nih.gov/medlineplus/nutrition.html>

MedlinePlus: Vitamin and Mineral Supplements: <http://www.nlm.nih.gov/medlineplus/vitaminandmineral supplements.html>

MedlinePlus: Weight Loss/Dieting: <http://www.nlm.nih.gov/medlineplus/weightlossdieting.html>

National Center for Chronic Disease Prevention and Health Promotion: Nutrition and Physical Activity: Healthy Eating Tips: <http://www.cdc.gov/nccdphp/dnpa/heal_eat.htm>

National Institute of Nutrition/L'Institut National de la Nutrition (Canada): <http://www.nin.ca/>

U.S. Department of Agriculture (USDA): *Nutrition and Your Health: Dietary Guidelines for Americans,* 5th ed.: <http://www.health.gov/dietaryguidelines/>

Nutrition.gov: <http://www.nutrition.gov/>

Nutrition Cafe: <http://www.exhibits.pacsci.org/nutrition/>

U.S. Department of Agriculture (USDA): USDA for Kids: <http://www.usda.gov/news/usdakids/>

Office of Nutrition Policy and Promotion (Canada): <http://www.hc-sc.gc.ca/hppb/nutrition/pube/food guid/>

Partnership for Healthy Weight Management: <http://www.consumer.gov/weightloss/>

Tufts University: Nutrition Navigator: <http://navigator.tufts.edu/>

University of Nebraska: Institute of Agriculture and Natural Resources: Index: Food and Nutrition: <http://www.ianr.unl.edu/pubs/Foods/>

Vegetarian Society (UK): Health and Nutrition: <http://www.vegsoc.org/health/>

University of California Berkeley: Wellness Letter: 14 Keys to a Healthy Diet: <http://www.berkeleywellness.com/html/fw/fwNut01HealthyDiet.html>

Hotlines

American Dietetic Association:
1-800-877-1600
Beech-Nut Nutrition Hotline:
1-800-523-6633
U.S. Department of Agriculture (USDA):
(301) 436-7725
Weight Control Information Network:
1-877-946-4627, or e-mail: <win@info.niddk.nih.gov>

FAQs

Calorie Control Council (CCC): FAQs: <http://www.caloriecontrol.com/faqs.html>

Food and Drug Administration (FDA): Food, Nutrition, and Cosmetics Questions and Answers: <http://vm.cfsan.fda.gov/~dms/qa-top.html>

Food and Nutrition Information Center (FNIC): Food Guide Pyramid: <http://www.nal.usda.gov/fnic/Fpyr/pyramid.html>

Medical Specialty

Dietetics

Professional Organizations

American Dietetic Association: <http://www.eatright.org/>

International and American Associations of Clinical Nutritionists (IAACN): <http://www.iaacn.org/>

4. Exercise, Fitness, and Physical Activity

Recommended Search Terms

- "Exercise program"
- Fitness exercise ".gov"
- Fitness exercise ".org"
- Fitness exercise sports ".org"
- "Personal exercise program"
- "Personal fitness training"
- "Physical fitness" ".gov"
- "Physical fitness" ".org"
- "Work out program"

Important Sites

American Council on Exercise (ACE): <http://www.acefitness.org/>

American Fitness Alliance: <http://www.americanfitness.net/>

American Heart Association: Just Move! Fitness Center: <http://www.justmove.org/home.cfm>

Canada's Healthy Workplace Week: Resource Well: <http://www.nqi.ca/chww/well.htm>

Centers for Disease Control and Prevention (CDC): Body and Mind (BAM!) (Teens): <http://www.bam.gov/>

Federal Citizen Information Center (FCIC): Consumer Focus: Combat Winter Weight Gain: <http://www.pueblo.gsa.gov/cfocus/cfweight02/focus.htm>

Federal Citizen Information Center (FCIC): Life Advice About…Fitness and Exercise: <http://www.pueblo.gsa.gov/cic_text/health/fitnexer/fitnexer.htm>

Federal Citizen Information Center (FCIC): Walking for Exercise and Pleasure: <http://www.pueblo.gsa.gov/cic_text/health/walking/walking.htm>

FiftyPlus Fitness Association: <http://www.50plus.org/>

HealthierUS.gov: <http://healthierus.gov/>

Food and Nutrition Information Center (FNIC): Fitness, Sports, and Sports Nutrition: <http://www.nal.usda.gov/fnic/etext/000054.html>

KidsHealth: Parents: Nutrition and Fitness: <http://www.kidshealth.org/>

MedlinePlus: Exercise for Seniors: <http:/www./nlm.nih.gov/medlineplus/exerciseforseniors.html>

MedlinePlus: Exercise/Physical Fitness: <http://www.nlm.nih.gov/medlineplus/exercisephysicalfitness.html>

MedlinePlus: Sprains and Strains: <http://www.nlm.nih.gov/medlineplus/sprainsandstrains.html>

Michigan Electronic Library (MeL): Health Information Resources: Health Aspects of Exercise, Sport and Athletic Fitness: <http://mel.lib.mi.us/health/health-exercise-health.html>

National Association for Health and Fitness (NAHF): <http://www.physicalfitness.org/>

National Institute of Diabetes and Digestive and Kidney Diseases (NIDDK): Active at Any Size: <http://www.niddk.nih.gov/health/nutrit/activeatanysize/active.html>

Native American Fitness Instructors Network (NAFINN)/ Native American Fitness Alliance (NAFA): <http://pages.prodigy.net/ceduncan/>

President's Council for Physical Fitness and Sports (PCPFS): <http://www.fitness.gov/>

Recreation.gov: <http://www.recreation.gov/>

Shape Up America: <http://www.shapeup.org/>

SIRCMedical: <http://www.sportdiscus.com/sircmedical.html>

SPORTQuest: Sports Science Resources: Associations— National: <http://www.sportquest.com/resources/sportscience2.cfm?scat=Assocations%20%20National%StartRow=1>

VERB (Youth): <http://www.verbnow.com/>

HOTLINES

President's Council for Physical Fitness and Sports: (202) 690-9000

FAQS

American Council on Exercise (ACE): Fit Facts: <http://www.acefitness.org/fitfacts/>

American Heart Association: Fitness News: Frequently Asked Questions: <http://www.justmove.org/fitnessnews/faqbodyframe.htm>

Big Folks Exercise and Fitness Resources FAQ: <http://www.faqs.org/faqs/fat-acceptance-faq/fitness/>

MEDICAL SPECIALTY

Sports medicine; Recreational therapy; Sports therapy

PROFESSIONAL ORGANIZATIONS

American College of Sports Medicine (ACSM): <http://www.acsm.org/>

American Council on Exercise (ACE): <http://www.acefitness.org/>

American Therapeutic Recreation Association (ATRA): <http://www.atra-tr.org/atra.htm>

PATIENT SUPPORT ORGANIZATIONS/ DISCUSSION GROUPS

Family Health Center: Fit and Trim: <http://www.families-first.com/fitandtrim/>

Shape Up America: <http://www.shapeup.org/>

5. PREVENTION

Recommended Search Terms

- "Health promotion"
- Prevention preventive health medicine
- "Disease prevention"

Important Sites

American Institute for Preventive Medicine: Health at Home: Your Complete Guide to Symptoms, Solutions, and Self-Care: <http://www.mcare.org/healthathome/>

American Social Health Association (ASHA): <http://www.ashastd.org/>

Centers for Disease Control and Prevention (CDC): <http://www.cdc.gov/>

Centers for Disease Control and Prevention (CDC): National Center for Infectious Diseases: Travelers' Health: <http://www.cdc.gov/travel/>

Centers for Disease Control and Prevention (CDC): National Prevention Information Network (NPIN): <http://www.cdcnpin.org/>

Centers for Disease Control and Prevention (CDC): Public Health Emergency Preparedness and Response: <http://www.bt.cdc.gov/>

Clinician's Handbook of Preventive Services, 2nd ed.: <http://www.ahrq.gov/clinic/ppiphand.htm>

U.S. Army: HOOAH4Health: <http://www.hooah4health.com/>

Injury Prevention Web (IPW): <http://www.injuryprevention.org/>

National Eating Disorders Association (NEDA): <http://www.nationaleatingdisorders.org/>

Office of Disease Prevention and Health Promotion (ODPHP): <http://odphp.osophs.dhhs.gov/>

Prevention Report: <http://odphp.osophs.dhhs.gov/pubs/prevrpt/Default.htm>

SafetyAlerts: <http://www.safetyalerts.com/>

University of Michigan Health System: Health Education Resource Center: <http://www.med.umich.edu/mfit/herc/>

U.S. Army Center for Health Promotion and Preventive Medicine (USACHPPM): <http://chppm-www.apgea.army.mil/>

U.S. Preventive Services Task Force (USPSTF): <http://www.ahcpr.gov/clinic/uspstfix.htm>

MEDICAL SPECIALTIES

Preventive medicine; Preventive dentistry; Aerospace medicine; Environmental medicine; Occupational medicine; Public health

6. RISK FACTORS AND CHOICES

Recommended Search Terms

- "Health risk appraisal"
- "Health risk assessment"
- "Health status indicators"
- Personal risk factors
- Personal risk profile
- Individual risk factors

Important Sites

Agency for Healthcare Research and Quality (AHRQ): Put Prevention into Practice (PPIP): *A Step-by-Step Guide to Delivering Clinical Preventive Services*: Appendix C: Health Risk Profiles and Flow Sheets: <http://www.ahcpr.gov/ppip/manual/appendc.htm>

Canadian Center for Occupational Health and Safety: OSH Answers: Personal or Individual Risk Factors: <http://www.ccohs.ca/oshanswers/ergonomics/office/risk_individual.html>

Indiana University: Adolescence Directory On-Line (ADOL): Health Risk Factors for Adolescents: <http://education.indiana.edu/cas/adol/risk.html>

LifeScan: Health Risk Appraisal: <http://wellness.uwsp.edu/Health_Service/Services/lifescan/lifescan.htm>

Public Health Foundation: <http://www.phf.org/>

Risk World: Health Risks: <http://www.riskworld.com/Websites/Webfiles/ws5aa009.htm>

You First: Health Risk Assessment: <http://www.youfirst.com/>

FAQs

National Health Service (NHS [UK]): National Electronic Library for Health: Heart Diseases: QandA: <http://wmrlheart.directional.co.uk/faq.htm>

7. HEALTH INSURANCE

[*See also* "Tools and Support," p. (133, vol. 1).]

Recommended Search Terms

- "Access to care"
- Access "health care"
- Access "health care" [use with name of special population, such as African American, Asian-American, Hispanic, Latino, children, women]
- "Free health screenings"
- "Free health services"
- "Subsidized clinic" [use with name of your state or region]
- Uninsured children
- Uninsured "health risks"
- Uninsured "risk factor"

Important Sites

American College of Physicians (ACP): Internal Medicine/Doctors for Adults: Decision 2000 Campaign: No Health Insurance? It's Enough to Make You Sick: <http://www.acponline.org/uninsured/lack-contents.htm>

Covering Kids and Families: <http://www.coveringkids.org/>

Insure Kids Now!: <http://www.insurekidsnow.gov/>

Kaiser Commission on Medicaid and the Uninsured: Uninsured in America: <http://www.kff.org/docs/sections/kcmu/uninsuredmay2000.html>

Kaiser Family Foundation (KFF): Partnership for Children's Health Coverage: <http://www.kff.org/cbs/>

National Center for Policy Analysis: Questions and Answers about Uninsured Children: <http://www.ncpa.org/ba/ba225.html>

National Women's Health Information Center: 4woman.gov: Health Care Access and African American Women: <http://www.4woman.gov/faq/hca-aa.htm>

National Women's Health Information Center: 4woman.gov: Health Care Access and Hispanic American Women: <http://www.4woman.gov/faq/hca-ha.htm>

Quality Interagency Coordination Task Force (QuIC): Health Care Quality: <http://www.consumer.gov/qualityhealth/>

U.S. Census Bureau: Low Income Uninsured Children: <http://www.census.gov/hhes/hlthins/lowinckid.html>

8. HEALTH SCREENING

Recommended Search Terms

- Why "health screening"
- "Health screening" benefits

- "Screening tests" benefits
- "Health screening"
- "Screening tests" labs
- "Home tests" health
- "Home testing" screening

Recommended Search Terms for Specific Screening Tests

- Mammogram
- "Screening mammogram"
- Mammography
- Sigmoidoscopy
- "Fecal occult blood test"
- FOBT
- "Faecal occult blood test"
- "Stool occult blood"
- Hemoccult
- Haemoccult
- "Guaiac smear test"
- PSA test
- "Total PSA"
- "Free-PSA"
- "Prostate-specific antigen"
- CA125
- "Cancer antigen 125"
- OCA125
- "Ovarian cancer antigen 125"

Important Sites

Agency for Healthcare Research and Quality (AHRQ): Recommendations and Rationale: Screening for Cervical Cancer: <http://www.ahrq.gov/clinic/3rduspstf/cerv can/cervcanrr.htm>

CA: A Cancer Journal for Clinicians: "American Cancer Society Guideline for the Early Detection of Cervical Neoplasia and Cancer": <http://caonline.amcancersoc .org/cgi/content/short/52/6/342>

Harvard University: Family Health Guide: Diagnostic Tests: Fecal Occult Blood Test: <http://www.health .harvard.edu/fhg/diagnostics/fecal/fecal.shtml>

Lab Tests Online: <http://www.labtestsonline.org/>

Lab Tests Online: CA-125 Test at a Glance: <http://www .labtestsonline.org/understanding/analytes/ca125/ glance.html>

Lab Tests Online: Fecal Occult Blood Test at a Glance: <http://www.labtestsonline.org/understanding/ analytes/fobt/glance.html>

Lab Tests Online: PSA (Prostate-Specific Antigen) at a Glance: <http://www.labtestsonline.org/understanding/ analytes/psa/glance.html>

Lab Tests Online: Screening Tests for Adults (Age 30 to 49): <http://www.labtestsonline.org/understanding/ wellness/d_adult.html>

Lab Tests Online: Screening Tests for Children (Up to 12): <http://www.labtestsonline.org/understanding/ wellness/b_children.html>

Lab Tests Online: With Home Testing, Consumers Take Charge of their Health: <http://www.labtestsonline .org/understanding/features/hometesting.html>

National Cancer Institute (NCI): Cancer.gov: Finding Ovarian Cancer Early in High-Risk Women: Risk of Ovarian Cancer Algorithm (ROCA) Study: <http://epi .grants.cancer.gov/ovarian/>

National Cancer Institute (NCI): Cancer.gov: Screening and Testing for Cancer: <http://www.nci.nih.gov/ cancerinfo/screening/>

National Cancer Institute (NCI): Cancer.gov: Testing for Cancer: Types of Tests: <http://www.nci.nih.gov/ cancerinfo/screening/types-of-tests/>

National Cancer Institute (NCI): Cancer Information Service: Cancer Facts: Colorectal Cancer Screening: Questions and Answers: <http://cis.nci.nih.gov/fact/5 _31.htm>

National Cancer Institute (NCI): Cancer Information Service: Cancer Facts: Mamografías selectivas de detección: preguntas y respuestas (Spanish): <http://cis.nci .nih.gov/fact/5_28s.htm>

National Cancer Institute (NCI): Cancer Information Service: Cancer Facts: Questions and Answers about the Prostate, Lung, Colorectal, and Ovarian Cancer Screening Trial: <http://cis.nci.nih.gov/fact/5_12 .htm>

National Cancer Institute (NCI): Cancer Information Service: Cancer Facts: Questions and Answers about the Prostate-Specific Antigen (PSA) Test: <http://cis.nci .nih.gov/fact/5_29.htm>

National Cancer Institute (NCI): Cancer Information Service: Cancer Facts: Screening Mammograms: Questions and Answers: <http://cis.nci.nih.gov/fact/ 5_28.htm>

National Cancer Institute (NCI): Cancer Information Service: Cancer Facts: The Pap Test: Questions and Answers: <http://cis.nci.nih.gov/fact/5_16.htm>

9. IMMUNIZATION AND VACCINATION

[See also "Children's Health Issues: Immunization," p. 122; "Infectious Diseases," p. 98, vol. 2.]

Recommended Search Terms

- Immunization "benefits of"
- Immunize "importance of"
- Vaccination "benefits of"
- "Vaccination injuries"
- Vaccine "risks of"

Important Sites

All Kids Count: Immunization Registry Benefits: <http://www.allkidscount.org/>

Centers for Disease Control and Prevention (CDC): National Immunization Program (English/Spanish): <http://www.cdc.gov/nip/>

Centers for Disease Control and Prevention (CDC): Vaccines for Children Program (English/Spanish): <http://www.cdc.gov/nip/vfc/>

MedlinePlus: Immunization/Vaccination: <http://www.nlm.nih.gov/medlineplus/immunizationvaccination.html>

National Academies Press: *Setting the Course: A Strategic Vision for Immunization*: Part 2 Summary of the Austin Workshop: <http://books.nap.edu/books/0309085179/html/>

National Immunization Information Hotline: <http://www.vaccines.ashastd.org/>

National Vaccine Injury Compensation Program (VICP): <http://www.hrsa.gov/ osp/vicp/>

HOTLINE

Centers for Disease Control and Prevention (CDC): National Immunization Information Hotline:
1-800-232-2522; 1-800-232-0233 (Spanish); 1-800-243-7889 (TTY)

10. OVERWEIGHT AND OBESITY

Recommended Search Terms

- Healthy weight
- Obesity health
- Overweight "health risks"
- "Weight control"
- "Weight loss" benefits
- "Weight management"

Important Sites

Aim for a Healthy Weight: <http://www.nhlbi.nih.gov/health/public/heart/obesity/lose_wt/>

National Institute of Diabetes and Digestive and Kidney Diseases (NIDDK): Weight-control Information Network (WIN): <http://www.niddk.nih.gov/health/nutrit/win.htm>

Partnership for Healthy Weight Management: <http://www.consumer.gov/weightloss/>

Partnership for Healthy Weight Management: Setting Goals for Weight Loss: <http://www.consumer.gov/weightloss/setgoals.htm>

11. POVERTY

[*See also* "Tools and Support," p. 133, vol. 1.]

Recommended Search Terms

- "Low income" "at risk" disease
- "Low income" "health risk"
- "Low income" health "risk factor" "gov"
- Poor "at risk" health
- Poor "risk factor" illness
- Poverty "at risk" disease
- Poverty "at risk" health
- Poverty "health risk"
- Underserved "risk factor" illness

Important Sites

Agency for Healthcare Research and Quality (AHRQ): Minority Health: <http://www.ahcpr.gov/research/minorix.htm>

Cabinet Office (UK): Tackling the Diseases of Poverty: A Report by the Performance and Innovation Unit (PIU): <http://www.number-10.gov.uk/su/health/default.htm>

Centers for Disease Control and Prevention (CDC): Chronic Disease Prevention: The Burden of Chronic Diseases and Their Risk Factors—2002: <http://www.cdc.gov/nccdphp/burdenbook2002/>

Centers for Disease Control and Prevention (CDC): WISEWOMAN: <http://www.cdc.gov/wisewoman/>

ContentBank: <http://www.contentbank.org/>

National Center for Chronic Disease Prevention and Health Promotion: Behavioral Risk Factor Surveillance System (BRFSS): <http://www.cdc.gov/brfss/>

Regional Municipality of Peel (Canada): Health and Wealth: A Fundamental Link: <http://www.region.peel.on.ca/health/health-status-report/pdfs/health_wealth.pdf>

Society of Actuaries: Factors Affecting Retirement Mortality (FARM): <http://www.soa.org/sections/farm/farm.html>

United Nations (UN): Population Fund (FPA): *State of the World Population 2002*: Health and Poverty: <http://www.unfpa.org/swp/2002/english/ch5/>

12. STRESS AND ANXIETY

Recommended Search Terms

- Anxiety ".gov"
- Anxiety ".org"
- Anxiety "risk factor"
- Anxiety "health risk"
- "Panic disorders"

- "Post traumatic stress disorder"
- PTSD
- Stress "health risk" ".org"
- "Stress assessment"

Important Sites

Anxiety Busters: <http://www.anxietybusters.com/>

Anxiety Disorders Association of America (ADAA): <http://www.adaa.org/>

Anxiety Network International: <http://www.anxiety network.com/>

The Anxiety Panic Internet Resource (tAPir): <http://www.algy.com/anxiety/>

Anxiety Self Help: <http://www.anxietyselfhelp.com/>

Center for Mental Health Services: Managing Anxiety in Times of Crisis: <http://www.mentalhealth.org/cmhs/childrenanxiety/>

FranklinCovey: Stress Assessment Quiz: <http://www.franklincovey.com/promotion/stressedout/>

MedlinePlus: Anxiety: <http://www.nlm.nih.gov/medline plus/anxiety.html>

MedlinePlus: Panic Disorder: <http://www.nlm.nih.gov/medlineplus/panicdisorder.html>

MedlinePlus: Post-Traumatic Stress Disorder: <http://www.nlm.nih.gov/medlineplus/posttraumaticstressdisorder.html>

MedlinePlus: Stress: <http://www.nlm.nih.gov/medlineplus/stress.html>

Mind Tools (UK): Stress Management Techniques: <http://mindtools.com/smpage.html>

National Anxiety Foundation (NAF): <http://www.lexington-on-line.com/naf.html>

National Cancer Institute (NCI): Anxiety Disorder (PDQ): <http://www.nci.nih.gov/cancerinfo/pdq/supportivecare/anxiety/patient/>

National Cancer Institute (NCI): Cancer Facts: Psychological Stress and Cancer: <http://cis.nci.nih.gov/fact/3_17.htm>

National Center for Post-Traumatic Stress Disorder (NCPTSD): PTSD and Physical Health: <http://www.ncptsd.org/facts/specific/fs_physical_health.html>

National Institute of Mental Health (NIMH): Anxiety Disorders: <http://www.nimh.nih.gov/anxiety/anxiety menu.cfm>

New York University (NYU) School of Medicine, Department of Psychiatry: Online Screening for Anxiety: <http://www.med.nyu.edu/Psych/screens/anx.html>

Pax (UK): <http://www.panicattacks.co.uk/>

Surgeon General's Office: *Mental Health: A Report of the Surgeon General*: <http://www.surgeongeneral.gov/library/mentalhealth/toc.html>

Wellness.net: <http://www.wellnessnet.com/teststrs.htm>

Hotlines

National Alliance for the Mentally Ill: 1-800-799-0208

National Institute of Mental Health: 1-800-647-2642

National Mental Health Association: 1-800-969-6642

National Mental Heath Consumers Self-Help Clearinghouse: 1-800-553-4539

Panic Disorder Information Hotline: 1-800-64-PANIC

13. Tobacco and Smoking

Recommended Search Terms

- "Chewing tobacco"
- "Lung cancer" prevention
- "Lung cancer" "risk factor"
- Nicotine risks
- Quit smoking
- Smoking pregnancy
- "Smoking cessation"
- "Smokeless tobacco"
- Snuff tobacco
- "Spit tobacco"
- Stop smoking tobacco
- Tobacco "health risk"
- Tobacco smoking risks

Important Sites

50+Health (UK): Health topics: Smoking: Health risks: <http://www.50plushealth.co.uk/index.cfm?articleid=903>

Action on Smoking and Health (UK): <http://www.ash.org.uk/>

American Lung Association: Freedom From Smoking Online: <http://www.lungusa.org/ffs/>

Centers for Disease Control and Prevention (CDC): Smoking and Health Database: <http://www.cdc.gov/tobacco/search/>

Centers for Disease Control and Prevention (CDC): Tobacco Information and Prevention Source (TIPS): <http://www.cdc.gov/tobacco/>

Foundation for a Smokefree America: <http://www.anti-smoking.org/>

Giving Up Smoking (UK): <http://www.givingupsmoking.co.uk/>

MedlinePlus: Smokeless Tobacco: <http://www.nlm.nih.gov/medlineplus/smokelesstobacco.html>

MedlinePlus: Smoking: <http://www.nlm.nih.gov/medline plus/smoking.html>

MedlinePlus: Smoking Cessation: <http://www.nlm.nih.gov/medlineplus/smokingcessation.html>

National electronic Library for Health (NeLH): Heart Diseases: Q and As: What Are the Absolute Risks Associated with Nicotine Replacement Therapy (NRT) of Developing Cancer?: <http://wmrlheart.directional.co.uk/faq7.htm>

National Institute on Drug Abuse (NIDA): Research Report Series: Nicotine Addiction: <http://www.nida.nih.gov/ResearchReports/Nicotine/Nicotine.html>

QuitNet: Quit Smoking All Together: <http://www.quitnet.org/>

Trytostop.org: Quit Smoking and Make Smoking History: <http://www.trytostop.org/>

Wellness.net: Stop Smoking and Stress: <http://www.wellnessnet.com/stopsmoking-quiz-stress.htm>

WELLNESS AND LIFESTYLE PUBLICATIONS ON THE INTERNET

American Academy of Family Physicians: News and Publications: <http://www.aafp.org/afp/>

AARP (American Association of Retired Persons): Email Newsletters: <http://www.aarp.org/newsletters/home.html>

American College of Physicians (ACP): Internal Medicine/Doctors for Adults: *ACP Observer*: <http://www.acponline.org/journals/news/obstoc.htm>

British Medical Journal (BMJ): <http://www.bmj.com/>

Canadian Medical Association Journal (CMAJ): *eCMAJ*: <http://www.cma.ca/cmaj/>

Food and Drug Administration (FDA): *FDA Consumer Magazine*: <http://www.fda.gov/fdac/>

GoInside: Health: <http://goinside.com/health.html>

Health and Fitness Sports Magazine: <http://www.healthandfitnessmag.com/>

Health Canada: REAL Health: <http://www.hc-sc.gc.ca/real/>

JAMA and Archives: <http://pubs.ama-assn.org/>

Journal of the American Medical Women's Association (JAMWA): <http://jamwa.amwa-doc.org/>

Journey to Wellness: African American Health Radio: <http://www.journeytowellness.com/>

Medical Reporter: <http://medicalreporter.health.org/>

National Health Service (NHS [UK]: Electronic Quality Information for Patients (EQUIP): <http://www.equip.nhs.uk/>

StudentHealth.co.uk (UK): <http://www.unimed.co.uk/health/>

University of California Berkeley: Wellness Letter: Newsletter of Nutrition, Fitness, and Self-Care: <http://www.berkeleywellness.com/>

U.S. Public Health Service: Environmental Health Policy Committee: Subcommittee on Risk Communication and Education: Health Risk Communicator: <http://www.atsdr.cdc.gov/HEC/HRC/hrchome.html>

BEST ONE-STOP SHOPS

Aetna InteliHealth: <http://www.intelihealth.com/>

American Academy of Family Physicians (AAFP): Family Doctor: <http://familydoctor.org/>

Best Practice of Medicine: Patient Guide: <http://praxis.md/index.asp?page=bhg/>

British Broadcasting Corporation (BBC): Health: <http://www.bbc.co.uk/health/>

C-Health: <http://chealth.canoe.ca/>

Centers for Disease Control and Prevention (CDC): CDC en Español: Temas de Salud A–Z: <http://www.cdc.gov/spanish/indice.htm>

Centers for Disease Control and Prevention (CDC): Health Topics A to Z: <http://www.cdc.gov/health/>

Consumer and Patient Health Information Section (CAPHIS): For Health Consumers: <http://caphis.mlanet.org/consumer/>

Columbia University: College of Physicians and Surgeons: *Complete Home Medical Guide*: <http://cpmcnet.columbia.edu/texts/guide/>

Health Care Information Resources: Wellness (English/French): <http://www-hsl.mcmaster.ca/tomflem/well.html>

healthfinder: <http://www.healthfinder.gov/>

healthfinder Español: <http://www.healthfinder.gov/Espanol/>

healthfinder: Health Library: Prevention and Wellness: <http://www.healthfinder.gov/scripts/>

Health on the Net (HON): MedHunt: <http://www.hon.ch/medhunt/>

KidsHealth: <http://www.kidshealth.org/>

KidsHealth en Español: <http://www.kidshealth.org/parent/en_espanol/>

MayoClinic.com: Healthy Living Center: <http://www.mayoclinic.com/findinformation/healthylivingcenter/index.cfm>

MedlinePlus: Health Information: <http://www.medlineplus.gov/>

MedlinePlus: Informacion de salud (Spanish): <http://medlineplus.gov/esp/>

Merck Manual of Medical Information, 2nd home ed: <http://www.merckhomeedition.com/home.html>

NetWellness: <http://www.netwellness.org/>

New York Online Access to Health (NOAH): <http://www.noah-health.org/>

Preguntale a NOAH sobre temas de salud y recursos: <http://www.noah-health.org/spanish/spqksearch.html>

Part II: Safety

P. F. Anderson

SPECIAL SEARCHING ISSUES FOR THIS TOPIC

The idea of safety is a bit contradictory, including both concepts of risk, prevention, and protection. To find quality information on safety, the most effective strategy is to combine a specific area of concern with a variety of safety, risk, defense, prevention, and protection words. One of the most consistently useful words is "safely," which is just as useful and sometimes more useful than "safety" itself. If you want a wider variety of information than the strings or sources listed in this chapter, try some of these other safety terms.

- defense
- freedom
- invulnerable
- prevention
- protection
- refuge
- risk
- safeness
- sanctuary
- security
- shelter

Many of these topics tended to retrieve large numbers of sites devoted to commercial security or protection services or sites selling products, but including very little information. Many of these sites tended to include stories intended to alarm the reader into feeling threatened and purchasing the services. Some of the commercial sites, however, had very good information and were designed specifically for the purposes of helping to protect the public by providing information. For this reason, you may wish to begin your search by including one of the following search strings, and then browse their links or recommended sites to see what other similar sites are being recommended by several of the better sources.

- ".gov"
- ".org"
- ".info"
- ".net"
- ".edu"

As a general rule of thumb, the best information tended to come from the government sites. The safety of the public is one of the government's top priorities, and the information was both available, well designed, well written, and covered all topics.

ABBREVIATIONS USED IN THIS SECTION

AAFP = American Academy of Family Physicians
AAOS = American Academy of Orthopaedic Surgeons
AARP = American Association of Retired Persons
ACP = American College of Physicians
AHRQ = Agency for Healthcare Research and Quality
AMA = American Medical Association
BBC = British Broadcasting Corporation
CDC = Centers for Disease Control and Prevention
CDRH = Center for Devices and Radiological Health
CFSAN = Center for Food Safety and Applied Nutrition
CPSC = Consumer Product Safety Commission
DHHS = Department of Health and Human Services
DOE = Department of Energy
DOEd = Department of Education
DOT = Department of Transportation
EPA = Environmental Protection Agency
FBI = Federal Bureau of Investigation
FCIC = Federal Consumer Information Center
FDA = Food and Drug Administration
FEMA = Federal Emergency Management Administration
FSIS = Food Safety Information Service
HHS = Health and Human Services
NCEH = National Center for Environmental Health
NHTSA = National Highway Traffic Safety Administration
NIH = U.S. National Institutes of Health
NIOSH = National Institute for Office Safety and Health
PBS = Public Broadcasting Service
USDA = U.S. Department of Agriculture
USFA = U.S. Fire Administration

PROCEDURES AND SPECIAL TOPICS

14. GENERAL

Recommended Search Terms

- Accident prevention
- Injury prevention
- Safe
- Safely
- Safety

Important Sites

American Civil Liberties Union (ACLU): Safe and Free: <http://www.aclu.org/safeandfree/>

Canadian Centre for Occupational Health and Safety: Transportation Health and Safety Association of Ontario: <http://www.thsao.on.ca/>

Insurance Institute for Highway Safety (IIHS)/Highway Loss Data Institute (HLDI): <http://www.hwysafety.org/>

International Consumer Product Health and Safety Organization (ICPHSO): <http://www.icphso.org/>

Kids Safety Society Coalition: <http://www.ksscoalition.org/>

National Highway Traffic Safety Administration (NHTSA): <http://www.nhtsa.dot.gov/>

National SAFE KIDS Campaign: <http://www.safekids.org/>

National Safety Council: <http://www.nsc.org/>

Occupational Safety and Health Administration (OSHA): <http://www.osha.gov/>

S.A.F.E. Alternatives (Self-Abuse Finally Ends): <http://www.selfinjury.com/>

WorldSafety.com: <http://www.WorldSafety.com/>

15. BIOTERRORISM

Recommended Search Terms

- Bioterrorism
- Biological weapons
- Biologics protection
- Chemical weapons
- Nerve agents
- Nuclear emergencies
- Radiological emergencies

Important Sites

Agency for Healthcare Research and Quality (AHRQ): Bioterrorism and Emerging Infections: <http://www.bioterrorism.uab.edu/>

American Academy of Pediatrics: Anthrax/Bioterrorism Q and A: <http://www.aap.org/advocacy/releases/anthraxqa.htm>

American College of Physicians (ACP): Internal Medicine/Doctors for Adults: Bioterrorism Resources: <http://www.acponline.org/bioterro/?hp/>

American Medical Association (AMA): Center for Disaster Preparedness and Medical Response: <http://www.ama-assn.org/ama/pub/category/6206.html>

American Red Cross: Terrorism—Preparing for the Unexpected: <http://www.redcross.org/services/disaster/0,1082,0_589_,00.html>

Association for Professionals in Infection Control and Epidemiology (APIC): Bioterrorism Resources: <http://www.apic.org/bioterror/>

Centers for Disease Control and Prevention (CDC): Página Principal del Terrorismo Biológico [Spanish]: <http://www.cdc.gov/spanish/bt/>

Centers for Disease Control and Prevention (CDC): Public Health Emergency Preparedness and Response: <http://www.bt.cdc.gov/>

Centers for Disease Control and Prevention (CDC): Public Health Emergency Preparedness and Response: Biological Agents/Diseases: <http://www.bt.cdc.gov/Agent/agentlist.asp>

Centers for Disease Control and Prevention (CDC): Public Health Emergency Preparedness and Response: Chemical Agents: <http://www.bt.cdc.gov/Agent/agentlistchem.asp>

Food and Drug Administration (FDA): Counterbioterrorism: <http://www.fda.gov/oc/opacom/hottopics/bioterrorism.html>

Global Security: Textbook of Military Medicine: War Psychiatry: <http://www.globalsecurity.org/military/library/report/1995/wp/>

healthfinder: Health Library: Bioterrorism: <http://www.healthfinder.gov/scripts/SearchContext.asp?topic=14337andrefine=1>

JAMA and Archives: Bioterrorism Articles: <http://pubs.ama-assn.org/cgi/collection/bioterrorism/>

MedlinePlus: Anthrax: <http://www.nlm.nih.gov/medlineplus/anthrax.html>

MedlinePlus: Chemical Weapons: <http://www.nlm.nih.gov/medlineplus/chemicalweapons.html>

Virtual Naval Hospital: Textbook of Military Medicine: Medical Aspects of Chemical and Biological Warfare: <http://www.vnh.org/MedAspChemBioWar/>

FAQs

Countering Bioterrorism: Frequently Asked Questions (FAQs): <http://www.fda.gov/cber/faq/cntrbfaq.htm>

Federal Emergency Management Administration (FEMA): About FEMA: Frequently Asked Questions: <http://www.fema.gov/about/faq1.shtm>

Food and Drug Administration (FDA): Center for Biologics Evaluation and Research: Public Health Emergency Preparedness and Response: Questions and Answers about Anthrax: Frequently Asked Questions (FAQs): <http://www.bt.cdc.gov/agent/anthrax/faq/index.asp>

16. DISASTER PLANNING AND EMERGENCY PREPAREDNESS

Recommended Search Terms

- "Disaster management"
- "Disaster planning"
- "Disaster preparedness"
- "Emergency management"
- "Emergency preparedness"
- "Emergency response"
- "Natural disasters" planning
- "Natural hazards" prepare

Important Sites

American Red Cross: Disasters: Be Prepared: <http://www.redcross.org/services/disaster/0,1082,0_500_,00.html>

Canadian Centre for Emergency Preparedness: <http://www.ccep.ca/>

Department of Energy (DOE): Smart Communities Network: Disaster Planning Introduction: <http://www.sustainable.doe.gov/disaster/disintro.shtml>

Department of Transportation (DOT): 2000 Emergency Response Guidebook: <http://hazmat.dot.gov/gydebook.htm>

Disaster Center: <http://www.disastercenter.com/>

Disaster Preparedness and Emergency Response Association (DERA): DERA International: <http://www.disasters.org/>

Disaster Relief: Disaster Preparedness Materials: <http://www.disasterrelief.org/Library/Prepare/>

EmergencyNet: <http://www.emergency.com/>

Emergency Preparedness Information Exchange (EPIX): <http://epix.hazard.net/>

Federal Emergency Management Agency (FEMA): <http://www.fema.gov/>

Federal Emergency Management Agency (FEMA): FEMA for KIDS Homepage: <http://www.fema.gov/kids/>

Federal Emergency Management Agency (FEMA): Your Family Disaster Supplies Kit: <http://www.fema.gov/library/diskit.shtm>

MedlinePlus: Disasters and Emergency Preparedness: <http://www.nlm.nih.gov/medlineplus/disastersandemergencypreparedness.html>

Office of Critical Infrastructure Protection and Emergency Preparedness (OCIPEP): Safe Guard/Sauve Garde Network (Canada): <http://www.safeguard.ca/>

17. ENVIRONMENTAL SAFETY

Recommended Search Terms

- "Air pollution"
- "Environmental chemicals"
- "Environmental health"
- "Environmental illness"
- "Environmental safety"
- "Environmental tobacco smoke"
- "Hazardous waste"
- "Indoor air quality"
- "Multiple chemical sensitivity"
- "Noise pollution"
- "Passive smoking"
- "Sick building syndrome"

Important Sites

BELLE (Biological Effects of Low-Level Exposures) Online Newsletter: <http://www.belleonline.com/>

Centers for Disease Control and Prevention (CDC): National Center for Environmental Health (NCEH): <http://www.cdc.gov/nceh/>

Centers for Disease Control and Prevention (CDC): National Center for Environmental Health (NCEH): Basic Housing Inspection: <http://www.cdc.gov/nceh/publications/books/housing/housing.htm>

Centers for Disease Control and Prevention (CDC): National Center for Environmental Health (NCEH): CDC Childhood Lead Poisoning Prevention Program: <http://www.cdc.gov/nceh/lead/lead.htm>

Chartered Institute of Environmental Health (CIEH) Today (UK): <http://www.cieh.org.uk/>

Children's Environmental Health Network (CEHN): <http://www.cehn.org/>

Consumer Product Safety Commission (CPSC): CPSC Finds Lead Poisoning Hazard for Young Children on Public Playground Equipment: <http://www.cpsc.gov/cpscpub/prerel/prhtml97/97001.html>

Department of Energy (DOE): Office of Environment, Safety, and Health: <http://tis.eh.doe.gov/portal/home.htm>

Environmental Protection Agency (EPA): Indoor Air-IAQ Tools for Schools: Frequent Questions: <http://www.epa.gov/iaq/schools/scfaqs.html>

Environmental Protection Agency (EPA): Radon Frequent Questions: <http://www.epa.gov/iedweb00/radon/radonqa1.html>

healthfinder: Health Library: Environmental Health: <http://www.healthfinder.gov/scripts/SearchContext.asp?topic=290>

Health.gov: Report on Multiple Chemical Sensitivity: <http://www.health.gov/environment/mcs/toc.htm>

MedlinePlus: Air Pollution: <http://www.nlm.nih.gov/medlineplus/airpollution.html>

MedlinePlus: Electromagnetic Fields (EMF): <http://www.nlm.nih.gov/medlineplus/electromagneticfields.html>

MedlinePlus: Environmental Health: <http://nlm.nih.gov/medlineplus/environmentalhealth.html>

MedlinePlus: Noise: <http://nlm.nih.gov/medlineplus/noise.html>

MedlinePlus: Radiation Exposure: <http://www.nlm.nih.gov/medlineplus/radiationexposure.html>

MedlinePlus: Radon <http://www.nlm.nih.gov/medlineplus/radon.html>

MedlinePlus: Secondhand Smoke: <http://www.nlm.nih.gov/medlineplus/secondhandsmoke.html>

National Environmental Health Association (NEHA): <http://www.neha.org/>

National Institute of Environmental Health Sciences (NIEHS): <http://www.niehs.nih.gov/>

National Institute of Environmental Health Sciences (NIEHS): Kids' Pages: <http://www.niehs.nih.gov/kids/home.htm>

National Safety Council: Environmental Health Center: <http://www.nsc.org/ehc.htm>

S.A.F.E. Smokefree Air for Everyone: <http://www.pacificnet.net/~safe/>

FAQs

Health, Environment and Work: FAQs: <http://www.agius.com/hew/faqhew.htm>

National Institute of Environmental Health Sciences (NIEHS): Alphabetical Index of Health Topics: <http://www.niehs.nih.gov/external/faq/alpha.htm>

MEDICAL SPECIALTIES

Occupational medicine; Clinical ecology; Environmental health; Environmental medicine; Health physics; Sanitary engineering; Sanitation

HOTLINE

National Institute of Environmental Health Sciences (NIEHS):
1-800-435-9617

18. FIRE SAFETY

Recommended Search Terms

- "Fire prevention"
- "Fire safety"
- "Home fire safety"
- Preventing fires

Important Sites

Sites for Adults

Fire Kills You Can Prevent It (UK): <http://www.firekills.gov.uk/>

Fire Safe Council: <http://www.firesafecouncil.org/>

FireSafe: Fire and Safety Directory: <http://www.firesafe.com/>

FireWise: <http://www.firewise.org/>

MedlinePlus: Fire Safety: <http://www.nlm.nih.gov/medlineplus/firesafety.html>

National Fire Protection Association (NFPA) Online: <http://www.nfpa.org/>

Residential Fire Safety Institute (RFSI): <http://www.firesafehome.org/>

SafeUSA: Fire Safety: <http://www.safeusa.org/fire/firesafe.htm>

U.S. Fire Administration (USFA): Home Fire Safety: Factsheets: <http://www.usfa.fema.gov/dhtml/public/safety.cfm>

Sites for Kids

Fire PALS: Fire Prevention and Life Safety: <http://www.firepals.org/>

Smoky Bear (Only You Can Prevent Wildfires): <http://www.smokeybear.com/>

Sparky the Fire Dog: <http://www.sparky.org/>

U.S. Fire Administration (USFA): USFA's Kid's Page: <http://www.usfa.fema.gov/kids/>

19. FOOD AND BEVERAGE SAFETY

[*See also* "Diet and Nutrition," p. 4.]

Recommended Search Terms

- "Beverage safety"
- Botulism
- Campylobacter
- "Food additives"
- "Food allergy"
- "Food contamination"
- "Food poisoning"

- "Food safety"
- "Food spoilage"
- "Rotten food" risks
- Safe cooking
- "Safe food"
- "Safe water"
- "Spoiled food" risks
- "Spoiled food" prevention
- Yersinia

Important Sites

American Council on Science and Health (ACSH): Feeding Baby Safely: <http://www.acsh.org/publications/booklets/feedingbaby.html>

Eat Well, Eat Safe (Canada): <http://www.eatwelleatsafe.ca//>

Food and Drug Administration (FDA): Center for Food Safety and Applied Nutrition (CFSAN): <http://www.cfsan.fda.gov/>

Food and Drug Administration (FDA): Center for Food Safety and Applied Nutrition (CFSAN): Consumer Advice: <http://www.cfsan.fda.gov/~lrd/advice.html>

U.S. Department of Agriculture (USDA): Food Safety and Inspection Service (FSIS): Food Safety for Persons with AIDS: <http://www.fsis.usda.gov/OA/pubs/aids.htm>

FoodHACCP.com: Food Safety Information Website: <http://www.foodhaccp.com/>

Food Safety Network (Canada): <http://www.foodsafetynetwork.ca/>

FoodSafety.gov: Gateway to Government Food Safety Information: <http://www.foodsafety.gov/>

FoodSafety.gov: Consumer Advice: <http://www.foodsafety.gov/~fsg/fsgadvic.html>

Home Food Safety: Frequently Asked Questions: <http://www.homefoodsafety.com/faqs.html>

IFT InfoSource: <http://infosource.ift.org/>

MedlinePlus: Drinking Water: <http://www.nlm.nih.gov/medlineplus/drinkingwater.html>

MedlinePlus: Food Allergy: <http://www.nlm.nih.gov/medlineplus/foodallergy.html>

MedlinePlus: Food Contamination/Poisoning: <http://nlm.nih.gov/medlineplus/foodcontaminationpoisoning.html>

MedlinePlus: Food Safety: <http://www.nlm.nih.gov/medlineplus/foodsafety.html>

MedlinePlus: Salmonella Infections: <http://www.nlm.nih.gov/medlineplus/salmonellainfections.html>

Michigan State University: Preserving Food Safely: <http://www.msue.msu.edu/msue/imp/mod01/master01.html>

Mothers for Natural Law (M4NL): Dangers of Genetic Engineering Campaign: <http://www.safe-food.org/>

Proctor & Gamble: Science in the Box: Hygiene Tips for the Kitchen: <http://scienceinthebox.com/en_UK/rd/cleaningthe21stcentury/theeraofpersonalhygiene/10tipsforbetterkitchenhygiene.shtml>

Safe Tables Our Priority (STOP): <http://www.stop-usa.org/>

Food and Nutrition Information Center (FNIC): Food Preservation at Home: <http://www.nal.usda.gov/fnic/etext/000028.html>

U.S. Department of Agriculture (USDA): Food Safety and Inspection Service (FSIS): <http://www.fsis.usda.gov/>

U.S. Department of Agriculture (USDA): Food Safety and Inspection Service (FSIS): Frequently Asked Questions about Food Safety from the USDA Meat and Poultry Hotline: <http://www.fsis.usda.gov/OA/FAQ/hotlinefaq.htm>

U.S. Department of Agriculture (USDA): Food Safety and Inspection Service (FSIS): Food Safety Publications: <http://www.fsis.usda.gov/OA/pubs/consumerpubs.htm>

U.S. Department of Agriculture (USDA): Meat and Poultry Hotline: <http://www.fsis.usda.gov/

HOTLINES

American Institute for Cancer Research (AICR): Education Services: Nutrition Hotline:
1-800-843-8114

Eat Well, Eat Safe (Canada):
1-866-50FSNET/1-866-503-7638, or e-mail <fsnrsn@uoguelph.ca>

FDA: Center for Food Safety and Applied Nutrition (CFSAN):
1-888-SAFEFOOD/1-888-723-3366

FAQs

Food Allergy and Anaphylaxis Network (FAAN): Answers to Frequently Asked Questions: <http://www.foodallergy.org/questions.html>

Foodsafety.gov: Frequently Asked Questions: <http://www.foodsafety.gov/~fsg/fsgfaq.html>

Food and Beverage Safety Publications on the Internet

Food and Drug Administration (FDA): Center for Food Safety and Applied Nutrition (CFSAN): Bad Bug Book: Foodborne Pathogenic Microorganisms and Natural Toxins Handbook: <http://vm.cfsan.fda.gov/~mow/intro.html>

Food and Drug Administration (FDA): Center for Food Safety and Applied Nutrition (CFSAN): Food Safety at Home, School and When Eating Out: An Activity

Book for You to Color: <http://www.foodsafety.gov/
~dms/cbook.html>

Food Australia: <http://www.foodaust.com.au/>

FoodHACCP.com: Internet Journal of Food Safety:
<http://www.foodhaccp.com/journal1.html>

Food Safety Forum (FSF): Media Resource Guide:
<http://www.wnpa.com/foodsafetyforum/contents
.html>

World of Food Science: An Online Food Science and
Technology Magazine: <http://www.worldfoodscience
.org/>

Professional Organizations

Australian Institute of Food Science and Technology
(AIFST): <http://www.aifst.asn.au/>

Canadian Institute of Food Science and Technology
(CIFST): <http://www.cifst.ca/>

Council for Agricultural Science and Technology (CAST):
<http://www.cast-science.org/>

European Society on Agricultural and Food Ethics (Eur-
Safe): <http://www.eursafe.org/>

Institute of Food Science and Technology (IFST) (UK):
<http://www.ifst.org/ifsthp3.htm>

Institute of Food Technologists: <http://www.ift.org/>

International Association for Food Protection (IAFP):
<http://www.foodprotection.org/>

National Food Processors Association: The Food Safety
People: <http://www.nfpa-food.org/>

New Zealand Institute of Food Science and Technology
(NZIFST): <http://www.nzifst.org.nz/>

20. Health Safety and Health Advisories

Recommended Search Terms

- "Health advisories"
- "Health advisory"
- "Health advisory" [you may use this with
  another term of interest]
- "Health alert"
- "Patient safety"
- "Public health advisories"
- "Safety alert"

Important Sites

Agency for Healthcare Research and Quality (AHRQ):
Health Care: Medical Errors and Patient Safety:
<http://www.ahcpr.gov/qual/errorsix.htm>

Agency for Toxic Substances and Disease Registry
(ATSDR): Public Health Advisories: <http://www
.atsdr.cdc.gov/HAC/healthad.html>

American Red Cross: Health and Safety Services: Living
Well, Living Safely: <http://www.redcross.org/services/
hss/lifeline/>

American Society of Health System Pharmacists (AHSP):
SafeMedication.com: <http://www.safemedication
.com/>

Australian Patient Safety Foundation: <http://www.apsf
.net.au/>

Center for Patient Advocacy: <http://www.patient
advocacy.org/>

Centers for Disease Control and Prevention (CDC):
Health Alert Network (HAN): <http://www.bt.cdc
.gov/documentsapp/HAN/han.asp>

Communications New Brunswick (CNB) Online: Public
Alerts (Canada): <http://www.gnb.ca/0053/issues/
Advisory-e.asp>

Consumers' Health Forum of Australia: <http://www.chf
.org.au/>

CyberGrrl: HealthGrrl: <http://www.cybergrrl.com/views/
healthgrrl/>

Environmental Protection Agency (EPA): Health Advisories: <http://www.epa.gov/waterscience/health/>

European Commission: Health and Consumer Protection
Directorate: <http://europa.eu.int/comm/dgs/health
_consumer/index_en.htm>

Food and Drug Administration (FDA): Center for Devices
and Radiological Health (CDRH): Safety Alerts, Public Health Advisories and Notices from CDRH:
<http://www.fda.gov/cdrh/safety.html>

Food and Drug Administration (FDA): Losing Weight
Safely: <http://www.fda.gov/opacom/lowlit/weightls
.html>

Health and Safety Executive (HSE) (UK): <http://www
.hse.gov.uk/>

Health Consumers' Council (Western Australia): <http://
www.hcc-wa.global.net.au/index2.html>

HealthSafetyInfo: <http://www.healthsafetyinfo.com/>

Institute For Safe Medication Practices (ISMP): <http://
www.ismp.org/>

National Institute for Aging: Age Page: Health Information: Medicines: Use Them Safely: <http://www.nia
.nih.gov/health/agepages/medicine.htm>

National Patient Safety Agency (NPSA) (UK): <http://
www.npsa.nhs.uk/>

National Patient Safety Foundation: <http://www.npsf
.org/>

National Resource Centre for Consumer Participation in
Health (Australia): <http://www.participateinhealth
.org.au/>

Partnership for Patient Safety (P4PS): <http://www.p4ps
.org/>

Patient Advocate Foundation (PAF): <http://www.patient advocate.org/>

Patient Safety Institute (PSI): <http://www.ptsafety.org/>

Veterans Administration: A National Center for Patient Safety (NCPS): <http://www.patientsafety.gov/>

HOTLINES

Patient Advocate Foundation (PAF):

1-800-532 5274; (757) 873-8999 (FAX), or e-mail <help@ patientadvocate.org>

21. HOME SAFETY

[*See also* "First Aid and Survival Medicine," p. 29.]

Recommended Search Terms

- "Child safety"
- "Crib safety"
- "Electrical safety"
- Family safety
- Home safety
- "Home safety"
- "Home fire safety"
- "Home electrical safety"
- Home accident prevention
- Home injury prevention
- Household accident prevention
- Household injury prevention
- Household safety
- "Infant safety"
- "Injuries in the home" prevention
- "Residential safety"
- Safe home

Important Sites

American Academy of Orthopaedic Surgeons (AAOS): Home Safety Checklist: <http://orthoinfo.aaos.org/>

Association of Trial Lawyers of America (ATLA): Keep Our Families Safe: <http://www.atla.org/famsafe/>

Childhood Injury Prevention Coalition: <http://www .cchealth.org/prevention/coalitions/cipc/>

Children's Safety Network (CSN): Links: Residential Safety: <http://www.childrenssafetynetwork.org/links/ ressafe.asp>

Children's Safety Network (CSN): National Injury and Violence Prevention Resource Center: <http://www .childrenssafetynetwork.org/>

Consumer Product Safety Commission (CPSC): <http:// www.cpsc.gov/>

Consumer Product Safety Commission (CPSC): Crib Safety and SIDS Reduction: <http://www.cpsc.gov/ cpscpub/pubs/cribsafe.html>

Consumer Product Safety Commission: Household Products Safety Publications: <http://www.cpsc.gov/cpsc pub/pubs/house.html>

Electrical Safety Foundation International (ESFi): Home Electrical Safety Tips: <http://www.esfi.org/sub.php ?l0=hs&l1=hest>

FirstGov for Consumers: Home and Community: <http:// www.cpsc.gov/cpscpub/pubs/house.html>

Google: Directory: Home: Emergency Preparation: <http://directory.google.com/Top/Home/Emergency _Preparation/>

Home Safety Council: <http://www.homesafetycouncil .org/>

MedlinePlus: Accidents: <http://www.nlm.nih.gov/medline plus/accidents.html>

MedlinePlus: Asbestos/Asbestosis: <http://www.nlm.nih .gov/medlineplus/asbestosasbestosis.html>

MedlinePlus: Household Poisons: <http://www.nlm.nih .gov/medlineplus/householdpoisons.html>

MedlinePlus: Lead Poisoning: <http://www.nlm.nih.gov/ medlineplus/leadpoisoning.html>

MedlinePlus: Mercury: <http://www.nlm.nih.gov/medline plus/mercury.html>

MyPrimetime: Family: Family Checklists: <http://www.my primetime.com/family/tool/content/checklist _jumpage/index.shtml>

National Fire Protection Agency (NFPA): RiskWatch: Kids Only!: <http://www.nfpa.org/riskwatch/kids.html>

National Fire Protection Agency (NFPA): RiskWatch: Unintentional Injuries: <http://www.nfpa.org/risk watch/>

National Safety Council (NSC): Family Safety and Health: <http://www.nsc.org/pubs/fsh.htm>

Oregon Health and Science University (OHSU): Health: Household and Common Emergencies: Household Safety Checklist: <http://www.ohsuhealth.com/ ntrauma/check.asp>

Parenthood.com: Child/Household Safety: <http://www .links.parenthood.com/links_display.html?cat=64>

Proctor & Gamble: Science in the Box: <http://sciencein thebox.com/home.html>

Safe Motherhood: <http://www.safemotherhood.org/>

SafeUSA: Safe at Home: <http://www.safeusa.org/home/ safehome.htm>

St John Ambulance Centre (Australia): Home Safe: <http://www.stjohn.org.au/emergency/homesafe.pdf>

22. INTERNET SAFETY

Recommended Search Terms

- "Internet safety"
- "Safe surfing"
- "Internet safety" children parent

- "Internet safety" -kid -parent
- Cyberstalking

Important Sites

American Bar Association: Safeshopping.org: <http://www.safeshopping.org/>

CyberAngels.org: <http://www.cyberangels.org/>

CyberAngels.org: Internet 101: <http://www.cyberangels.org/101/>

Department for Education and Safety (DfES) Superhighway Safety (UK): <http://safety.ngfl.gov.uk/>

Department for Education and Safety (DfES) Superhighway Safety (UK): Using Technology Safety in Schools (UK): <http://safety.ngfl.gov.uk/schools/>

Department of Education: ED.gov: Technology: Internet Safety: <http://www.ed.gov/about/offices/list/os/technology/safety.html>

ePublicEye.com: <http://www.thepubliceye.com/>

Federal Bureau of Investigation (FBI): A Parent's Guide to Internet Safety: <http://www.fbi.gov/publications/pguide/pguidee.htm>

Internet Education Foundation: GetNetWise: <http://www.getnetwise.org/>

Internet Safety Awareness: <http://www.internet-safety.org/>

Kid Safety on the Internet: The Police Notebook: <http://www.ou.edu/oupd/kidsafe/start.htm>

NetSafe: The Internet Safety Group: <http://www.netsafe.org.nz/>

Organization for Internet Safety: <http://www.oisafety.org/>

SafeKids.com: <http://www.safekids.com/>

SafeTeens.com: <http://www.safeteens.com/>

Science Fiction and Fantasy Writers of America (SFWA): Cyberstalking and Internet Safety FAQ: <http://www.sfwa.org/gateway/stalking.htm>

WiredPatrol: <http://www.wiredpatrol.org/>

WiredPatrol: Cyberstalking Index: <http://www.wiredpatrol.org/stalking/>

Working to Halt Online Abuse (WHOA): <http://www.haltabuse.org/>

23. Office and Workplace Safety

[*See also* "Home Safety," p. 18; "Environmental Safety," p. 14.]

Recommended Search Terms

- Chemical handling safety
- Chemical safety
- Employee injury prevention

- "Employee safety"
- Ergonomics
- "Materials safety"
- MSDS [include name of a product or vendor]
- "Occupational health"
- "Occupational safety"
- Office evacuation planning
- Office injury prevention
- "Office safety"
- "Work place" safety
- "Work safety"
- Workplace safety

Important Sites

Centers for Disease Control and Prevention (CDC): National Institute for Occupational Safety and Health (NIOSH): Emergency Preparedness for Business: <http://www.cdc.gov/niosh/topics/prepared/>

Chemical Safety at Work: <http://chemicalsafetybook.com/>

Cumulative Trauma Disorder (CTD) News: <http://www.ctdnews.com/>

Google: Health: Occupational Health and Safety: <http://directory.google.com/Top/Health/Occupational_Health_and_Safety/>

Howard Hughes Medical Institute. Laboratory Safety Program: Online Safety Course: <http://www.practicingsafescience.org/>

MedlinePlus: Occupational Health: <http://www.nlm.nih.gov/medlineplus/occupationalhealth.html>

National Institute for Occupational Safety and Health (NIOSH): <http://www.cdc.gov/niosh/homepage.html>

Nolo. Law for All: Health and Safety FAQ: <http://www.nolo.com/encyclopedia/articles/emp/emp5.html>

Occupational Health and Safety Magazine: <http://www.ohsonline.com/>

Occupational Health (OH) Net: <http://www.occupational-health.net/>

Occupational Safety and Health Act (OSHA): OSHA Bulletin: <http://www.oshabulletin.com/>

Occupational Safety and Health Administration (OSHA.): <http://www.osha.gov/>

Safe Supervisor: <http://www.safesupervisor.com/>

Workplace Safety Services (Australia): <http://www.worksafety.com.au/>

WorkSafeBC.com: Health and Safety Centre: <http://www.healthandsafetycentre.org/>

WorkSafeBC.com: Health and Safety Centre: Injury Prevention Resources: <http://tourism.healthandsafetycentre.org/s/InjuryPreventionResources.asp>

MEDICAL SPECIALTIES

Occupational therapy; Occupational medicine; Vocational rehabilitation

24. OUTDOOR SAFETY

[*See also* "First Aid: Survival Medicine," p. 29.]

Recommended Search Terms

- "Camp safely"
- "Camping safety"
- "Climb safely"
- "Climbing safety"
- "Dehydration" "hot weather" prevention
- "Extreme cold" "first aid"
- "Hiking safety"
- Hypothermia
- Hypothermia prevention
- "Outdoor recreation" safety
- Outdoor safety
- "Poison Ivy" prevention
- "Poison Oak" treatment
- "Safe camping"
- "Safe climbing"
- "Safe hiking"

Important Sites

American Safe Climbing Association (ASCA): <http://www.safeclimbing.org/>

Centers for Disease Control and Prevention (CDC): National Center for Environmental Health. Outdoor Safety: <http://www.cdc.gov/nceh/hsb/extremecold/outdoorsafety.htm>

eMedicine:. Wilderness Emergencies—Medical References: <http://www.emedicine.com/wild/>

HikerCentral.com: Safety: <http://www.hikercentral.com/safety/>

KidsHealth: Woods and Camping Safety for the Whole Family: <http://kidshealth.org/parent/firstaid_safe/outdoor/woods.html>

MedlinePlus: Hypothermia: <http://www.nlm.nih.gov/medlineplus/hypothermia.html>

Outdoor Action (OA): First Aid and Safety: <http://www.princeton.edu/~oa/safety/>

OutdoorEd: Outdoor Safety Management: <http://www.outdoored.com/Articles/Article.asp?ArticleID=121>

Princeton University Outdoor Action: Outdoor Action Guide to Outdoor Safety Management: <http://www.princeton.edu/~oa/safety/safeman.html>

Search and Rescue Society of British Columbia (SARBC): Outdoor Recreation and Safety: <http://www.sarbc.org/sar-rec.html>

U.S. Geological Services (USGS): Viewing Lava Safely: Common Sense Is Not Enough: <http://geopubs.wr.usgs.gov/fact-sheet/fs152-00/>

U.S. Scouting Service Project: Climb On Safely: <http://www.usscouts.org/safety/ClimbOnSafely.html>

U.S. Scouting Service Project: Health and Safety: <http://www.usscouts.org/usscouts/safety.asp>

25. PERSONAL SAFETY AND DOMESTIC VIOLENCE

Recommended Search Terms

- Assault prevention
- Battering
- "Battered child"
- "Battered spouse"
- "Battered wife"
- "Child abuse" prevention
- "Child neglect"
- "Child sexual abuse"
- "Date rape"
- "Domestic violence"
- "Domestic violence" stop
- "Elder abuse"
- "Family violence"
- Incest
- "Model mugging"
- Rape
- Rape defense
- Rape prevention
- "Parent battering"
- "Personal safety"
- Refuges violence
- "Safe house"
- "Self defense"
- "Self protection"
- "Senior abuse" prevention
- "Sexual assault"
- "Sexual assault" prevention
- "Sexual violence"
- "Spousal abuse"
- "Spouse abuse" stop

Important Sites

AdvocateWeb: <http://www.advocateweb.org/>

American Institute on Domestic Violence: <http://www.aidv-usa.com/>

American Medical Association (AMA): Violence Prevention: <http://www.ama-assn.org/ama/pub/category/3242.html>

American Women Overseas: Domestic Violence Crisis Line: <http://www.awoscentral.com/>

Arming Women against Rape and Endangerment (AWARE): <http://www.aware.org/>

Arming Women against Rape and Endangerment (AWARE): Self-Protection Quiz: <http://www.aware.org/quizzes/quizselfprot.shtml>

British Broadcasting Corporation (BBC): Health: Relationships: Hitting Home—Domestic Violence: <http://www.bbc.co.uk/hittinghome/>

British Columbia Institute against Family Violence (BCIAFV): BCIAFV Newsletter: <http://www.bcifv.org/resources/newsletter/>

Centers for Disease Control and Prevention (CDC): National Center for Injury Prevention and Control (NCIPC): Sexual Violence against People with Disabilities: <http://www.cdc.gov/ncipc/factsheets/disabvi.htm>

Childline (UK): <http://www.childline.org.uk/>

City of Fullerton, CA: Crime Prevention Tips for the Disabled: <http://www.ci.fullerton.ca.us/police/tips/crimeprv.html>

City of Fullerton, CA: Rape Prevention Tips: <http://www.ci.fullerton.ca.us/police/tips/rapeprev.html>

Cybergrrl Safety Net: <http://www.cybergrrl.com/fs.jhtml?/views/dv/>

Department of Justice (DOJ), Office on Violence against Women: <http://www.ojp.usdoj.gov/vawo/>

Domestic Violence and Incest Resource Centre (Australia): <http://home.vicnet.net.au/~dvirc/>

Faith Trust Institute (previously Center for the Prevention of Sexual and Domestic Violence): <http://www.cpsdv.org/>

Family Violence Prevention Fund: <http://www.fvpf.org/>

Health Canada: National Clearinghouse on Family Violence: <http://www.hc-sc.gc.ca/hppb/familyviolence/>

Hidden Hurt (UK): Domestic Abuse Information: Helpline Telephone Numbers: <http://www.geocities.com/nosiris126/helplines.htm>

MaleSurvivor: National Organization on Male Sexual Victimization: <http://www.malesurvivor.org/>

McGruff the Crime Dog: <http://www.mcgruff-safe-kids.com/>

MedlinePlus: Domestic Violence: <http://www.nlm.nih.gov/medlineplus/domesticviolence.html>

MedlinePlus: Rape: <http://www.nlm.nih.gov/medlineplus/rape.html>

Men Can Stop Rape: <http://www.mencanstoprape.org/>

National Center on Elder Abuse (NCEA): <http://www.elderabusecenter.org/>

National Clearinghouse on Child Abuse and Neglect Information: <http://www.calib.com/nccanch/>

National Coalition against Domestic Violence: <http://www.ncadv.org/>

National Coalition against Sexual Assault (NCASA): Guidelines for Choosing a Self-Defense Course: <http://www.karatevid.com:80/article-SDguidelines.html>

National Committee for the Prevention of Elder Abuse (NCPEA): <http://www.preventelderabuse.org/>

National Council on Child Abuse and Family Violence (NCCAFV): <http://nccafv.org/>

National Domestic Violence Hotline: <http://www.ndvh.org/>

National Institute on Aging (NIA): The National Elder Abuse Incidence Study: <http://www.aoa.gov/abuse/report/>

National Society for the Prevention of Cruelty to Children (NSPCC) (UK): <http://www.nspcc.org.uk/>

No Nonsense Self Defense: <http://www.nononsenseselfdefense.com/>

Public Broadcasting Service (PBS): No Safe Place: <http://www.pbs.org/kued/nosafeplace/>

Rape101.com: <http://www.rape101.com/>

Rape Abuse and Incest National Network (RAINN): <http://www.rainn.org/>

Rape Aggression Defense (RAD) Systems: <http://www.rad-systems.com/>

Rape and Sexual Abuse Counselling (RASAC) (UK): <http://www.rasac.org.uk/>

Rape Crisis Federation Wales and England (UK): <http://www.rapecrisis.co.uk/>

Rape Prevention Information and Resources: <http://www4.nau.edu/fronske/brochures/rape.html>

Safe Child Program: <http://www.safechild.org/>

Safe Haven: <http://www.safehaven-uk.org/>

Safe Horizon: <http://www.safehorizon.org/>

Self Defense Tips, Tricks and Advice for Women: <http://www.safetyforwomen.com/>

Self Defense IMPACT Chicago: Self-Defense Resources: <http://www.impactchicago.org/resource.html>

SouthCoast Today: Shattered Love Broken Lives: Domestic Violence: <http://www.s-t.com/projects/DomVio/domviohome.html>

State University of New York at Buffalo, Counseling Services: Sexual Assertiveness Questionnaire and Date Rape Prevention: <http://ub-counseling.buffalo.edu/rapeprevent.shtml>

Stop Abuse for Everyone (SAFE): <http://www.safe4all.org/>

Stop It Now: <http://www.stopitnow.com/>

Toolkit to End Violence against Women: <http://toolkit.ncjrs.org/>

Trauma Treatment Manual: <http://amsterdam.park.org/Guests/Stream/trauma_manual.htm>

V-Day: Until the Violence Stops: <http://www.vday.org/>

Violence against Women Online Resources (VAWOR): <http://www.vaw.umn.edu/>

Women against Violence against Women (WAVAW) (Canada): Rape Crisis Centre: <http://www.wavaw.ca/index2.htm>

Women against Violence Europe (WAVE): <http://www.wave-network.org/>

Women Lawyers: Domestic Violence Notepad: <http://www.womenlawyers.com/domestic.htm>

Women's Aid Federation of England (UK): <http://www.womensaid.org.uk/>

World Health Organization (WHO): Injuries and Violence Prevention: <http://www.who.int/violence_injury_prevention/>

YMCA Safe Place: <http://www.safeplaceservices.org/>

The Zero: Domestic Violence International Resources: <http://www.vachss.com/help_text/domestic_violence_intl.html>

The Zero: Resources: <http://www.vachss.com/help_text/>

HOTLINES

Australia

Adelaide Rape Crisis Centre:
(008) 188-095 (toll free); (08) 293-8666 (crisis line)
DOCS Domestic Violence Line Phone:
1-800-656-463
Domestic Violence Helpline:
1-800-800-098
Kids Helpline:
1-800-551-800
Sydney Rape Crisis Centre:
1-800-424-017
Rape and Sexual Assault Services:
1-800-817-421

Canada

Canadian National Clearinghouse on Family Violence:
1-800-267-1291; (613) 941-8930 (Fax)
Child Abuse Hotline:
1-800-387-KIDS
Kids Help Phone:
1-800-668-6868
National Domestic Violence Hotline (English/French):
1-800-363-9010
Sexual Assault Support and Crisis:
1-800-909-7007
Women against Violence against Women (WAVAW): Rape Crisis Centre:
1-877-392-7583 or e-mail <wavaw@shaw.ca>

United Kingdom

British Broadcasting Corporation (BBC) free helpline:
08000 934-934
Childline:
0800-1111
National Society for the Prevention of Cruelty to Children (NSPCC):
Child Protection Helpline: 0808-800-5000
Rape and Abuse Line:
0808-800-0123
Rape/Indecent Assault Crisis Counselling:
0800-735-0567
Refuge 24-Hour National Crisis Line:
0990-995-443 / 0870-599-5443
Women's Aid National Domestic Violence Helpline (UK):
08457-023-468

United States

American Women Overseas: International Crisis Line:
1-866-USWOMEN/(866) 879-6636; (503) 907-6554; (Fax) or e-mail <awos@awoscentral.com>
National Domestic Violence Hotline:
1-800-799-SAFE/1-800-799-7233;
1-800-787-3224 (TDD)
Rape, Abuse, and Incest National Network (RAINN):
1-800-656-HOPE

26. PRODUCT AND SHOPPING SAFETY

Recommended Search Terms

- "Consumer safety"
- "Customer safety"
- "Product recalls"
- "Product safety"
- "Safe climbing"

Important Sites

American Bar Association: Safeshopping.org: <http://www.safeshopping.org/>

Better Business Bureau: <http://www.bbb.org/>

Complaints.com: <http://www.complaints.com/>

Consumer Alert: <http://www.consumeralert.org/>

Consumer Product Safety Commission (CPSC): <http://www.cpsc.gov/>

Consumer Product Safety Commission (CPSC): Toy Hazard Recalls: <http://www.cpsc.gov/cpscpub/prerel/category/toy.html>

Consumer Product Safety Commission (CPSC): Toy Product Publications: <http://www.cpsc.gov/cpscpub/pubs/toy_sfy.html>

Consumer Reports Online for Kids: <http://www.zillions.org/>

Consumer Watchdog (Australia): <http://www.watchdog.com.au/>

Consumer World: <http://www.consumerworld.org/>

ePublicEye.com: <http://www.thepubliceye.com/>

International Consumer Product Health and Safety Organization (ICPHSO): <http://www.icphso.org/>

International Consumer Rights Protection Council: <http://icrpc.tripod.com/>

National Association of State Public Interest Research Groups (PIRGs): ToySafety.net: <http://www.pirg.org/toysafety/>

National Consumer Complaint Centre: <http://www.alexanderlaw.com/nccc/>

Recall Announcements: <http://www.recallannouncements.com/>

Recall Announcements: Your Health and Safety Matters: <http://www.recallannouncements.com/health_and_safety/>

Trading Standards Consumer Complaints (UK): <http://www.consumercomplaints.org.uk/>

U.S. Attorney General: Consumer Protection: <http://www.attorneygeneral.gov/pei/bcp.cfm>

27. School, Playground, and Campus Safety

Recommended Search Terms

- "Campus safety"
- "Playground safety"
- "Safe climbing"
- "School bus safety"
- "School safety"
- "Schoolbus safety"

Important Sites

American Academy of Orthopaedic Surgeons (AAOS): Playground Safety: <http://orthoinfo.aaos.org/fact/thr_report.cfm?Thread_ID=95&topcategory=Play-ground%20Safety/>

American Academy of Orthopaedic Surgeons (AAOS): Playground Safety Checklist: <http://orthoinfo.aaos.org/fact/thr_report.cfm?Thread_ID=180&topcategory=Play-ground%20Safety/>

American Academy of Orthopaedic Surgeons (AAOS): A Guide to Playground Safety: <http://orthoinfo.aaos.org/brochure/thr_report.cfm?Thread_ID=39&topcategory=Play-ground%20Safety/>

Center for Effective Collaboration and Practice: Early Warning, Timely Response: A Guide to Safe Schools: <http://cecp.air.org/guide/earlywarning.htm>

Childline (UK): Bullying: <http://www.childline.org.uk/Bullying.asp>

Consumer Product Safety Commission (CPSC): Handbook for Public Playground Safety: <http://www.cpsc.gov/cpscpub/pubs/325.pdf> (NOTE: Adobe Acrobat file)

Consumer Product Safety Commission (CPSC): Kidd Safety: <http://www.cpsc.gov/kids/kidsafety/>

Department of Education, Office of Safe and Drug-Free Schools (OSDFS): <http://www.ed.gov/offices/OESE/SDFS/>

Howard Hughes Medical Institute: Safety in the Lab: Online Safety Course: <http://www.practicingsafescience.org/>

McGruff the Crime Dog: <http://www.mcgruff-safe-kids.com/>

National Alliance for Safe Schools: <http://www.safeschools.org/>

National Education Association (NEA): School Safety: <http://www.nea.org/issues/safescho/>

Northwest Regional Educational Laboratory: Safetyzone: <http://www.safetyzone.org/>

Safe Kids Canada/SécuriJeunes Canada: <http://www.safekidscanada.ca/>

Safe Routes to Schools (UK): <http://www.saferoutestoschools.org.uk/>

Safe Schools Coalition: <http://www.safeschools-wa.org/>

Safe Schools Coalition, Inc.: <http://www.thesafeschools.org/>

SafeUSA: Safe at School: <http://www.safeusa.org/school/safescho.htm>

SafeUSA: Playground Safety: <http://www.safeusa.org/school/safescho.htm#Playground%20Safety/>

National Highway Traffic Safety (NHTSA): School Bus Safety Program: <http://www.nhtsa.dot.gov/people/injury/buses/>

School Bus Safety Rules (National Safety Council): <http://www.nsc.org/library/facts/schlbus.htm>

Security on Campus: <http://www.campussafety.org/>

Stay Alert Stay Safe (SASS) (Canada): <http://www.sass.ca/>

28. Sexual Safety

[*See also* "Sexual Health Issues," p. 178.]

NOTE: 1. Information in this section concerns making safe choices of sexual behavior. Information about sexual violence and rape prevention is in "Personal Safety and Domestic Violence," p. 20.

2. Because of the nature of this topic some of the Web sites listed contain graphic materials and information.

Most require that the viewer be at least 18 years of age. Sites that are intended for adolescent viewers are indicated with the word "teen," if it is not included in the title of the Web site.

Recommended Search Terms

- "AIDS/HIV" prevention
- "Birth control"
- Healthy sexuality
- "HIV/AIDS" prevention
- Pregnancy prevention
- "Reproductive health"
- Responsible "sexual choices"
- "Safe sex"
- "Safer sex"
- "Sex education"
- "Sex safety"
- "Sexual education"
- "Sexual risks"
- "Sexual safety"
- "Sexually transmitted diseases" prevention
- "STD" prevention

Important Sites

American Medical Women's Association (AMWA): Reproductive Health Initiative: <http://www.amwa-doc.org/RHI.htm>

American Social Health Association (ASHA): iwannaknow [Teen]: <http://www.iwannaknow.org/>

Avert (UK): AIDS, Sex and Teens: <http://www.avert.org/young.htm>

Avert (UK): Lesbians, Bisexual Women and Safe Sex: <http://www.avert.org/lesbiansafesex.htm>

The Body: An AIDS and HIV Information Resource: Safe Sex and HIV Prevention: <http://www.thebody.com/safesex.html>

California Abortion and Reproduction Rights Action League (CARAL): Research Center: <http://www.choice.org/researchcenter/>

CancerBACUP (UK): Sexuality and Cancer: Healthy Sexuality: <http://www.cancerbacup.org.uk/info/sex/sex-8.htm>

Disability Online (Australia): Condom for Women—Safe Sex and Contraception: <http://www.disability.vic.gov.au/dsonline/dsarticles.nsf/pages/Condom_for_women_safe_sex_and_contraception?OpenDocument/>

Families Are Talking: For Young People [Teen]: Talk about Sex: <http://www.familiesaretalking.org/teen/teen0000.html>

Family Health International (FHI) (Multilingual): <http://www.fhi.org/>

Go Ask Alice! [Teen]: <http://www.goaskalice.columbia.edu/>

International Centre for Reproductive Health: <http://www.icrh.org/>

International Planned Parenthood Federation (IPPF): <http://www.ippf.org/>

Kaiser Network: Daily Reports: Daily Reproductive Health Report: <http://report.kff.org/repro/>

National Campaign to Prevent Teen Pregnancy (NCPTP): <http://www.teenpregnancy.org/>

National Campaign to Prevent Teen Pregnancy (NCPTP): Information for Teens: <http://www.teenpregnancy.org/resources/teens/>

Oregon Health and Science University (OHSU): Health.com: Women's Health: Guidelines for Safer Sex: <http://www.ohsuhealth.com/woman/safesex.asp?sub=2>

Parents Place: Safe Sex during Pregnancy: 10 Things You Need to Know: <http://www.parentsplace.com/expert/midwife/articles/>

Pathfinder International: <http://www.pathfind.org/>

Planned Parenthood Federation of America: <http://www.plannedparenthood.org/>

Public Broadcasting Service (PBS), WGBH—Boston: American Experience: The Pill: <http://www.pbs.org/wgbh/amex/pill/>

Reproductive Health Outlook (RHO): <http://www.rho.org/>

Reproductive Health Outlook—Spanish (RHO): <http://www.rhoespanol.org/>

ReproLine (Reproductive Health Online): <http://www.reproline.jhu.edu/>

safersex.org: filchyboy safersex: <http://www.safersex.org/>

Scarleteen: Sex Education for the Real World [Teen]: <http://www.scarleteen.com/>

Sex! Life! (Australia): Sexuality and Sexual Health: Post-Partum Frequently Asked Questions: <http://www.sexlife.net.au/3_9_1.html>

Sexual Health Infocenter: <http://www.sexhealth.org/>

Sexuality Information and Education Council of the United States (SIECUS): <http://www.siecus.org/>

Sexuality Information and Education Council of the United States (SIECUS): Issues and Answers: Fact Sheet on Sexuality Education: <http://www.siecus.org/pubs/fact/fact0007.html>

Sexuality.org: Society for Human Sexuality: Guide to Safer Sex (Concise): <http://www.sexuality.org/concise.html>

Sexuality.org: Society for Human Sexuality: Guide to Safer Sex (Lengthy): <http://www.sexuality.org/safesex.html>

Safely Singles for Singles: <http://www.solosingles.com/ssafe/>

29. STREET SMARTS

Recommended Search Terms

- "Model mugging"
- Mugging prevention
- "Pedestrian safety"
- "Street-proof"
- "Street-proofing"
- "Street-safe"
- "Street safety" ".org"
- "Street smart" safe
- "Street smarts" safety
- "Walk safely"
- "Walking safety"

Important Sites

American Council of the Blind: Pedestrian Safety: <http://www.acb.org/pedestrian/>

Campus Outreach Services: Take Back the Night: <http://www.campusoutreachservices.com/tbtn2.htm>

Centers for Disease Control and Prevention (CDC): National Center for Injury Prevention and Control (NCIPC): National Strategies for Advancing Child Pedestrian Safety: <http://www.cdc.gov/ncipc/pedestrian/>

Children's Hospital of Pittsburgh: For Kids: Street Safety: <http://www.chp.edu/besafe/kids/01road_rules.php>

Children's Hospital of Pittsburgh: For Parents: Street Safety: <http://www.chp.edu/besafe/adults/02street.php>

Department for Transport (UK): The Kerbcraft Manual: Smart Strategies for Pedestrian Safety: <http://www.kerbcraft.org.uk/manual.htm>

Department for Transport (UK): Think! Driving Requires All Your Attention: <http://www.thinkroadsafety.gov.uk/>

Department for Transport (DOT) (UK): Think! Road Safety: Hedgehogs (For Kids): <http://www.hedgehogs.gov.uk/>

Department of Transportation (DOT): Federal Highway Administration (FHWA): Pedestrian Safety: <http://safety.fhwa.dot.gov/fourthlevel/ped.htm>

Department of Transportation (DOT): National Highway Traffic Safety Administration (NHTSA): Pedestrian Safety (Kids): <http://www.nhtsa.dot.gov/kids/biketour/pedsafety/>

Department of Transportation (DOT): Federal Highway Administration. Pedestrian Safety Campaign: <http://safety.fhwa.dot.gov/pedcampaign/>

Do2Learn. Games: Safety Games: Street Safety Activity Page: <http://www.dotolearn.com/games/safetygames/activity_sheets/activity_streetsafety.htm>

Federal Highway Administration: Pedestrian and Bicycle Safety Research: <http://www.tfhrc.gov/safety/pedbike/pedbike.htm>

Injury Prevention Web (IPW): Internet Injury Prevention Resources: Bicycle and Pedestrian Safety: <http://www.injuryprevention.org/links/links-bikeped.htm>

KidsHealth: Do You Know How to Be Street Smart?: <http://kidshealth.org/kid/watch/out/street_smart.html>

National Fire Protection Agency (NFPA): RiskWatch: Bike and Pedestrian Safety: <http://www.nfpa.org/riskwatch/parent_bike.html>

National Highway Traffic Safety Administration (NHTSA): People: Injury Prevention: Pedestrian Safety: <http://www.nhtsa.dot.gov/people/injury/pedbimot/ped/>

National Network for Child Care (NNCC): Look to the Left, Look to the Right: <http://www.nncc.org/Health/look.left.right.html>

New Orleans Police Department: Street Smart: Tips for Working, Living and Playing Downtown: <http://www.nopdonline.com/tips.htm>

New York State (NYS): Department of Motor Vehicles: Traffic Sign Quiz for Kids: <http://www.nysgtsc.state.ny.us/kidssign.htm>

Pedestrians Educate Drivers about Safety (PEDS): <http://www.peds.org/>

Pedestrians Educate Drivers about Safety (PEDS): Kids Page: What Is KidsWalk: <http://www.peds.org/prog_kids.htm>

Safe Campuses Now: Safety When Walking on Streets: <http://www.safecampusesnow.org/Safety/StreetSafety.htm>

Safe Kids Canada: Pedestrian Safety: <http://www.safekidscanada.ca/English/SKW/SKW_RoadSafety/SKW_Pedestrian.html>

Safe Routes to Schools (UK): <http://www.saferoutestoschools.org.uk/>

Stay Alert Stay Safe (SASS) (Canada): <http://www.sass.ca/>

Virtual Children's Hospital: Pediatrics Common Questions, Quick Answers: Pedestrian Safety: <http://www.vh.org/pediatric/patient/pediatrics/cqqa/pedestriansafety.html>

30. TRAVEL HEALTH AND SAFETY

Recommended Search Terms

- Hotel safety
- Travel medicine
- Travel safety
- Traveler health
- Traveler safety

Important Sites

Airsafety.com. Airport and Airline Security: <http://www.airsafe.com/>

Centers for Disease Control and Prevention (CDC): National Center for Infectious Diseases: Traveler's Health: <http://www.cdc.gov/travel/>

Consumer Product Safety Commission (CPSC): Hotel and Motel Crib and Play Yard Safety Checklist: <http://www.cpsc.gov/cpscpub/pubs/5136.html>

Department of State: The Bureau of Consular Affairs: <http://travel.state.gov/>

eMedicine: Wilderness and Travel Medicine: <http://www.emedicine.com/emerg/topic838.htm>

FirstGov.gov: Travel Safely: <http://www.firstgov.gov/Topics/Usgresponse/Travel_Safely.shtml>

International Society of Travel Medicine: <http://www.istm.org/>

Medical College of Wisconsin: Healthlink: Travel Health Links: <http://healthlink.mcw.edu/travel-links.html>

MedlinePlus: Traveler's Health: <http://www.nlm.nih.gov/medlineplus/travelershealth.html>

Michigan.gov: Department of Management and Budget: Travel: Tips on Hotel Safety: <http://www.Michigan.gov/>

Virtual Hospital: Emporiatrics: An Introduction to Travel Medicine: <http://www.vh.org/adult/provider/internalmedicine/TravelMedicine/TravelMedHP.html>

World Health Organization (WHO): International Travel and Health: <http://www.who.int/ith/>

Related Sites

AARP (American Association of Retired Persons): Global Aging: Achieving Its Potential: <http://www.aarp.org/international/Articles/a2003-04-15-globalaging.htm>

AARP (American Association of Retired Persons): International Affairs: <http://www.aarp.org/international/>

Global Health: Frequently Asked Questions (FAQs): <http://www.globalhealth.gov/faq.shtml>

31. VEHICLE AND TRAFFIC SAFETY

[*See also* "Traffic Accidents," p. 41.]

NOTE: This section deals only with ground traffic vehicles. Air traffic safety is included in "Travel Health and Safety," p. 25; water vehicle safety is included in "Water Safety," p. 27.

HOTLINE

Department of Transportation (DOT), National Highway Traffic Safety Administration (NHTSA): Auto Safety Hotline:
1-888-DASH-2-DOT/1-888-327-4236

Recommended Search Terms

- Auto safety
- Automobile maintenance
- Automobile repair guidelines
- Automobile safety
- Bicycle safety
- Bicycling safety
- Biking safety
- Car maintenance
- Car safety
- Cycling safety
- Cyclist safety
- Defensive cycling
- Defensive driving
- Defensive motorcycling
- Driver safety
- Driving safety
- Driving safely
- Motorcycle safety
- Motorcycling safety
- Passenger safety
- "Road rage"
- Safe driving
- Traffic safety
- Transportation safety

Important Sites

Car Maintenance Safety Tips: <http://www.nsc.org/issues/idrive/drivtips.htm>

Car-Safety.org: Carseat FAQ: <http://www.car-safety.org/faq.html>

Citizens for Safe Cycling (CfSC) (Canada): <http://www.cfsc.ottawa.on.ca/>

Department for Transport (UK): THINK! Driving Requires All Your Attention: <http://www.thinkroadsafety.gov.uk/>

Department of Transportation (DOT [U.S.]): Federal Motor Carrier Safety Administration (FMCSA): Share the Road Safely: <http://www.sharetheroadsafely.org/>

Drive Home Safe: A Teen Driving Website Center: <http://www.drivehomesafe.com/>

Fatality Analysis Reporting System (FARS) Web-Based Encyclopedia: <http://www-fars.nhtsa.dot.gov/>

Insurance Institute for Highway Safety (IIHS)/Highway Loss Data Institute (HLDI): Crash Testing and Highway Safety: <http://www.hwysafety.org/>

McGruff the Crime Dog: <http://www.mcgruff-safe-kids.com/>

National Highway Traffic Safety Administration (NHTSA): <http://www.nhtsa.dot.gov/>

National Highway Traffic Safety Administration (NHTSA): Child Passenger Safety: <http://www.nhtsa.dot.gov/people/injury/childps/>

National Highway Traffic Safety Administration (NHTSA): DOT Auto Safety Hotline: <http://www.nhtsa.dot.gov/hotline/>

National Highway Traffic Safety Administration (NHTSA): Driving Safely While Aging Gracefully: <http://www.nhtsa.dot.gov/people/injury/olddrive/Driving%20Safely%20Aging%20Web/>

National Highway Traffic Safety Administration (NHTSA): Injury Prevention: <http://www.nhtsa.dot.gov/people/injury/>

National Highway Traffic Safety Administration (NHTSA): Office of Defects Investigation (ODI): <http://www-odi.nhtsa.dot.gov/cars/problems/recalls/index.cfm>

National Highway Traffic Safety Administration (NHTSA): School Bus Safety Program: <http://www.nhtsa.dot.gov/people/injury/buses/>

National Highway Traffic Safety Administration (NHTSA): Spanish: <http://www.nhtsa.dot.gov/multicultural/hispanicamerican/hispanic-index.html>

National SAFE KIDS Campaign: <http://www.safekids.org/>

National Safety Council (NSC): Driver Safety: <http://www.nsc.org/issues/drivsafe.htm>

National Safety Council: Fact Sheet Library: Schoolbus Safety Rules: <http://www.nsc.org/library/facts/schlbus.htm>

National Transportation Safety Board (NTSB): <http://www.ntsb.gov/>

North America Railway Foundation: Crossing Safely: <http://www.crossingsafely.com/>

Oregon Health and Science University (OHSU) Health: Household and Common Emergencies: Bicycle Safety: <http://www.ohsuhealth.com/ntrauma/bike.asp>

Oregon Health and Science University (OHSU) Health: Household and Common Emergencies: Seat Belts and Car Seats: <http://www.ohsuhealth.com/ntrauma/seatbelt.asp>

Safe Routes to Schools (UK): <http://www.saferoutestoschools.org.uk/>

SafetyBeltSafe USA: Safe Ride Helpline for Child Passenger Safety: <http://www.carseat.org/>

SafeUSA: Bike Safety: <http://safeusa.org/bike/bike.htm>

SafeUSA: Safe on the Move: <http://www.safeusa.org/move/safemove.htm>

32. WATER SAFETY

Recommended Search Terms

- Aquatic safety
- Boat accident prevention
- Boat safe
- "Boat safety"
- "Boating safety"
- Drowning prevention
- "Fishing safely"
- "Fishing safety"
- "Flood safety"
- Lifeguard
- Lifesaver water safety
- "Pool safety"
- Safe boating
- Swim safe
- Swim safely
- Swim safety
- "Swimming safety"
- "Water safety"

Important Sites

American Academy of Orthopaedic Surgeons (AAOS): Make Your Summer Safe: Tips for the Pool: <http://orthoinfo.aaos.org/fact/thr_report.cfm?Thread_ID=106&topcategory=Playground%20Safety/>

American Red Cross: Disaster Services. Disaster Safety: Flood and Flash Flood (English/ Spanish): <http://www.redcross.org/services/disaster/>

American Red Cross: Swimming and Lifeguarding: <http://www.redcross.org/services/hss/aquatics/>

Boat Safe: Boating Courses, Boating Tips, Boating Safety, Boating Contests: <http://www.boatsafe.com/>

Boat Safe Kids: <http://www.boatsafe.com/kids/>

Centers for Disease Control and Prevention (CDC): National Center for Injury Prevention: Water-Related Injuries: <http://www.cdc.gov/ncipc/factsheets/drown.htm>

Consumer Product Safety Commission (CPSC): Pool and Spa Safety Publications: <http://www.cpsc.gov/cpscpub/pubs/chdrown.html>

Epilepsy Action: Epilepsy and Swimming: <http://www.epilepsy.org.uk/info/swimming.html>

Epilepsy Foundation of Victoria (Australia): Epilepsy Information: Swimming Safely: <http://www.epinet.org.au/info/swim.html>

Federal Emergency Management Agency (FEMA): National Flood Insurance Program (NFIP): Flood Safety: <http://www.fema.gov/nfip/floodsaf.shtm>

MedlinePlus: Drowning: <http://www.nlm.nih.gov/medlineplus/drowning.html>

National Safe Boating Council: <http://www.safeboating council.org/>

SafeUSA: Water Safety: <http://safeusa.org/water/water.htm>

U.S. Coast Guard (USCG): Office of Boating Safety: <http://www.uscgboating.org/>

USA Swimming: Best of Safety Quarterly: What Is Safety?: <http://www.usswim.org/coaches/sq_whatis.htm>

The Weather Channel: Weather Safety: Flood: <http://www.weather.com/safeside/flood/>

WeatherEye: Flash Flood!: <http://weathereye.kgan.com/cadet/flood/>

SAFETY PUBLICATIONS ON THE INTERNET

Canadian Occupational Safety Magazine: <http://www.cos-mag.com/>

ConsumerReports.org: <http://www.consumerreports.org/main/home.jsp>

EurOhs: European *Occupational Health and Safety Magazine*: <http://www.eurohs.eu.com/training2.htm>

Food and Drug Administration (FDA): *FDA Consumer Magazine*: <http://www.fda.gov/fdac/>

Health!Canada Features: <http://www.hc-sc.gc.ca/english/feature/>

Occupational Health and Safety (Canada): <http://www.ohsonline.com/>

Occupational Health and Safety Magazine (Canada): <http://www.ohscanada.com/>

Safe Supervisor: <http://www.safesupervisor.com/>

HOTLINES

Selected Web Sites Listing Safety Hotlines

Department of Health and Human Services (DHHS): HHS Information and Hotline Directory: <http://www.hhs.gov/about/referlst.html>

Environmental Protection Agency (EPA): Hotlines: <http://www.epa.gov/epahome/hotline.htm>

Federal Citizen Information Center (FCIC): National Contact Center: Federal Toll-free Numbers: <http://www.info.gov/toll-free.htm>

U.S. Blue Pages: <http://bp.fed.gov/>

Selected Safety Hotline Numbers

Centers for Disease Control and Prevention (CDC): Public Health Emergency Preparedness and Response: 1-888-246-2675; 1-888-246-2857 (Spanish); 1-866-874-2646 (TTY)

Department of Energy (DOE): Health and Safety Hotline: 1-877-447-9756

Department of Transportation (DOT): Auto Safety Hotline: 1-888-DASH-2-DOT/1-888-327-4236

U.S. Department of Transportation (DOT). Safety Hotline 1-888-DOT-SAFT

Eat Well, Eat Safe (Canada): 1-866-50FSNET/1-866-503-7638 or e-mail <fsnrsn@uoguelph.ca>

Food Safety and Inspection Service (FSIS). Food Safety Education Staff Meat and Poultry Hotline: 1-800-535-4555/1-800-256-7072 (TDD/TTY) or e-mail <mphotline.fsis@usda.gov>

National Domestic Violence Hotline: 1-800-799-SAFE /1-800-787-3224 (TDD)

National Safety Council: Radon Hotline: 1-800-SOS-RADON/1-800-767-7236

Nuclear Safety Hotline: 1-800-626-6376

U.S. Consumer Product Safety Commission: 1-800-638-CPSC/1-800-638-8270 (TTY) or e-mail <info@cpsc.gov>

FAQS

American College of Physicians (ACP): Internal Medicine/Doctors for Adults: Patient Safety: Frequently Asked Questions: <http://www.acponline.org/ptsafety/faq.htm>

American Red Cross: FAQs: Health and Safety FAQs: <http://www.redcross.org/faq/0,1096,0_381_,00.html>

Electrical Safety Foundation International (ESFi): Home Safety FAQ: <http://www.esfi.org/sub.php?l0=hs&l1=hsfaq/>

Institute of Food Science and Technology (UK): Frequently Asked Questions about Food Science, Nutrition and Safety: <http://www.ifst.org/ifstfaq.htm>

MEDICAL SPECIALTIES

Occupational health; Occupational medicine; Public health; Safety engineering;

PROFESSIONAL ORGANIZATIONS

American Association of Occupational Health Nurses (AAOHN): <http://www.aaohn.org/>

American Industrial Hygiene Association (AIHA): <http://www.aiha.org/>

American Public Health Association (APHA): <http://www.apha.org/>

American Society of Safety Engineers (ASSE): <http://www.asse.org/>

Association of Societies for Occupational Safety and Health (ASOSH): <http://www.asosh.org/>

Board of Canadian Registered Safety Professionals (BCRSP): <http://www.acrsp.ca/>

Board of Certified Safety Professionals: <http://www.bcsp.org/>

Canadian Association of Road Safety Professionals/L'Association Canadienne des Professionnels de la Sécurité Routière (CARSP/ACPSER): <http://www.carsp.ca/>

Canadian Public Health Association/Association Canadienne de Santé Publique (CPHA-ACSP): <http://www.cpha.ca/>

Education Safety Association of Ontario (ESAO) (Canada): <http://www.esao.on.ca/>

Farm and Ranch Safety and Health Association (Canada): <http://www.farsha.bc.ca/>

Farm Safety Association (Canada): <http://www.farmsafety.ca/>

Firearms Safety Society: <http://huntingsociety.org/nevers.html>

International Commission on Occupational Health (ICOH): <http://www.icoh.org.sg/>

International Ergonomics Association (IEA): <http://www.iea.cc/>

International Occupational Hygiene Association (IOHA): <http://www.ioha.com/>

Ontario Occupational Health Nurses Association (Canada): <http://www.oohna.on.ca/>

UK Public Health Association: <http://www.ukpha.org.uk/>

World Safety Organization (WSO): <http://www.worldsafety.org/>

CONSUMER SUPPORT ORGANIZATIONS/ DISCUSSION GROUPS

Consumer Gateway (UK): <http://www.consumer.gov.uk/consumer_web/index_v4.htm>

Consumers Union: <http://www.consumersunion.org/>

BEST ONE-STOP SHOPS

American College of Physicians (ACP): Internal Medicine/Doctors for Adults: Patient Safety: <http://www.acponline.org/ptsafety/?idx/>

American Red Cross: <http://www.redcross.org/>

Consumer Product Safety Commission (CPSC): <http://www.cpsc.gov/>

Consumers Union: <http://www.consumersunion.org/>

healthfinder: Health Library: Prevention and Wellness: Safety: <http://www.healthfinder.gov/scripts/SearchContext.asp?topic=762&super=112&Branch=5>

MedlinePlus: Safety (General): <http://www.nlm.nih.gov/medlineplus/safetygeneral.html>

National Fire Protection Agency (NFPA): RiskWatch: <http://www.nfpa.org/riskwatch/>

National Safety Council: <http://www.nsc.org/>

Oregon Health and Science University (OHSU): Health: Household and Common Emergencies: Preventing

Unintentional Injuries: <http://www.ohsuhealth.com/ntrauma/prepare.asp>

SafeUSA: <http://www.safeusa.org/index.htm>

Part III: First Aid and Survival Medicine

P. F. Anderson

[*See also* "Safety," p. 12.]

SPECIAL SEARCHING ISSUES FOR THIS TOPIC

The core concepts of this chapter imply urgency or emergency. If there is an immediate situation to be addressed, do not read this chapter or go to Web sites, but rather phone the U.S. emergency number (911) or your local health care provider. The topics and sources discussed in this chapter are intended for preparation and prevention, and should be consulted in advance of any true emergency. Hopefully, they will help you identify the types of situations or concerns most likely and how to be prepared or prevent those.

The term "first aid," as meaning immediate care or emergency care for an acute illness or injury, is almost universal in the English language. Most of the searching ideas in this chapter reflect the general success in locating information by using "first aid" with the injury or illness term. Many of the injuries described in this chapter can occur in a variety of locations in the body. In your search, try combining terms such as "strain" or "fracture" with a more specific body location. For accurate body terms, refer to a medical dictionary or the anatomy resources mentioned in "Basic Health Concepts" (p. 119, vol. 1).

The main difficulty encountered in searching for first aid information is the large quantity of marginal health information pages provided by companies and firms providing first aid supplies and services. Because this can be a major problem in retrieving high quality information, we recommend limiting your search to sites that are either provided by government or nonprofit organizations, or that link to them. You may do this by including either one of the following search strings at the end of your topic search:

- ".gov"
- ".org"

If you really are having trouble finding good information on a specific topic, you may wish to use the local search engine provided at many of our Best One-Stop

Shops for this chapter, or exclude commercial sites altogether by using -".com"

PROCEDURES AND SPECIAL TOPICS

33. GENERAL

Recommended Search Terms

- "First aid" ".com"
- "First aid" ".gov"
- "First aid" ".org"
- "First aid" ".com" ".co.uk"
- "Emergency care"

Important Sites

American Red Cross: Santa Clara Valley Chapter: First Aid Station Medical Protocols: <http://chapters.red cross.org/ca/scv/medprot.html>

Children's Hospital of Pittsburgh: Injury Prevention: <http://www.chp.edu/besafe/>

Health and Safety Executive: First Aid at Work: <http://www.hse.gov.uk/pubns/firindex.htm>

MayoClinic.com: First-Aid Guide: <http://www.mayo clinic.com/home?id=SP5.6>

National Ag Safety Database (NASD): AgSafe: Basic First Aid: Script: <http://www.cdc.gov/nasd/docs/d000101 -d000200/d000105/d000105.html>

University of Maryland Medicine (UMM): First Aid: Household Safety Checklist: <http://www.umm.edu/ non_trauma/check.htm>

U.S. Scouting Service Project: First Aid: <http://www .usscouts.org/usscouts/mb/mb008.html>

Virtual Naval Hospital: First Aid for Soldiers [FM 21-11]: <http://www.vnh.org/FirstAidForSoldiers/fm2111 .html>

Virtual Naval Hospital: Hospital Corpsman Sickcall Screeners Handbook [BUMEDINST 6550:9A]: <http://www.vnh.org/SickcallScreeners/Contents .html>

Virtual Naval Hospital: Standard First Aid Course [NAVEDTRA 13119]: <http://www.vnh.org/Standard FirstAid/toc.html>

Walgreens: Health Library: First Aid and Emergency Care: <http://www.walgreens.com/library/firstaid/>

Wilderness Survival: First Aid and Health: <http://www .bcadventure.com/adventure/wilderness/survival/first .htm>

34. FIRST AID INITIAL ASSESSMENT TOOLS

Recommended Search Terms

- Assessing "first aid"
- Assessment "first aid"
- "Injury assessment"
- Triage "first aid"

Important Sites

American Academy of Family Physicians (AAFP): Self-Care on familydoctor.org: <http://www.familydoctor .org/flowcharts/>

Columbia University: College of Physicians and Surgeons: *Complete Home Medical Guide*: Summoning Help: Victim Assessment and Goals of First Aid Transporting the Victim: <http://cpmcnet.columbia.edu/texts/ guide/toc/toc14.html>

Locators-Online: First Aid: <http://www.locators-online .org/firstaid.htm>

The Physician and Sportsmedicine: On-Field Examination and Care: An Emergency Checklist: <http://www.phys sportsmed.com/issues/1998/11nov/stuart.htm>

Rescue Training Resource and Guide: Casualty Assessment: <http://www.techrescue.org/firstaid/firstaid -ref3.html>

Rescue Training Resource and Guide: Simple Triage and Rapid Treatment (START): <http://www.techrescue .org/firstaid/firstaid-ref2.html>

Sierra Club: Standard First Aid-Patient Assessment System: <http://sanfranciscobay.sierraclub.org/backpacking/ Leaders_Corner/StandardFirstAid.htm>

St. John Ambulance Centre (Australia): Emergency First Aid—A Quick Guide: <http://www.stjohn.org.au/ emergency/guide.htm>

Virtual Naval Hospital: First Aid for Soldiers [FM 21-11]: <http://www.vnh.org/FirstAidForSoldiers/fm2111 .html>

Virtual Naval Hospital: Hospital Corpsman Sickcall Screeners Handbook [BUMEDINST 6550:9A]: <http://www.vnh.org/SickcallScreeners/Contents .html>

35. FIRST AID SKILLS

Recommended Search Terms

- "Basic life support"
- "Cardiopulmonary resuscitation" basics
- CPR training
- "First aid" bandaging person ".gov"
- "First aid" bandaging person ".org"
- "First aid" splint "how to" ".org"
- "First aid" sling "how to" ".gov"
- "Heimlich maneuver"
- "Heimlich manoeuvre"

Important Sites

American Heart Association (AHA): Heimlich Maneuver: <http://www.americanheart.org/presenter.jhtml?identifier=4605>

British Broadcasting Corporation (BBC): Health: First Aid Action: Essential Skills: DR. ABC: The Letters That Save Lives!: <http://www.bbc.co.uk/health/first_aid_action/es_index.shtml>

Harvard Medical School: Family Health Guide: Emergencies and First Aid: Cardiopulmonary Resuscitation: <http://www.health.harvard.edu/fhg/firstaid/CPR.shtml>

Harvard Medical School: Family Health Guide: Emergencies and First Aid: Choking: <http://www.health.harvard.edu/fhg/firstaid/choking.shtml>

Harvard Medical School: Family Health Guide: Emergencies and First Aid: Moving a Person with a Suspected Back Injury: <http://www.health.harvard.edu/fhg/firstaid/backInj.shtml>

Harvard Medical School: Family Health Guide: Emergencies and First Aid: Removing a Fishhook: <http://www.health.harvard.edu/fhg/firstaid/fishhook.shtml>

Harvard Medical School: Family Health Guide: Emergencies and First Aid: Removing a Speck from the Eye: <http://www.health.harvard.edu/fhg/firstaid/eyeSpeck.shtml>

Harvard Medical School: Family Health Guide: Emergencies and First Aid: Removing a Stuck Ring: <http://www.health.harvard.edu/fhg/firstaid/ring.shtml>

Johns Hopkins University: Bloomberg School of Public Health: Center for Communication Programs: Africa: Tools for Life: First Aid: Cleaning and Bandaging Wounds: <http://www.jhuccp.org/africa/tools/info/27.shtml>

MedlinePlus: First Aid/Emergencies: <http://www.nlm.nih.gov/medlineplus/firstaidemergencies.html>

MedlinePlus: Medical Encyclopedia: How to Make a Sling: <http://www.nlm.nih.gov/medlineplus/ency/article/000017.htm>

MedlinePlus: Medical Encyclopedia: How to Make a Splint: <http://www.nlm.nih.gov/medlineplus/ency/article/000040.htm>

Rescue Training Resource and Guide: First Aid: Quiz #1: Basic Life Support: <http://www.techrescue.org/firstaid/firstaid-test1.html>

Resuscitation Council (UK): Basic Life Support: Resuscitation Guidelines 2000: <http://www.resus.org.uk/pages/bls.htm>

Resuscitation Council (UK): Paediatric Basic Life Support: Resuscitation Guidelines 2000: <http://www.resus.org.uk/pages/pbls.htm>

36. First Aid Supplies for Home, Office, and Travel

Recommended Search Terms

- "First aid" kit camping
- "First aid" kit children
- "First aid" kit farm
- "First aid" kit hiking
- "First aid" kit home
- "First aid" kit office
- "First aid" kit travel
- "First aid" kit traveler
- "First aid" kit wilderness
- "First aid" kit workplace
- "First aid" kits ".gov"
- "First aid" kits ".org"

Important Sites

Alberta Agriculture Food and Rural Development (Canada): How to Make Your Own Farm First Aid Kit: <http://www.agric.gov.ab.ca/ruraldev/safefarm/trained.html>

American College of Emergency Physicians (ACEP): Health Information: Travel Tips: Be Prepared for the Unexpected: <http://www.acep.org/1,240,0.html>

American College of Emergency Physicians (ACEP): Health Information: Travelers' First Aid Kit: <http://www.acep.org/download.cfm?resource=566>

American College of Emergency Physicians (ACEP): Health Information: Your Home First Aid Kit: <http://www.acep.org/download.cfm?resource=567>

National Ag Safety Database (NASD): First Response to Farm Accidents: <http://www.cdc.gov/nasd/docs/d000901-d001000/d000931/d000931.html>

National Ag Safety Database (NASD): Safe Farm: Promoting Agricultural Health and Safety Farm Emergency and First Aid Kits: <http://www.cdc.gov/nasd/docs/d001001-d001100/d001080/d001080.html>

Cincinnati Children's Hospital Medical Center: Travel: First Aid Kit for Traveling: <http://www.cincinnatichildrens.org/health/info/safety/travel/firstaid-travel.htm>

Colorado Mountain Club: What to Bring Hiking: <http://www.cmc.org/cmc/hike_eqp.html>

eMedicine: First Aid Kit Preparation: <http://www.emedicine.com/aaem/topic205.htm>

KidsHealth: First-Aid Kit: <http://kidshealth.org/parent/firstaid_safe/home/firstaid_kit.html>

NetDoctor (UK): First-Aid Kit: <http://www.netdoctor.co.uk/health_advice/facts/firstaidkit.htm>

NetDoctor (UK): First-Aid Kit for Traveling Abroad: <http://www.netdoctor.co.uk/travel/diseases/first_aid_kit_for_travelling_abroad.htm>

Oregon Health and Science University (OHSU) Health: Household/Common Emergencies: First-Aid Kit: <http://www.ohsuhealth.com/ntrauma/firstaid.asp>

Princeton University Outdoor Action: First Aid Kit: <http://www.princeton.edu/~oa/firstaid.html>

Ready.gov: Make a Kit: First Aid Kit: <http://www.ready.gov/first_aid_kit.html>

University of Maryland Medicine (UMM): First Aid: <http://www.umm.edu/non_trauma/firstaid.htm>

37. Information Resources for First Responders

Recommended Search Terms

- "Emergency medical services" guidelines
- "Emergency medical technician" guidelines
- EMT hazards
- "Emergency responders"
- "First aiders" resources
- "First responder" safety
- "Life savers" guidelines
- Paramedic resources
- Rescuer guidelines
- "Wilderness first responder" hazards

Important Sites

Center for Research on Occupational and Environmental Toxicology (CROET): Emergency Responder: <http://www.croetweb.com/outreach/croetweb/links.cfm?topicID=46>

Centers for Disease Prevention and Control (CDC): National Institute for Occupational Safety and Health (NIOSH): Emergency Response Resources: <http://www.cdc.gov/niosh/topics/emres/>

Department of Transportation (DOT): Office of Hazardous Materials Safety: Emergency Response Guidebook: <http://hazmat.dot.gov/gydebook.htm>

Emergency Responder Safety and Health Database: <http://www.ershfocus.com/search_results.php?all=2&type=a>

Fire and EMS Network: <http://www.fire-ems.net/>

Harvard Medical School: Family Health Guide: Emergencies and First Aid: Moving a Person with a Suspected Back Injury: <http://www.health.harvard.edu/fhg/firstaid/backInj.shtml>

Harvard Medical School: Family Health Guide: Emergencies and First Aid: Recovery Position: <http://www.health.harvard.edu/fhg/firstaid/recovery.shtml>

National Interagency Fire Center (NIFC): Safety: <http://www.nifc.gov/safety_study/>

Occupational Safety and Health Administration (OSHA): Emergency Preparedness and Response: <http://www.osha.gov/SLTC/emergencyresponse/>

Rand Corporation: Protecting Emergency Responders: Lessons Learned from Terrorist Attacks: <http://www.rand.org/publications/CF/CF176/>

Virtual Naval Hospital: Standard First Aid Course [NAVEDTRA 13119]: Chapter Ten: Medical Injuries: <http://www.vnh.org/StandardFirstAid/chapter10.html>

Virtual Naval Hospital: Standard First Aid Course [NAVEDTRA 13119]: Chapter Eleven: Rescue and Transportation: <http://www.vnh.org/StandardFirstAid/chapter11.html>

38. First Aid Information for and about Children

["Children's Health Issues," p. 119; "Safety," p. 12; and other specific topics under "Health and Wellness."]

Recommended Search Terms

- "First aid" children
- "First aid" child
- "First aid" kids

Important Sites

American Academy of Pediatrics: Section on Injury and Poisoning Prevention: <http://www.aap.org/sections/ipp/>

American College of Emergency Physicians (ACEP): Health Information: Medical Forms: Emergency Information Form for Children with Special Health Cares Needs: <http://www.acep.org/1,374,0.html>

American College of Emergency Physicians (ACEP): Health Information: Monthly Health Columns: How to Childproof Your Home: <http://www.acep.org/1,275,0.html>

Centers for Disease Prevention and Control (CDC): *Morbidity and Mortality Weekly Report (MMWR)*: The Management of Acute Diarrhea in Children: Oral Rehydration, Maintenance, and Nutritional Therapy: <http://www.cdc.gov/epo/mmwr/preview/mmwrhtml/00018677.htm>

Children's Emergency Care Alliance: <http://www.cecatenn.org/>

Children's Hospital of Pittsburgh: Injury Prevention: <http://www.chp.edu/besafe/>

Children's Safety Network: <http://www.edc.org/HHD/csn/>

Federal Emergency Management Agency (FEMA): FEMA 'Zine: <http://www.fema.gov/kids/zine.htm>

Hug-a-Tree National Headquarters: <http://www.tbt.com/hugatree/>

Kidd Safety: <http://www.cpsc.gov/kids/kidsafety/>

KidsHealth: First Aid and Safety: <http://kidshealth.org/parent/firstaid_safe/>

KidsHealth: Bites and Scratches: <http://kidshealth.org/parent/firstaid_safe/emergencies/bites.html>

KidsHealth: CPR: <http://kidshealth.org/parent/firstaid_safe/emergencies/cpr.html>

KidsHealth: Dehydration: <http://kidshealth.org/parent/firstaid_safe/emergencies/dehydration.html>

KidsHealth: Emergency Contact Sheet: <http://kidshealth.org/parent/firstaid_safe/sheets/emergency_contact.html>

KidsHealth: Everyday Illness and Injuries: <http://www.kidshealth.org/kid/ill_injure/>

KidsHealth: Teaching Your Child How to Use 911: <http://kidshealth.org/parent/firstaid_safe/emergencies/911.html>

KidsHealth: When to Call Your Child's Doctor: <http://kidshealth.org/parent/firstaid_safe/emergencies/call_doc.html>

MayoClinic.com: Children's Health Center: Keeping Your Child Safe: Prevent Accidents and Injuries: <http://www.mayoclinic.com/>

National Safe Kids Campaign: <http://www.safekids.org/>

Oregon Health and Science University (OHSU) Health: Child Health A–Z: Common Injuries and Poisonings: <http://www.ohsuhealth.com/dch/health/poison/>

Oregon Health and Science University (OHSU) Health: Child Health A–Z: Safety and Injury Prevention: <http://www.ohsuhealth.com/dch/health/safety/>

Search and Rescue Society of British Columbia (SARBC): Lost in the Woods: Child Survival K–7: <http://www.sarbc.org/litw.html>

U.S. Scouting Service Project: First Aid: <http://www.usscouts.org/usscouts/mb/mb008.html>

39. First Aid for Animals

Recommended Search Terms

- Animal health
- Animal safety
- "Animal safety" "disaster planning"
- "Companion animals" health
- "Farm animals" "first aid"
- "Emergency care" [name of animal type (dog, cat) or breed (terrier, Siamese)]
- "Emergency care" pets

- "First aid" [name of animal type (dog, cat) or breed (terrier, Siamese)]
- "First aid" avian
- "First aid" bird
- "First aid" birds
- "First aid" canine
- "First aid" cat
- "First aid" dog
- "First aid" feline
- "Health advice" [name of animal type (dog, cat) or breed (terrier, Siamese)]
- "Healthcare" [name of animal type (dog, cat) or breed (terrier, Siamese)]
- Healthy pets ".org"
- Injury [name of animal type (dog, cat) or breed (terrier, Siamese)]
- Livestock "first aid"
- Pets "first aid"
- Pet health
- Pet protection

Important Sites

American Pet Association: <http://www.apapets.com/>

American Red Cross: Prepare.org: California Preparedness Materials: First Aid for Animals: <http://www.redcross.org/disaster/safety/fa-anim.html>

American Red Cross: Services: Disaster Services: Be Prepared: Animal Safety <http://www.redcross.org/services/disaster/beprepared/animalsafety.html>

American Red Cross: Services: Disaster Services: Be Prepared: Animal Safety: Farm Animals: Preparedness: <http://www.redcross.org/services/disaster/beprepared/barnyard.html>

American Red Cross: Services: Disaster Services: Be Prepared: Animal Safety: First Aid for Pets: <http://www.redcross.org/services/disaster/beprepared/firstaid.html>

American Red Cross: Services: Disaster Services: Be Prepared: Animal Safety: Pets and Disaster: <http://www.redcross.org/services/disaster/beprepared/animalsafety.html>

American Society for the Prevention of Cruelty to Animals (ASPCA): Animal Poison Control Center (APCC): <http://www.napcc.aspca.org/>

American Veterinary Medical Association (AVMA): Care for Animals: <http://www.avma.org/careforanimals/default.asp>

American Veterinary Medical Association (AVMA): NetVet: <http://netvet.wustl.edu/vet.htm>

Christchurch City Council (Australia): Animals and Pets: <http://www.ccc.govt.nz/animals/>

Christchurch City Council (Australia): First Aid for Your Dog: <http://www.ccc.govt.nz/animals/DogFirstAid.asp>

Cornell Feline Health Center: <http://web.vet.cornell.edu/Public/FHC/>

Dog-First-Aid.com: Contents for your Canine First Aid Kit: <http://www.dog-first-aid.com/html/what_you_need.html>

Federal Emergency Management Agency (FEMA): Pets and Disasters: <http://www.fema.gov/library/petsf.shtm>

HealthWeb: Veterinary Medicine: <http://healthweb.org/browse.cfm?subjectid=95>

Horse Information Center: Frequently Asked Questions: First Aid Index: <http://www.horseinfo.com/info/faqs/faqfirstaidindex.html>

MedlinePlus: Pets and Pet Health: <http://www.nlm.nih.gov/medlineplus/petsandpethealth.html>

National Agricultural Library: Animal Welfare Information Center: <http://www.nalusda.gov/awic/>

National Library of Medicine: Pet and Animal Diseases: Where Can I Find Information about My Pet?: <http://www.nlm.nih.gov/services/animal.html>

Pet Bird FAQ Files: <http://rec.pets.birds.org/>

PetEducation: Emergencies and First Aid for Birds: <http://www.peteducation.com/category_summary.cfm?cls=15&cat=1912>

Prepare.org: Disaster Preparedness Information: First Aid for Animals: <http://www.prepare.org/animal/petaid.htm>

Provet: Animal Health Information (UK): <http://www.provet.co.uk/>

VetInfo: A Veterinary Information Service: <http://www.vetinfo.com/>

VetInfo4Cats: Cat Info—Alphabetical Index: <http://www.vetinfo4cats.com/catindex.html>

VetInfo4Dogs: Alphabetical Index—Dog Info: <http://www.vetinfo4dogs.com/dogindex.html>

VETS411: <http://www.vets411.com/>

40. COMMON ILLNESSES AND HEALTH EMERGENCIES

Recommended Search Terms

- Common health emergencies
- "Common illnesses" "first aid"
- "First aid" diarrhea
- "First aid" diarrhoea
- "First aid" vomiting
- "First aid" [name of specific concern, such as vomiting, fever, or other concern]

Important Sites

American Academy of Family Physicians (AAFP): Family Doctor: Self-Care: Cold and Flu: <http://www.familydoctor.org/flowcharts/517.html>

American Academy of Family Physicians (AAFP): Family Doctor: Self-Care: Cough: <http://www.familydoctor.org/flowcharts/516.html>

Centers for Disease Control and Prevention (CDC): *Morbidity and Mortality Weekly Report* (*MMWR*): The Management of Acute Diarrhea in Children: <http://www.cdc.gov/epo/mmwr/preview/mmwrhtml/00018677.htm>

Johns Hopkins University: Center for Communication Programs: Information Cards: Preventing Common Illnesses and Diseases, First Aid: Cleaning and Bandaging Wounds: <http://www.jhuccp.org/africa/tools/info/27.shtml>

Johns Hopkins University: Center for Communication Programs: Tools for Life: Information Cards: Preventing Common Illnesses and Diseases: <http://www.jhuccp.org/africa/tools/info/disease.shtml>

KidsHealth: Dehydration: <http://kidshealth.org/parent/firstaid_safe/emergencies/dehydration.html>

KidsHealth: Vomiting: <http://kidshealth.org/parent/firstaid_safe/emergencies/vomit.html>

MedlinePlus: Common Cold: <http://www.nlm.nih.gov/medlineplus/commoncold.html>

MedlinePlus: Diarrhea: <http://www.nlm.nih.gov/medlineplus/diarrhea.html>

MedlinePlus: Influenza: <http://www.nlm.nih.gov/medlineplus/influenza.html>

MedlinePlus: Nausea and Vomiting: <http://www.nlm.nih.gov/medlineplus/nauseaandvomiting.html>

Oregon Health and Science University (OHSU) Health: Household/Common Emergencies: <http://www.ohsuhealth.com/ntrauma/>

Sonning Common Health Centre (UK): Emergencies and Accidents: <http://www.sonningcommonhealthcentre.co.uk/pages/emergencies.html>

University of Maryland Medicine (UMM): First Aid for Minor Emergencies: Appendicitis: <http://www.umm.edu/non_trauma/append.htm>

University of Maryland Medicine (UMM): First Aid for Minor Emergencies: Asthma Attacks: <http://www.umm.edu/non_trauma/asthma.htm>

University of Maryland Medicine (UMM): First Aid for Minor Emergencies: Chest Pain / Heart Attack Symptoms: <http://www.umm.edu/non_trauma/chespain.htm>

University of Maryland Medicine (UMM): First Aid for Minor Emergencies: Dehydration and Heat Stroke: <http://www.umm.edu/non_trauma/dehyrat.htm>

University of Maryland Medicine (UMM): First Aid for Minor Emergencies: Fever: <http://www.umm.edu/non_trauma/fever.htm>

University of Maryland Medicine (UMM): First Aid for Minor Emergencies: Influenza: <http://www.umm.edu/non_trauma/flu.htm>

University of Maryland Medicine (UMM): First Aid for Minor Emergencies: Stroke/Brain Attack: <http://www.umm.edu/non_trauma/stroke.htm>

Virtual Hospital: Health Topics A–Z: First Aid/Emergencies: <http://www.vh.org/navigation/vh/topics/pediatric_patient_first_aid_emergencies.html>

41. ANIMAL AND INSECT BITES OR STINGS:

Recommended Search Terms

- "Animal bites"
- "Bee stings"
- "Bug bites"
- "Cat bites"
- "Dog bites"
- "Ehrlichiosis"
- "Flea bites"
- "Mosquito bites"
- "Spider bites"
- "Tick bites"

Important Sites

American Academy of Family Physicians (AAFP): Family Doctor: Cat and Dog Bites: <http://familydoctor.org/handouts/203.html>

MedlinePlus: Bites and Stings: <http://www.nlm.nih.gov/medlineplus/bitesandstings.html>

MedlinePlus: Insect Bites and Stings: <http://www.nlm.nih.gov/medlineplus/insectbitesandstings.html>

University of Maryland Medicine (UMM): First Aid for Minor Emergencies: Animal Bites and Rabies: <http://www.umm.edu/non_trauma/bites.htm>

University of Maryland Medicine (UMM): First Aid for Minor Emergencies: Bee Stings: <http://www.umm.edu/non_trauma/bee.htm>

University of Maryland Medicine (UMM): First Aid for Minor Emergencies: Spider Bites: <http://www.umm.edu/non_trauma/spider.htm>

42. BLEEDING AND BRUISING

Recommended Search Terms

- "Black eye" "first aid"
- "Blunt trauma" "emergency care"
- Bruises "first aid"

- Bruising swelling "first aid"
- Contusion "emergency care"
- Cuts "first aid"
- Scrapes "first aid"
- Bleeding "first aid"
- "External bleeding" "first aid"
- "Internal bleeding" "first aid"
- "Severe bleeding" "emergency care"
- "Soft tissue injuries" treatment

Important Sites

Harvard Medical School: Family Health Guide: Emergencies and First Aid: Bleeding: <http://www.health.harvard.edu/fhg/firstaid/bleed.shtml>

KidsHealth: Bleeding: <http://kidshealth.org/parent/firstaid_safe/emergencies/bleeding.html>

KidsHealth: Nosebleeds: <http://kidshealth.org/parent/firstaid_safe/emergencies/nose_bleed.html>

The Physician and Sportsmedicine: Blunt-Trauma Carotid Artery Injury: Mild Symptoms May Disguise Serious Trouble: <http://www.physsportsmed.com/issues/feb_96/troop.htm>

Virtual Naval Hospital: Standard First Aid Course [NAVEDTRA 13119]: Chapter Three: Bleeding: <http://www.vnh.org/StandardFirstAid/chapter3.html>

Virtual Naval Hospital: Standard First Aid Course [NAVEDTRA 13119]: Chapter Five: Soft Tissue Injuries: <http://www.vnh.org/StandardFirstAid/chapter5.html>

43. BROKEN BONES AND FRACTURES

[*See also* "Musculoskeletal Disorders and Injuries," p. 120.]

Recommended Search Terms

- "First aid" "broken bone"
- "First aid" fracture
- "First aid" fracture
- "First aid" fractures
- "First aid" musculoskeletal

Important Sites

British Broadcasting Corporation (BBC): Health: First Aid Action: Home Skills: Caring for Adults: Fracture: <http://www.bbc.co.uk/health/first_aid_action/hs_adult/hs_fracture.shtml>

Captain Dave's Survival Center: First Aid Fractures, Sprains, Strains and Dislocations: <http://www.survival-center.com/firstaid/fracture.htm>

Harvard Medical School: Family Health Guide: Emergencies and First Aid: Broken Bones: <http://www.health.harvard.edu/fhg/firstaid/broken.shtml>

KidsHealth: Broken Bones, Sprains, and Strains: <http://kidshealth.org/parent/firstaid_safe/emergencies/broken_bones.html>

MedlinePlus: Fractures (Broken Bones): <http://www.nlm.nih.gov/medlineplus/fractures.html>

Virtual Naval Hospital: First Aid Anatomy: Fracture of an Extremity: <http://www.vnh.org/FirstAidAnatomy/FractureExtremity.html>

Virtual Naval Hospital: Standard First Aid Course [NAVEDTRA 13119]: Chapter Six: Bones, Joints, and Muscles: <http://www.vnh.org/StandardFirstAid/chapter6.html>

44. Burns

Recommended Search Terms

- Burns "first aid"
- "Chemical burn"
- "Electric burns"
- "Electrical burn"
- Scalds
- "Water burns"

Important Sites

National Ag Safety Database (NASD): First Aid for Electrical Accidents: <http://www.cdc.gov/nasd/docs/d000801-d000900/d000813/d000813.html>

eMJA (Medical Journal of Australia): First-Aid Management of Minor Burns in Children: <http://www.mja.com.au/public/issues/178_01_060103/mcc10517_fm.html>

Food and Drug Administration (FDA): FDA Consumer: OTC Options: Help for Cuts, Scrapes and Burns: <http://www.fda.gov/fdac/features/496_cuts.html>

KidsHealth: Burns: <http://kidshealth.org/parent/firstaid_safe/emergencies/burns.html>

MedlinePlus: Burns: <http://www.nlm.nih.gov/medlineplus/burns.html>

MedlinePlus: Medical Encyclopedia: Chemical Burn or Reaction: <http://www.nlm.nih.gov/medlineplus/ency/article/000059.htm>

National Safety Council: The Do's and Don'ts of Teaching Home Fire Safety: <http://www.nsc.org/issues/firstaid/homefire.htm>

Oregon Health and Science University (OHSU) Health: Child Health A–Z: Burns: <http://www.ohsuhealth.com/dch/health/burns/index.asp>

Shriners Hospitals for Children: Prevention: Burn Prevention Tips: <http://www.shrinershq.org/prevention/burntips/>

Shriners Hospitals for Children: Prevention: Emergency Treatment for Burns: <http://www.shrinershq.org/prevention/burntips/treatment.html>

U.S. Fire Administration (USFA): Burn/Scald Prevention: Handout: First Aid for Burns: <http://www.usfa.fema.gov/public/bur_a83.cfm>

45. Falls

Recommended Search Terms

- Accident prevention falling
- Falls "first aid"
- Falls prevention

Important Sites

American Academy of Orthopaedic Surgeons (AAOS): Prevent Falls: Don't Let a Fall Be Your Last Trip: <http://orthoinfo.aaos.org/>

American Academy of Orthopaedic Surgeons (AAOS): Prevent Falls: Getting Up from a Fall: <http://orthoinfo.aaos.org/>

American Academy of Orthopaedic Surgeons (AAOS): Prevent Falls: Home Safety Checklist: <http://orthoinfo.aaos.org/>

American Academy of Orthopaedic Surgeons (AAOS): Prevent Falls: How to Reduce Your Risk of Falling: <http://orthoinfo.aaos.org/>

American Academy of Orthopaedic Surgeons (AAOS): Prevent Falls: Ladder Safety Tips: <http://orthoinfo.aaos.org/>

American Academy of Orthopaedic Surgeons (AAOS): Prevent Falls: To keep Seniors Living Independently, Prevent Falls: <http://orthoinfo.aaos.org>

American Academy of Orthopaedic Surgeons (AAOS): Prevent Falls: Climb It Safe!: <http://orthoinfo.aaos.org/>

American College of Emergency Physicians (ACEP): Help the Elderly Cope with Falls: <http://www.acep.org/1,309,0.html>

MedlinePlus: Accidents: <http://www.nlm.nih.gov/medlineplus/accidents.html>

MedlinePlus: Fainting: <http://nlm.nih.gov/medlineplus/fainting.html>

National Safety Council: Falls in the Home: <http://www.nsc.org/issues/fallstop.htm>

National Safety Council: National Alliance to Prevent Falls As We Age: <http://www.nsc.org/fallsalliance.htm>

46. FEVERS

Recommended Search Terms

- "First aid" fever ".gov"
- "First aid" fever ".org"
- "First aid" fevers
- "High fever" "see a doctor"
- "High fever" "emergency room"
- "High temperature" "ask a doctor"

Important Sites

American Academy of Family Physicians (AAFP): Family Doctor: Self-Care: Fever: <http://www.familydoctor.org/flowcharts/503.html>

American Academy of Family Physicians (AAFP): Family Doctor (AAFP): Self-Care: Fever in Infants and Children: <http://www.familydoctor.org/flowcharts/504.html>

American College of Emergency Physicians (ACEP): Children and Fevers: What Parents Should Know: <http://www.acep.org/1,245,0.html>

KidsHealth: Fever: <http://kidshealth.org/parent/firstaid_safe/emergencies/fever.html>

MedlinePlus: Fever: <http://www.nlm.nih.gov/medlineplus/fever.html>

47. HEAD AND SPINAL CORD INJURIES:

Recommended Search Terms

- "Brain injury" "first aid"
- Concussion "first aid"
- "Head injury" "first aid"
- "Traumatic brain injury"

Important Sites

Brain Injury Resource Center: <http://www.headinjury.com/>

Dartmouth College Sports Medicine: Head Injury: Concussion Injury Information Guide: <http://www.dartmouth.edu/~sportmed/concussion.html>

Missouri Head Injury Guide: "What Everyone Should Know about Brain Injury": <http://www.oa.state.mo.us/gs/hi/tbi/HIGUIDE/index.html>

National Health Service (NHS) Direct Online: Self-Help Guide: Head Injury in Children: <http://www.nhsdirect.nhs.uk/SelfHelp/symptoms/childheadinjury/start.asp>

St. John Ambulance Australia: A Quick Guide to First Aid: Head Injury: <http://www.stjohn.org.au/emergency/html/head_injury.htm>

South Carolina Department of Disabilities and Special Needs: Head Injury: A Family Guide: <http://www.state.sc.us/ddsn/pubs/hinjury/sec1.htm>

Traumatic Brain Injury Survival Guide: <http://www.tbiguide.com/>

48. POISONS

Recommended Search Terms

- Ipecac "first aid"
- Fungicide poisoning
- Herbicide poison prevention
- Household poisons
- Insecticide ingestion
- Pesticide poison "first aid"
- Rodenticide overdose

Important Sites

Agency for Toxic Substances and Disease Registry (ATSDR): <http://www.atsdr.cdc.gov/>

American Academy of Pediatrics: Section on Injury and Poisoning Prevention: <http://www.aap.org/sections/ipp/>

American Association of Poison Control Centers (AAPCC): <http://www.aapcc.org/>

American Association of Poison Control Centers (AAPCC): Find Your Poison Center: <http://www.aapcc.org/findyour.htm>

American College of Emergency Physicians (ACEP): How to Protect Your Child from Poison: <http://www.acep.org/1,194,0.html>

Environmental Protection Agency (EPA): About Pesticides: Frequently Asked Questions: <http://www.epa.gov/pesticides/about/faqs.htm>

MedlinePlus: Carbon Monoxide Poisoning: <http://www.nlm.nih.gov/medlineplus/carbonmonoxidepoisoning.html>

MedlinePlus: Household Poisons: <http://www.nlm.nih.gov/medlineplus/householdpoisons.html>

MedlinePlus: Pesticides: <http://www.nlm.nih.gov/medlineplus/pesticides.html>

MedlinePlus: Poisoning: <http://www.nlm.nih.gov/medlineplus/poisoning.html>

National Ag Safety Database (NASD): Symptoms and First Aid for Poisonings: <http://www.cdc.gov/nasd/docs/d000801-d000900/d000817/d000817.html>

National Safety Council: National Poison Prevention Week: <http://www.nsc.org/poison.htm>

Oregon Health and Science University (OHSU): Center for Research on Occupational and Environmental Toxicology (CROET): Toxicology Information Center: <http://www.ohsu.edu/croet/outreach/tic/journals.html>

Oregon Health and Science University (OHSU) Health: Household/Common Emergencies: Alcohol-Related Injury Statistics: <http://www.ohsuhealth.com/ntrauma/alcohol_stats.asp>

Queensland Poisons Information Centre (Australia): First Aid: <http://www.health.qld.gov.au/Poisons InformationCentre/firstAid.htm>

University of Maryland Medicine (UMM): First Aid: Carbon Monoxide Poisoning: <http://www.umm.edu/non _trauma/carbon.htm>

University of Maryland Medicine (UMM): Child Safety: First Aid: Poison First Aid: <http://www.umm.edu/ childsafety/first_aid/ency/poison/poisonfirstaid.htm>

Virtual Naval Hospital: Standard First Aid Course [NAVEDTRA 13119]: Chapter Nine: Poisoning: <http://www.vnh.org/StandardFirstAid/chapter9.html>

HOTLINES

Agency for Toxic Substances and Disease Registry (ATSDR): 1-888-42-ATSDR/1-888-422-8737

American Association of Poison Control Centers (AAPCC): 1-800-222-1222

MEDICAL SPECIALTY

Toxicology

49. SEIZURES

[*See also* "Epilepsy," p. 68.]

Recommended Search Terms

- Convulsion "first aid"
- Epilepsy "first aid"
- Epilepsy "safety"
- Seizure "first aid"

Important Sites

Children's Hospital and Regional Medical Center (Seattle, Washington): Center for Children with Special Needs: Seizure First Aid (Plain Language) (English/Spanish): <http://www.cshcn.org/resources/ seizure-first-aid_eng_PL.htm>

Epilepsy Action (UK): First Aid—What to Do When Someone Has a Seizure: <http://www.epilepsy.org.uk/ info/firstaid.html>

KidsHealth: Seizures: <http://kidshealth.org/parent/first aid_safe/emergencies/seizure.html>

MedlinePlus: Seizures: <http://www.nlm.nih.gov/medline plus/seizures.html>

50. SHOCK
Recommended Search Terms

- Anaphalactic shock "emergency care"
- Allergic shock "first aid"
- Electric shock "first aid"
- Shock "first aid"
- Shock "treatment"

Important Sites

eMedicine: Excerpt from Shock, Cardiogenic: <http://www.emedicine.com/emerg/byname/shock-cardiogenic.htm>

eMedicine: Shock, Hemorrhagic: <http://www.emedicine.com/EMERG/topic531.htm>

National Ski Patrol: Outdoor Emergency Care: Emergency Care of Shock: <http://www.patrol.org/instructor/oec/ shock/sld007.htm>

U.S. Army: Common Core: Perform First Aid to Prevent or Control Shock: <http://www.atsc.army.mil/dld/ comcor/md1005s.htm>

Virtual Naval Hospital: Standard First Aid Course [NAVEDTRA 13119]: Chapter Four: Shock: <http://www.vnh.org/StandardFirstAid/chapter4.html>

Walgreens: Health Library: First Aid: Shock: <http://www.walgreens.com/library/firstaid/Shock.jhtml>

51. SPRAINS, STRAINS, AND MINOR INJURIES
Recommended Search Terms

- Cuts bandaging "first aid"
- Cuts "first aid" ".gov"
- Sprain "first aid" ".gov"
- Sprains treatment ".org"
- Strain treatment ".gov"
- Strains "first aid" ".org"
- Torn ligament "first aid"

Important Sites

American Academy of Family Physicians (AAFP): Family Doctor: Self-Care Flowcharts: Knee Problems: <http://familydoctor.org/flowcharts/542.html>

BetterHealth (Australia): Sprains and Strains: <http://www.betterhealth.vic.gov.au/bhcv2/bhcpdf.nsf/ByPdf/ vut_Sprains_and_strains/$File/Sprains_and_strains.pdf>

KidsHealth: Broken Bones, Sprains, and Strains: <http://kidshealth.org/parent/firstaid_safe/emergencies/broken_bones.html>

MedlinePlus Medical Encyclopedia: Muscle strain treatment: <http://www.nlm.nih.gov/medlineplus/ency/article/002116.htm>

MedlinePlus Medical Encyclopedia: Sprains: <http://www.nlm.nih.gov/medlineplus/ency/article/000041.htm>

MedlinePlus Medical Encyclopedia: Strains—First Aid: <http://www.nlm.nih.gov/medlineplus/ency/article/000042.htm>

National Institute of Arthritis and Musculoskeletal and Skin Diseases (NIAMS): Health Topics: Questions and Answers about Knee Problems: <http://www.niams.nih.gov/hi/topics/kneeprobs/kneeqa.htm>

University of Tasmania (UTAS): Guide for Emergencies: First Aid: Fracture, Dislocation, Sprain: <http://www.chem.utas.edu.au/safety/Safety_Manual/main/Guide%20for%20Emergencies/guide2/f18.html>

Virtual Naval Hospital: Standard First Aid Course [NAVEDTRA 13119]: Chapter Six: Bones, Joints, and Muscles: <http://www.vnh.org/StandardFirstAid/chapter6.html>

Walgreens: Health Library: First Aid: Sprain: <http://www.walgreens.com/library/firstaid/Sprain.jhtml>

52. Survival Medicine

Recommended Search Terms

- "Extreme cold" "first aid"
- Hypothermia
- Hypothermia prevention
- "Poison ivy"
- "Poison oak"
- Survival medicine
- Wilderness medicine
- Wilderness survival

Important Sites

American College of Emergency Physicians (ACEP): Know Your Stuff Before Taking It Rough: Safety Tips for Your Next Adventure Trip: <http://www.acep.org/1,305,0.html>

Captain Dave's Survival Center: First Aid Tutorial: <http://www.survival-center.com/firstaid/book.htm#toc>

Centers for Disease Control and Prevention (CDC): National Center for Environmental Health: Outdoor Safety: Extreme Cold: <http://www.cdc.gov/nceh/hsb/extremecold/outdoorsafety.htm>

eMedicine: Wilderness Emergencies Medical Reference: <http://www.emedicine.com/wild/>

Hiker Central: Survival Links: <http://www.hikercentral.com/survival/>

Interactive Broadcasting Corporation (IBC) (Canada): BC Adventure: Wilderness Survival Guide: <http://www.bcadventure.com/adventure/wilderness/survival/>

MedlinePlus: Hypothermia: <http://www.nlm.nih.gov/medlineplus/hypothermia.html>

Outdoor Action: First Aid and Safety: <http://www.princeton.edu/~oa/safety/index.shtml>

Outdoor Action: Guide to Outdoor Safety Management: <http://www.princeton.edu/~oa/safety/safeman.html>

Outdoor Action: First Aid and Safety: <http://www.princeton.edu/~oa/safety/>

OutdoorEd.com: Outdoor Safety Management: <http://www.outdoored.com/Articles/Article.asp?ArticleID=121>

Survival Bible 2001 Freeware (Canada): <http://www.icomm.ca/survival/>

Survival Medical FAQ: <http://www.survival-center.com/med-faq/>

WannaLearn.com: Sports and Leisure: Outdoor Activities: Wilderness Survival: <http://www.wannalearn.com/Sports_and_Leisure/Outdoor_Activities/Wilderness_Survival/>

Wilderness Medical Society (WMS): <http://www.wms.org/>

Wilderness Survival: <http://www.wilderness-survival.net/>

Wilderness Survival Guide: Outdoor Educators and Training: <http://www.bcadventure.com/adventure/wilderness/survival/>

Wilderness Survival: First Aid and Health: <http://www.bcadventure.com/adventure/wilderness/survival/first.htm>

53. Weather and Exposure

Recommended Search Terms

- "Altitude sickness"
- "Cold injury" "first aid"
- Frostbite prevention
- "Heat exposure" "first aid"
- "Heat illness"
- "Heat prostration"
- "Heat sickness"
- "Heat stroke"
- Hypothermia "emergency care"
- "Outdoor health" "first aid"
- "Storm safety"
- "Sun exposure" "first aid"
- "Sun poisoning"
- "Sun safety"
- "Sun stroke"

- Sunburn prevention
- Sunstroke treatment
- Weather "first aid"
- "Weather safety"
- "Winter safety"

Important Sites

American Red Cross: Project Safeside: Keeping You Ahead of the Storm: <http://www.redcross.org/services/disaster/keepsafe/safeside.html>

Family Caregiver Alliance: Hot Weather Tips: <http://www.caregiver.org/caregiver/jsp/content_node.jsp?nodeid=871>

MedlinePlus: Heat Illness: <http://www.nlm.nih.gov/medlineplus/heatillness.html>

MedlinePlus: Hypothermia: <http://www.nlm.nih.gov/medlineplus/hypothermia.html>

MedlinePlus: Sun Exposure: <http://www.nlm.nih.gov/medlineplus/sunexposure.html>

Outdoor Action: First Aid and Safety: <http://www.princeton.edu/~oa/safety/index.shtml>

SafeUSA: Winter Safety: <http://www.safeusa.org/winter.htm>

54. When to Go to the Emergency Room

NOTE: Check with your health care provider or clinic *and* your insurance company for guidelines on emergency care—now, before you need the information.

Recommended Search Terms

- "Emergency medical care" necessary
- "Emergency room" essentials
- "Emergency room" kit
- "Emergency room" "what to bring"
- "Emergency room" "what to pack"
- "Emergency room" "when should I"
- "Is this an emergency" hospital
- "What to do in an emergency"
- "When to call" emergency doctor
- "When to go" "emergency room"

Important Sites

American College of Emergency Physicians (ACEP): Health Information: Keep Important Health Information at Hand: <http://www.acep.org/1,1310,0.html>

American College of Emergency Physicians (ACEP): Health Information: Seconds Save Lives in Medical Emergencies: <http://www.acep.org/1,242,0.html>

American College of Emergency Physicians (ACEP): Health Information: The Emergency Department: What to Expect: <http://www.acep.org/1,241,0.html>

American College of Emergency Physicians (ACEP): Health Information: What to Do in an Emergency: <http://www.acep.org/1,243,0.html>

Health Services Executive (UK): What to Do in an Emergency: <http://www.hse.gov.uk/pubns/indg347.pdf>

KidsHealth: When to Call Your Child's Doctor: <http://kidshealth.org/parent/firstaid_safe/emergencies/call_doc.html>

MCare: Is It Urgent or Emergent Care?: <http://www.mcare.org/members/mprov_urgentcare.html>

Oregon Health and Science University (OHSU) Health: Household/Common Emergencies: Emergency Contact Information: <http://www.ohsuhealth.com/ntrauma/emerform.asp>

Oregon Health and Science University (OHSU) Health: Household/Common Emergencies: Potential Emergency Situations and Conditions: <http://www.ohsuhealth.com/ntrauma/condhub.asp>

Oregon Health and Science University (OHSU) Health: Household/Common Emergencies: When to Call for Help: <http://www.ohsuhealth.com/ntrauma/whento.asp>

Examples: Insurance Provider Guidelines

Blue Cross Blue Shield, Arizona: When to Go to the Emergency Room: <http://www.bcbsaz.com/vitality/emergencyroom.asp>

Gulfsouth: When Should I Go to the Emergency Room?: <http://www.gulfsouth.com/Emergency.html>

Example: Special Concerns: Lesbian, Gay, Bisexual, and Transgendered (LGBT)

CUFSmaine: "I'm Afraid to Go to the Emergency Room": Maine Hospital Procedures for Alternative Lifestylers in Need of Emergency Medical Care and Information for Hospital Personnel Regarding Alternative Lifestyle Patients and Their Injuries: <http://www.cufsmaine.org/imafraid.htm>

First Aid and Survival Medicine Hotline

911

FAQs

American College of Emergency Physicians (ACEP): Health Information: <http://www.acep.org/1,3,0.html>

American Red Cross: FAQs: Health and Safety FAQs: <http://www.redcross.org/faq/0,1096,0_381_,00.html>

National Safety Council (NSC): Frequently Asked Questions about First Aid: <http://www.nsc.org/home/articles/01sum22.htm>

SHOULD YOU SEE A DOCTOR?

American Academy of Family Physicians (AAFP): Self-Care on familydoctor.org: <http://www.familydoctor.org/flowcharts/>

MEDICAL SPECIALTIES AND PROFESSIONS

Emergency medical technicians (EMT); Emergency medicine; Emergency physicians; Paramedics; Trauma care; Trauma surgeons

Related Professions

Search and rescue

PROFESSIONAL ORGANIZATIONS

American Academy of Family Physicians (AAFP): <http://www.aafp.org/>

American Academy of Pediatrics (AAP): <http://www.aap.org/>

American Association of Poison Control Centers (AAPCC): <http://www.aapcc.org/>

American College of Emergency Physicians (ACEP): <http://www.acep.org/>

American Heart Association (AHA): <http://www.americanheart.org/>

American Trauma Society (ATS): <http://www.amtrauma.org/>

BEST ONE-STOP SHOPS

American Academy of Family Physicians (AAFP): Family Doctor: <http://www.familydoctor.org/flowcharts/>

American College of Emergency Physicians (ACEP): Health Information: <http://www.acep.org/1,3,0.html>

Americna Red Cross: FAQs: Health and Safety FAQs: <http://www.redcross.org/faq/0,1096,0_381_,00.html>

British Broadcasting Corporation (BBC) Health: First Aid Action: <http://www.bbc.co.uk/health/first_aid_action/>

Harvard Medical School: Family Health Guide: Emergencies and First Aid: <http://www.health.harvard.edu/fhg/firstaid/firstaid.shtml>

healthfinder: Health Library: Prevention and Wellness: First Aid: <http://www.healthfinder.gov/>

MayoClinic.com: First-Aid Guide: <http://www.mayoclinic.com/>

MedlinePlus: Accidents: <http://www.nlm.nih.gov/medlineplus/accidents.html>

MedlinePlus: Critical Care: <http://www.nlm.nih.gov/medlineplus/criticalcare.html>

MedlinePlus: Disasters and Emergency Preparedness: <http://www.nlm.nih.gov/medlineplus/disastersandemergencypreparedness.html>

MedlinePlus: First Aid/Emergencies: <http://www.nlm.nih.gov/medlineplus/firstaidemergencies.html>

Oregon Health and Science University (OHSU) Health: Household/Common Emergencies Index: <http://www.ohsuhealth.com/ntrauma/>

Outdoor Action First Aid and Safety: Outdoor Safety Information: <http://www.princeton.edu/~oa/safety/index.shtml>

University of Maryland Medicine: First Aid: <http://www.umm.edu/non_trauma/index.htm>

Virtual Naval Hospital: Standard First Aid Course [NAVEDTRA 13119]: <http://www.vnh.org/StandardFirstAid/toc.html>

Part IV: Traffic Accidents

Helen Look

[*See also* "Safety," p. 12.]

SPECIAL SEARCHING ISSUES FOR THIS TOPIC

Each year, there are more than 11 million traffic accidents ranging from minor "fender benders" that result in injuries to major crashes that result in fatalities. Motor vehicle accidents are the fifth leading cause of death in this country and the leading cause of death for people younger than 44 years old. Some of these deaths could have been prevented. At least 17 percent of the drivers in fatal traffic accidents were driving while under the influence of alcohol. Two-thirds of the children killed in traffic accidents were either not using seat belts or not using age-appropriate car restraints. With these types of staggering statistics, it is no surprise that most of the traffic accident related Web sites are focused on prevention. These Web sites focus on safety issues such as air bags, car seats or booster seats for children, and seat belts.[1]

What to Ask

When starting your research, it is important to determine whether you are interested in Web sites on traffic related injuries or Web sites on prevention.

Where to Start

Start your research by visiting some of the resources listed in the "Best One-Stop Shops" section of this topic. In general, it is best to consult Web sites maintained by the government or reputable organizations. Since traffic accident injuries can sometimes be difficult to diagnosis, it is always best to consult with your health care provider to confirm the information that you have found.

ADDITIONAL STRATEGIES

Searching for Web sites on traffic accidents can yield mixed results. If you are searching for traffic accident injuries, you may be deluged by Web sites for personal injury lawyers or auto insurance companies. Some of the sites can have valuable information but some are geared towards generating potential clients. You may want to modify your search strategies to specifically exclude these types of Web sites. See "Whiplash Injuries" (p. 43) for examples. Your choice of words can also yield different results. For example, health professions are more likely to use "whiplash syndrome" or "whiplash injuries" rather than just "whiplash." In government health resources, traffic accidents are often described as "motor vehicle accidents" or "motor vehicle related injuries" rather than "car accidents." Keep these tips in mind when doing your research on traffic accidents.

TOPIC PROFILE

Who

Anyone can be affected by traffic accidents. Some groups are at greater risks for sustaining motor vehicle-related injuries. These groups are infants, children, teenagers, seniors, and racial minorities.

What

Traffic accidents can result in fatality or injuries to the drivers, passengers, or pedestrians.

Where

The injuries can affect any part of the body (especially the head, neck, shoulder, and back).

When

Traffic accidents affect all age groups.

ABBREVIATIONS USED IN THIS SECTION

CDC = Centers for Disease Control and Prevention
DUI = Driving under the influence

DWI = Driving while intoxicated
MADD = Mothers Against Drunk Driving
NCICP = National Center for Injury Control and Prevention
NHTSA = National Highway Traffic Safety Administration
SADD = Students Against Drunk Driving/Students Against Destructive Decisions

PROCEDURES AND SPECIAL TOPICS

55. AIR BAGS
Recommended Search Terms

- "Air bag performance"
- "Air bag safety"
- "Air bag" "on-off switches"
- "Air bags" deactivated
- "Air bags" deployment
- "Air bags" depowered
- "Airbag safety"

Important Sites

National Highway Traffic Safety Administration (NHTSA): Air Bags: <http://www.nhtsa.dot.gov/airbags>
National Highway Traffic Safety Administration (NHTSA): Air Bag On-Off Switches: Questions and Answers: <http://www.nhtsa.dot.gov/airbags/airbgQandA.html>
Safety City's Airbag Safety Zone: <http://www.nhtsa.dot.gov/kids/research/airbag/index.html>

56. ALCOHOL-RELATED TRAFFIC ACCIDENTS
Recommended Search Terms

- Alcohol impaired driving
- "Drunk driving" victims
- "Driving under the influence" accidents
- DUI crashes
- DWI accidents
- Drinking driving crashes
- "Blood alcohol level" injuries
- "Blood alcohol concentration" accidents
- Alcohol "vehicle homicide"

Important Sites

Centers for Disease Control and Prevention (CDC): Alcohol-Related Traffic Crashes and Fatalities among Youth and Young Adults—United States, 1982-1994: <http://wonder.cdc.gov/wonder/prevguid/m0039652/m0039652.asp>

National Highway Traffic Safety Administration (NHTSA): Impaired Driving in the United States: Impaired Driving State Cost Fact Sheets: <http://www.nhtsa.dot.gov/people/injury/alcohol/page%202.htm>

Mothers Against Drunk Drivers (MADD): <http://www.madd.org/home/>

Students Against Destructive Decisions (SADD): <http://www.saddonline.com/>

57. CAR SEATS

Recommended Search Terms

- "Booster seat"
- "Booster seat" automobile
- "Car seats" types
- "Child passenger" auto safety
- "Child safety seat"
- "Forward facing" car seat
- "Infant car seat"
- "Infant safety seat"
- Newborn "car seat"
- "Rear facing" car seat

Important Sites

Centers for Disease Control and Prevention (CDC): National Center for Injury Prevention and Control: Research Update: CDC Recommends Booster Seats for Children: <http://www.cdc.gov/ncipc/duip/research/boosterseat.htm>

National Highway Traffic Safety Administration (NHTSA): Child Passenger Safety: <http://www.nhtsa.dot.gov/people/injury/childps>

Safety City's Car Seat Area: <http://www.nhtsa.dot.gov/kids/research/carseat/>

SeatCheck: <http://www.seatcheck.org/>

SeatCheck (in Spanish): <http://www.seatcheck.org/espanol/>

58. SEAT BELTS

Recommended Search Terms

- "Child safety belt"
- "Seat belts"
- "Seat belt" use

Important Sites

National Highway Traffic Safety Administration (NHTSA): Buckle Up America: News Service: <http://www.buckleupamerica.org/news/news_services.php>

National Safety Council: National Safety Belt Coalition: <http://www.nsc.org/traf/sbc.htm>

Safety City's Seat Belt Room: <http://www.nhtsa.dot.gov/kids/research/seatbelt/>

59. WHIPLASH INJURIES

Recommended Search Terms

- Automobile related "neck injuries"
- "Car accident" "back injuries"
- Car "spinal cord injury"
- Hyperextension
- Hyperflexion
- "Soft tissues" injury
- "Spinal fractures"
- Whiplash
- "Whiplash injury"
- "Whiplash injuries"
- whiplash -insurance
- whiplash -lawyer
- whiplash —legal
- "whiplash syndrome"

Important Sites

Headache Cybertext: Headaches/Neckaches from "Whiplash Injuries": <http://www.upstate.edu/neurology/haas/hpwhip.htm>

National Spinal Cord Injury Association ((NSCIA): Fact Sheets: Spinal Cord Injury: <http://www.spinalcord.org/html/factsheets/spin.php>

Spinal Injury Foundation: Whiplash101.com: What's Whiplash?: <http://www.whiplash101.com/what's.htm>

HOTLINES

SeatCheck (a service to find your local child safety seat inspection location):
1-866-SEAT CHECK/1-866-732-8243 (in both English and Spanish)

National Spinal Cord Injury Association Help Line:
1-800-962-9629

FAQs

Brain Injury Association of America: Frequently Asked Questions: <http://www.biausa.org/Pages/faqs.html>

National Safe Kids Campaign: Car: Frequently Asked Questions: <http://www.safekids.org/tier3_cd.cfm?content_item_id=6551&folder_id=170>

Spinal Injury Foundation: Whiplash101.com: Whiplash FAQ: <http://www.whiplash101.com/whiplash2.htm>

TRAFFIC ACCIDENT PUBLICATIONS ON THE INTERNET

National Academies Press (NAP): *Relative Risks of School Travel: A National Perspective and Guidance for Local Community Risk Assessment—Special Report 269 (2002) by the Transportation Research Board*: <http://www.nap.edu/html/SR269/SR269.pdf>

MEDICAL SPECIALTIES

Chiropractic; Internal medicine; Neurology; Orthopedics; Physical therapy

PROFESSIONAL ORGANIZATIONS

American Academy of Neurology: <http://www.aan.com/>

American Chiropractic Association: <http://www.amerchiro.org/>

American Medical Association: <http://www.ama-assn.org/>

American Physical Therapy Association: <http://www.apta.org/>

Brain Injury Association of America: <http://www.biausa.org/Pages/home.html>

PATIENT SUPPORT ORGANIZATION/ DISCUSSION GROUP

Whiplash Hurts Support Group: <http://www.network54.com/Forum/104157>

BEST ONE-STOP SHOPS

Centers for Disease Control and Prevention (CDC): Health Topics: Motor Vehicle-Related Injuries: <http://www.cdc.gov/health/motor.htm>

Centers for Disease Control and Prevention (CDC): National Center for Injury Control and Prevention: Motor Vehicle Related Injuries: <http://www.cdc.gov/ncipc/duip/duip.htm#mv>

Head Injury Hotline: Brain Injury Resource Center: <http://www.headinjury.com/welcome.htm>

MedlinePlus: Motor Vehicle Safety: <http://www.nlm.nih.gov/medlineplus/motorvehiclesafety.html>

National Highway Traffic Safety Administration (NHTSA): Child Passenger Safety: <http://www.nhtsa.dot.gov/people/injury/childps/>

National Highway Traffic Safety Administration (NHTSA): Injury Prevention: <http://www.nhtsa.dot.gov/people/injury/>

National Highway Traffic Safety Administration (NHTSA): Latino/Hispanic American Outreach (in Spanish): <http://www.nhtsa.dot.gov/multicultural/hispanicamerican/hispanic-index.html>

National Highway Traffic Safety Administration (NHSTA): Traffic Safety and Occupants Protection: <http://www.nhtsa.dot.gov/people/>

National Safe Kids Campaign: Car: <http://www.safekids.org/tier2_rl.cfm?folder_id=170>

National Safety Council: Driver Safety: <http://www.nsc.org/issues/drivsafe.htm>

Safety City's Research Laboratory: <http://www.nhtsa.dot.gov/kids/research/>

REFERENCES

1. *Statistical Abstract of the United States, 2001*: <http://www.census.gov/prod/2002pubs/01statab/stat-ab01.html>

Part V: Alternative/Complementary Health Sources

Faye K. Ogasawara

Alternative or complementary health sources provide information or treatment often used in place of, or in addition to, traditional Western medicine. These types of health sources often appeal to individuals who have terminal illnesses, who have tried traditional Western medical approaches with little or no results, or who find clinical settings or approaches unappealing. One research study reported that the majority of the individuals in their study, in addition to being better educated and reporting poorer health status, chose alternative medicine because it is more congruent with their values or beliefs.[1] Sources, therapies, treatments, or healing methods classified as complementary or alternative medicine (CAM) are often cultural, self-taught, or geographical in origin. CAM provides medical sources for therapy, healing, and improving the quality, healthy maintenance, and prolongation of life that are outside of the Western allopathic medical approach.

SPECIAL SEARCHING ISSUES FOR THIS TOPIC

Alternative or complementary health approaches often lack the rigorous clinical trials and professional certifications or licensure required for practitioners. While lack of supporting scientific data does not prevent an alternative or complementary approach from being effective, authenticity is questionable when there is not a known validation. On October 21, 2002, the National Council for Complementary and Alternative Medicine

(NCCAM) and 16 federal co-sponsors announced the launch of an Institute of Medicine (IOM) study of the scientific and policy implications of the American public's use of CAM,[2] thus demonstrating an awareness of the need for validation. Generally, reliable information is available on government Web sites such as NCCAM <http://nccam.nih.gov/>; higher education Web sites such as the Alternative Medicine HomePage <http://www.pitt.edu/~cbw/altm.html>, maintained by the University of Pittsburgh; and Web sites maintained by nationally recognized clinics such as M. D. Anderson <http://www.mdanderson.org/cimer/>.

What to Ask

Alternative or complementary health sources cover a very wide range of topics making it necessary to clarify what is desired in order to search effectively. Several questions may help narrow down a search: Is there a specific disease, condition, or illness of interest? Is there a particular CAM approach of interest (e.g. bodywork: smell, touch, sight, taste, movement, sound; nutrition/diet; mind/spirit; energy work/non-tactile; training; group support; cultural methods)?

Where to Start

If you are not familiar with alternative or complementary health sources or do not have a particular topic of interest, general searches will provide you with an overview of information you may find. For general information, use the key terms "alternative medicine," "alternative health sources," or "alternative healing." With general search engines, such as Google, Hotbot, Lycos, or AlltheWeb, these terms will retrieve helpful results. In medical databases such as PubMed, the terms "alternative medicine," "complementary medicine," "alternative therapies," and "complementary therapies" retrieve helpful results while MedlinePlus retrieves results primarily from terms starting with "alternative" not "complementary." With many search combinations, having a high number of results returned did not equate with quality Web sites. For general search engines, "alternative medicine" retrieved mainly government, university, or established hospital or treatment center results while "holistic healing" retrieved advertisements for individuals, organizations, or businesses. Other general searches retrieved an overwhelming majority of nongovernment or unrecognized authority results.

ADDITIONAL SEARCH STRATEGIES

Because the terms "alternative" or "complementary health sources" cover a variety of topics, it is often necessary to narrow your search. Start with the general sample search examples listed in "Procedures and Special Topics"

(p. 45). On general search engines, starting with "alternative medicine" retrieved the greatest number of results. Add words such as bodywork, dietary, energy, support groups, followed by a specific disease, such as cancer or heart disease; body part or symptom, such as back, skin, or headache; or a concern, such as fraud, professional organizations, training, or insurance coverage. Some examples of this strategy are "alternative medicine bodywork scam," "alternative medicine support groups cancer," or "alternative medicine energy work training." It may also be helpful to start with Web sites listed in the "Best One-Stop Shops" section followed by more detailed searches.

TOPIC PROFILE

Who

Everyone, especially individuals looking for non-clinical settings or approaches that reflect their values or beliefs, or who found little or no results with traditional Western medicine.

What

Promotes therapy, healing, and improved quality, healthy maintenance, and prolongation of life using medical sources that are outside of the allopathic medical approach currently dominant in European and North American medical culture.

Where

Entire body, mind, and spirit.

When

At all stages of life.

ABBREVIATIONS USED IN THIS SECTION

CAM = Complementary alternative medicine
IOM = Institute of Medicine
NCCAM = National Council for Complementary and Alternative Medicine
NOAH = New York Online Access to Health
TCM = Traditional Chinese medicine
UCSD = University of California San Diego

PROCEDURES AND SPECIAL TOPICS

60. GENERAL

Recommended Search Terms

- "Alternative health sources"
- "Alternative medicine"
- "Alternative healing"

- "Alternative therapies"
- "Complementary alternative medicine"
- "Complementary health sources"
- "Complementary medicine"
- "Complementary healing"
- "Complementary therapies"
- "Integrative therapies"
- "Holistic healing"

Important Sites

Alternative Medicine: Health Care Information Resources: <http://hsl.mcmaster.ca/tomflem/altmed.html>

Holistic Healing Web Page: Articles and Documents: <http://www.holisticmed.com/#docs>

M. D. Anderson Cancer Center: Complementary/Integrative Medicine: <http://www.mdanderson.org/departments/CIMER/>

MotherNature.com: Book Shelf: Natural Medicine for Arthritis: Choosing an Alternative: <http://library.mothernature.com/Library/bookshelf/Books/42/3.cfm>

Oregon Health and Science University: Complementary and Alternative Medicine: <http://www.ohsu.edu/ohmig/cam.html>

University of Michigan Health Systems: Complementary and Alternative Medicine Research Center (CAMRC): <http://www.med.umich.edu/camrc/index.html>

61. Deciding When to Use Complementary Alternative Medicine (CAM)

Recommended Search Terms

- Advantages "alternative medicine"
- Benefits "alternative medicine"
- Decide "complementary medicine"
- Risks "alternative medicine"
- Use "alternative medicine"
- +When use "alternative medicine"
- +Why use "alternative medicine"

Important Sites

Cancer Lynx: Making Health Decisions about Complementary Medicine: <http://www.cancerlynx.com/camdecisions.html/>

MediComm: How to Use Alternative and Complementary Medicine: <http://www.medicomm.net/Consumer%20Site/am/am_a3.htm>

National Cancer Institute (NCI): Cancer Facts: Complementary and Alternative Medicine: <http://cis.nci.nih.gov/fact/9_14.htm>

National Center for Complementary and Alternative Medicine (NCCAM): Health Information: <http://nccam.nih.gov/health/>

Richard and Hinda Rosenthal Center: Complementary and Alternative Medicine Resources: <http://www.rosenthal.hs.columbia.edu/CAM_Resources.html>

62. Selecting Complementary and Alternative Medicine (CAM) Practitioner

NOTE: Use the following link for assistance in understanding practitioner qualifications: By Region.net: Some Common Initials and Abbreviations for Licenses Holistic Practitioners: <http://www.byregion.net/glossary/initials.html>

Recommended Search Terms

- Choose "complementary medicine" doctor
- Find "herbalist"
- Locate "complementary medicine" therapist
- "Questions to ask" "acupuncturist"
- Select "alternative medicine" practitioner
- Select "massage therapist"

Important Sites

1UpHealth: Alternative Medicine: Considering Complementary and Alternative Medicine Therapies: <http://www.1uphealth.com/alternative-medicine/making-decisions-3.html>

National Center for Complementary and Alternative Medicine (NCCAM): Selecting a Complementary and Alternative Medicine (CAM) Practitioner: <http://nccam.nih.gov/health/practitioner/>

StopGettingSick.com: Considering CAM?: <http://www.stopgettingsick.com/templates/news_template.cfm/1563#approaching>

University of California, San Francisco (UCSF) Medical Center: Your Health Matters: Guidelines for Selecting a Complementary and Alternative Medicine Practitioner for Cancer Patients: <http://cc.ucsf.edu/crc/hm_CAM_and_cancer.pdf>

63. Deception and Fraud

Recommended Search Terms

- "Alternative medicine" deceit
- "Alternative medicine" evaluation
- "Alternative therapy" fraud

- "Chiropractic" Quacks
- "Holistic Healing" imposture
- Herbal fake
- Homeopathy cheat
- Naturopathy scams

Important Sites

Alternative Medicine Page: Fraud and Quackery: Internet Resources: Alternative Medicine: <http://www.pitt.edu/~cbw/fraud.html>

National Council against Health Fraud (NCAHF): <http://www.ncahf.org/>

National Fraud Information Center (NFIC): <http://www.fraud.org/welcome.htm>

Quackwatch: <http://www.quackwatch.org>

64. CLINICAL TRIALS

Recommended Search Terms

- "Alternative medicine" clinical trials
- "Alternative medicine" validation
- "Alternative healing" validating
- "Alternative therapy" validate
- Legitimate homeopathy

Important Sites

ClinicalTrials.gov: <http://www.clinicaltrials.gov/>

Department of Health and Human Services: Diseases and Conditions: Clinical Trials: <http://www.hhs.gov/diseases/index.shtml#clinical>

MedlinePlus: Alternative Medicine: Clinical Trials: <http://www.nlm.nih.gov/medlineplus/alternativemedicine.html#clinicaltrials>

National Center for Complementary and Alternative Medicine (NCCAM): Clinical Trials: <http://nccam.nih.gov/clinicaltrials/>

65. CRITICAL/TERMINAL ILLNESS

Recommended Search Terms

- "Alternative medicine" critical illness
- "Complementary therapies" terminal illness
- "Holistic healing" grave illness
- "Holistic therapies" acute disease
- "Integrative therapies" palliative care

Important Sites

Beyond Indigo: Caregiving and Terminal Illness: <http://www.beyondindigo.com/caregiving/>

Care of Dying: Supportive Voice: Supportive Care Model: A Philosophy of Care and Concepts of Care: <http://www.careofdying.org/>

Doctor Yourself: Terminal Illness: Ten Ways to Beat the Reaper: <http://www.doctoryourself.com/terminal.html>

RX.Magazine: End of Life Archive: Too Little, Too Late: Treating the Pain of the Terminally Ill: <http://rx.magazine.tripod.com/eol_20010328.htm>

University of Kentucky, Markey Cancer Center: Research Professional: Behavioral and Palliative Care: Integrative Medicine Program: <http://www.mc.uky.edu/markey/Research/im.shtml>

66. USING HERBALS WITH PRESCRIPTION MEDICATIONS

Recommended Search Terms

- "Alternative medicine" herbs
- "Alternative therapy" herbals
- "Complementary medicine" drug interactions
- "Complementary therapy" prescription medications

Important Sites

HerbMD: <http://www.herbmed.org/>

Holistic-Online: Herbal Medicine: <http://www.holistic-online.com/Herbal-Med/hol_herb.htm>

Memorial Sloan-Kettering Cancer Center: Information Resource: About Herbs, Botanicals and Other Products: <http://www.mskcc.org/aboutherbs>

Personal Health Zone: Side Effects, Interactions and Warnings About Herbs: <http://www.personalhealthzone.com/herbsafety.html>

RX List: RxList Alternatives: <http://www.rxlist.com/alternative.htm>

USA Drug: Drug Interaction Information: Interactions by Drug: <http://www.usadrug.com/IMCAccess/ConsLookups/InteractionsByDrug.shtml>

67. HEALTH CARE POLICY AND RESEARCH

Recommended Search Terms

- Acupuncture research
- "Alternative medicine" healthcare policy
- "Alternative medicine" "health care" policy
- "Complementary therapy" liability
- Homeopathic provider
- Massage "healthcare policy and research"
- "Naturopathy" insurance

Important Sites

Agency for Healthcare Research and Quality: <http://www.ahrq.gov/>

American Association for Health Freedom: Federal Affairs: <http://www.apma.net/federalaffairs.htm>

American Journal of Public Health: October 1, 2002: Volume 92, Issue 10: [Complementary and Alternative Medicine]: <http://www.ajph.org/content/vol92/issue10/index.shtml>

Annals of Internal Medicine: Academia and Clinic: Complementary and Alternative Medicine Series: Potential Physician Malpractice Liability Associated with Complementary and Integrative Medical Therapies: <http://www.annals.org/issues/v136n8/abs/200204160-00009.html>

Health Services Research Projects in Progress (HSRProj): Participating Organizations: <http://www.academyhealth.org/hsrproj/list.htm>

White House Commission on Complementary and Alternative Medicine Policy: Meetings: May 14-16, 2001: Understanding Coverage and Reimbursement, Washington, D.C.: Transcript: <http://www.whccamp.hhs.gov/meetings/transcript_5_14_01main.html>

White House Commission on Complementary and Alternative Medicine Policy: White House Commission on Complementary and Alternative Medicine Policy: Final Report, March 2002: <http://govinfo.library.unt.edu/whccamp/finalreport.html>

68. Chinese Medicine

Recommended Search Terms

- Chinese "alternative health sources"
- Chinese accupuncture
- "Chinese herbal medicine"
- Chinese qi
- TCM "alternative medicine"
- "Traditional Chinese medicine"

Important Sites

Health World Online: Traditional Chinese Medicine: <http://www.healthy.net/clinic/therapy/chinmed/>

MedlinePlus: Acupuncture: <http://www.nlm.nih.gov/medlineplus/acupuncture.html>

National Center for Complementary and Alternative Medicine: Treatment Information: Acupuncture: <http://nccam.nih.gov/health/acupuncture/>

National Parkinson Foundation (NPF): Complementary Therapies and Parkinson's Disease: <http://www.parkinson.org/therapies.htm>

Rebecca and John Moores University of California San Diego (UCSD) Cancer Center: Complementary and

Alternative Therapies for Cancer Patients: Traditional Chinese Medicine: <http://cancer.ucsd.edu/outreach/CAMs/traditionalchinese.asp>

RxList: RxList Alternatives: Chinese Herbal Remedies: <http://www.rxlist.com/chinese.htm>

69. Ayurvedic Medicine

Recommended Search Terms

- Ayurvedic "alternative medicine"
- Ayurvedic herbals
- Ayurvedic therapy
- Ayurvedic meditation

Important Sites

Ayurvedic Foundations: What is Ayurveda?: <http://www.ayur.com/about.html>

Health World Online: Ayurvedic Medicine: <http://www.healthy.net/clinic/therapy/ayurv/>

New York Online Access to Health (NOAH): Ask NOAH About: Ayurvedic Medicine: <http://www.noah-health.org/english/alternative/alternative.html#Aryuvedic>

70. Native American Medicine

Recommended Search Terms

- Aboriginal health wellness traditions
- "First people's" "traditional healing"
- "First nations" health medicine
- "Native American" "alternative medicine"
- "Native American" herbs
- "Native American" healing
- "Native American" "medicinal rituals"

Important Sites

American Cancer Society: Making Treatment Decisions: Native American Healing: <http://www.cancer.org/docroot/eto/content/eto_5_3x_native_american_healing.asp?sitearea=eto>

Navapache Regional Medical Center (NRMC): Integrative Health Services: Complementary and Alternative Modalities Offered at NRMC: <http://www.nrmc.org/Integrative%20Therapies.htm>

Rebecca and John Moores University of California San Diego (UCSD) Cancer Center: Complementary and Alternative Therapies For Cancer Patients: Native American Healing: <http://cancer.ucsd.edu/outreach/CAMs/nativeamerican.asp>

University of Michigan, Dearborn: Native American Ethnobotany: <http://herb.umd.umich.edu>

71. TRAINING

Recommended Search Terms

- Acupuncture certification
- Doula training
- Homeopathic certification
- "Massage therapy" schools
- Naturopathic degree

Important Sites

Alternative Medicine HomePage: Schools, Training and Licensure: Internet Resources: Alternative Medicine: <http://www.pitt.edu/~cbw/licen.html>

American Association of Naturopathic Physicians: Naturopathic Medicine: <http://www.naturopathic.org/education.htm>

Catalog of Federal Domestic Assistance: Research and Training in Complementary and Alternative Medicine: <http://www.cfda.gov/public/viewprog.asp?progid=1197>

ChiroWeb: Chiropractic and Other Related Links: <http://www.chiroweb.com/forum/important.html>

HealthWWWeb: Courses on Complementary Medicine and Alternative Therapies (CAM) Taught at Conventional U.S. Medical Schools: <http://www.healthwwweb.com/schools/CAM.html>

National Center for Complementary and Alternative Medicine (NCCAM): Training: <http://nccam.nih.gov/training/>

National Institutes of Health: Postdoctoral Research Training in Complementary and Alternative Medicine: <http://grants1.nih.gov/grants/guide/pa-files/PA-01-088.html>

72. BODYWORK

NOTE: The term "body work" retrieves Web sites related to cars. To retrieve sites on methods requiring a person to be touched by a therapist without sites on cars, use the minus sign before words for cars, as shown in a few of the sample searches below.

Recommended Search Terms

- "Alternative medicine" bodywork
- "Alternative therapies" bodywork
- Bodywork health -automotive
- Bodywork therapy -car -repair
- Lomilomi
- Lomi lomi
- Massage
- Rolfing
- "Thai massage"
- Traeger

Important Sites

BoMi (Body and Mind) Bodywork: Massage, Manipulation, Movement, Energy Work and Body Psychotherapies: <http://www.bomi.info/bodywork/>

Holistic Online: Back Pain: Bodywork: <http://www.holistic-online.com/Remedies/Backpain/back_bodywork.htm>

Lomilomi Somatic Healing Centre: What Is Lomilomi?: <http://www.lomi4life.com/what_is_lomilomi.htm>

New York Online Access to Health (NOAH): Ask NOAH About: Complementary and Alternative Medicine: Trager and Trager Mentastics <http://www.noah-health.org/english/alternative/alternative.html#Trager>

Open Directory Project (DMOZ): Health: Alternative: Massage Therapy and Bodywork: <http://dmoz.org/Health/Alternative/Massage_Therapy_and_Bodywork/>

Rolfing: Toward the Whole Human Being: What Is Rolfing?: <http://www.rolfnet.com/about.html>

73. DIETARY/INGESTED

NOTE: This refers both to alternative healing therapies that are eaten and to healing that results from ingesting particular substances.

Recommended Search Terms

- "Alternative health sources" dietary
- Digestive cleansing
- Fasting healing
- Ingested herbs
- Liver purge

Important Sites

1UpHealth: Alternative Medicine: Dietary Supplements Definition and Explanation: <http://www.1uphealth.com/alternative-medicine/dietary-supp-ex.html>

Alternative Medicine HomePage: Database: Alternative Medicine Resources: <http://www.pitt.edu/~cbw/database.html>

Body Therapy Alternative Healing: Naturopathic Alternative Healing Online Web Journal: <http://www.bodytherapy4u.com/alternative_healing/alternative_healing.htm>

D. A. Currie's Home Page: Health and Nutrition Links: <http://www.dacurrie.com/healthandnutrition.html>

Food and Drug Administration (FDA): Center for Food Safety and Applied Nutrition: Dietary Supplements: Warnings and Safety Information: <http://www.cfsan.fda.gov/%7Edms/ds-warn.html>

Holistic Online: Diabetes: Macrobiotic Approach: <http://www.holistic-online.com/Remedies/Diabetes/diabetes_macrobiotic.htm>

National Library of Medicine: Frequently Asked Questions: Dietary Supplements, Complementary or Alternative Medicines: <http://www.nlm.nih.gov/services/dietsup.html>

74. Energy Work

NOTE: The search term "energy" retrieves Web sites related to fuel. "Energy work" is the term for therapies that commence over a long distance or occur with or without any physical contact.

Recommended Search Terms

- "Alternative therapies" "energy work"
- "Alternative medicine" "energy work"
- "Energy work" modalities
- "Energy work" therapies
- Ki healing

Important Sites

Alternative Medicine Foundation: Energy Work: An Alternative and Complementary Medicine Resource Guide: <http://www.amfoundation.org/energywork.htm>

Complementary and Integrative Therapies: Manual and Energy Healing, Physical Touch: <http://cit.cancersource.com/therapy.cfm?CITTopicID=2>

CompWellness.org: Energy Work: <http://www.compwellness.org/eGuide/energy.htm>

Ki Health International: Healing with Vital Energy: <http://www.cdsb.org/>

Cranial Sacral

NOTE: Government and academic institutions generally list this under "craniosacral." This modality generally refers to therapy developed by William Sutherland, D.O., and involves light touch and interaction with the cerebral spinal fluid in the brain and spinal cord.

Recommended Search Terms

- Craniosacral
- Cranial sacral
- Biodynamic cranial sacral

Important Sites

Biodynamic Cranial Sacral: <http://www.biodynamiccranialsacral.com/index.htm>

BoMi (Body and Mind): Bodywork and Somatic Therapies Guide: Craniosacral Therapy: <http://homepage.tinet.ie/~bomi/bodywork/c.htm#Craniosacral%20Therapy>

Craniosacral Therapy Association of North America (CSTA/NA): <http://www.craniosacraltherapy.org/Whatis.htm>

The Upledger Institute: Therapies: CranioSacral Therapy: <http://www.upledger.com/therapies/cst.htm>

Polarity

NOTE: Searches using the term "polarity" by itself will also retrieve information on molecules.

Recommended Search Terms

- Polarity therapy
- Polarity energy
- Polarity balancing

Important Sites

American Polarity Therapy Association: About Polarity Therapy: <http://www.polaritytherapy.org/polarity/index.html>

American Cancer Society: Making Treatment Decisions: Polarity Therapy: <http://www.cancer.org/docroot/ETO/content/ETO_5_3X_Polarity_Therapy.asp?sitearea=ETO>

Mountain Valley Center: Polarity Energy Balancing is a Gentle Way to Internal Well Being: <http://www.mountainvalleycenter.com/politywb.htm>

Qi Gong

Recommended Search Terms

- Qigong
- Qi gong
- Qigong healing
- Chi Kung
- Ch'i Kung

Important Sites

Qigong Association of America: <http://www.qi.org/>

Acupuncture.com: Qi Gong (Chi Kung) Subject Index: <http://acupuncture.com/QiKung/QikunInd.htm>

The Qigong Institute: Qigong Healing: <http://pub21.ezboard.com/fqigonginstitutefrm2>

Reiki
Recommended Search Terms

- Reiki
- "Universal life energy"

Important Sites

ReikiAloha: <http://www.reikialoha.com/raymond/>
Reiki Ryoho: <http://www.angelfire.com/az/SpiritMatters/contents.html>
The Reiki Page: <http://reiki.7gen.com/>

Human Energy Field

NOTE: This topic refers to therapies that acknowledge the presence of human energy fields.

Recommended Search Terms

- Human energy field
- Bioenergetic therapy
- Therapeutic touch
- Energy field therapy

Important Sites

Chi: <http://chiexplorer.com/TT.html>
Energy Therapy: <http://energytherapy.net/>
Nurse-Healers Professional Associates International (NH-PAI): Therapeutic Touch: <http://www.therapeutic-touch.org/content/ttouch.asp>
Health World Online: Exploring the Human Energy System: <http://www.healthy.net/asp/templates/interview.asp?PageType=Interview&ID=165>

75. MIND/SPIRIT THERAPIES
Recommended Search Terms

- Buddhist meditation
- Meditation
- Psychedelic healing
- Spiritual healing
- Sweat lodge
- Transcendental meditation

Important Sites

American Meditation Institute: Frequently Asked Questions: <http://www.americanmeditation.org/faq.htm>
Holistic Online: Meditation: <http://holisticonline.com/meditation/hol_meditation.htm>

Rebecca and John Moores University of California San Diego (UCSD) Cancer Center: Complementary and Alternative Therapies for Cancer Patients: Meditation: <http://cancer.ucsd.edu/outreach/CAMs/meditation.asp>

Hypnotherapy
Recommended Search Terms

- Hypnotherapy
- Hypnosis
- Medical hypnosis

Important Sites

American Psychotherapy and Medical Hypnosis Association: Definition of the Process of Hypnosis and Trance States: <http://apmha.com/page8.htm>
Hypnosis: Your Frequently Asked Questions: <http://www.hypnosis.com/faq/>
Hypnotherapy: Medical Hypnosis—Uses, Techniques, and Contraindications of Hypnotherapy: <http://www.ncpamd.com/medical_hypnosis.htm>
The Permanente Journal: Medical Hypnosis: An Underutilized Treatment Approach: <http://www.kaiserpermanente.org/medicine/permjournal/Fall01/hypnosis.html>

Peptide Therapy
Recommended Search Terms

- Peptide therapy
- Candace Pert
- Protein therapy

Important Sites

Business Wire: Research into Peptide Therapy Offers Hope for Millions of Americans: <http://www.aegis.com/news/bw/1996/bw961115.html>
The Institute for New Medicine: <http://www.tinm.org/>
Karl Loren Home Page: Cancer Chemo (Toxico) Therapy Revisited and Alternative Ways of Healing: Cancer and Biopsy: <http://www.karlloren.com/biopsy/book/p9.htm>
The Seer: Candace Pert: <http://www.angelfire.com/hi/TheSeer/Pert.html>

76. SOUND/MUSIC

NOTE: This topic refers to therapies that focus on healing with sound, specific tones, or music.

Recommended Search Terms

- "Complementary therapy" sound
- "Crystal bowls"
- "Healing chant"
- Mantra healing
- "Music therapy"
- "Tibetan bowls"

Important Sites

American Music Therapy Association: <http://www.namt.com/>

Center for Spirituality and Healing: Research: Ongoing and Potential Investigations in Complementary Therapies and Healing Practices: <http://www.csh.umn.edu/Research/topics/>

Herald Sun: Columns: Mark Schultz: Ancient Practice Could Be Good for Both Body and Soul: <http://www.herald-sun.com/features/columns/schultz/>

Oregon Health and Science University (OHSU): Alternative Medicine: Art, Dance, and Music and CAM: <http://www.ohsuhealth.com/cam/art.asp>

77. VISIONS/LIGHT/COLOR

NOTE: This topic refers to therapies that focus on input from our eyes.

Recommended Search Terms

- "Alternative health sources" sight
- "Alternative medicine" vision
- "Color therapy"
- "Complementary therapies" eyes
- "Light therapy"

Important Sites

Healing About: Holistic Healing: Color Therapy—Chromotherapy: <http://healing.about.com/cs/colortherapy/a/aa_colortherapy.htm>

Holistic Online: Light Therapy: <http://www.holistic-online.com/Light_Therapy/hol_LightTherapy.htm>

International Iridology Association: <http://www.iridologyassn.org/>

Rebecca and John Moores University of California San Diego (UCSD) Cancer Center: Complementary and Alternative Therapies for Cancer Patients: Light Therapy: <http://cancer.ucsd.edu/outreach/CAMs/light.asp>

78. TOUCH

Recommended Search Terms

- "Alternative medicine" touch
- "Alternative therapies" touch
- "Cranial sacral"
- "Therapeutic touch"

Important Sites

BoMi (Body and Mind): Holistic Practitioner Listing and Clinics: <http://homepage.tinet.ie/~bomi/practitioners/main.htm>

New York Online Access to Health (NOAH): Ask NOAH About: Therapeutic Touch: <http://www.noah-health.org/english/alternative/alternative.html#touch>

Rebecca and John Moores University of California San Diego (UCSD) Cancer Center: Complementary and Alternative Therapies for Cancer Patients: Therapeutic Touch: <http://cancer.ucsd.edu/outreach/CAMs/touch.asp>

Yahoo! Health: Alternative Therapies: Therapeutic Touch: <http://health.yahoo.com/health/alternative_medicine/alternative_therapies/Therapeutic_Touch/>

Shiatsu
Recommended Search Terms

- Shiatsu
- Zen shiatsu
- Namikoshi shiatsu

Important Sites

Laughinghara: Zen Shiatsu: Keeping the World Naturally Healthy: <http://www.laughinghara.com/zen_shiatsu.htm>

Mike Flanagan's Shiatsu Pages: What's Here?: <http://homepage.ntlworld.com/mikeflanagan/shiatsu/>

Shiatsu: <http://www.geocities.com/CapeCanaveral/8538/shiatsuing.html>

Zen Shiatsu: The Legacy of Shizuto masunaga: <http://www.itmonline.org/arts/shiatsu.htm>

Reflexology

NOTE: Searches for "foot massage" by itself may retrieve sites unrelated to therapy.

Recommended Search Terms

- Reflexology
- Foot massage therapy

Important Sites

International Institute of Reflexology: History of Reflexology: <http://www.reflexology-usa.net/history.htm>

Massage and Bodywork: Reflexology: Footprint for Restoring Balance and Health: <http://www.abmp.com/copy pages/magazinepages/articles/FebMarch2002/Reflexology.html>

Modern Institute of Reflexology: Full Spectrum Reflexology: <http://www.reflexologyinstitute.com/reflex_def.php>

Myofascial Release

Recommended Search Terms

- Myofascial release
- Myofascial massage

Important Sites

Myofascial Release: <http://www.myofascial-release.com/>

Whole Health MD: Therapies: Myofascial Release Therapy: <http://www.wholehealthmd.com/refshelf/substances_view/1,1525,10156,00.html>

Hydrotherapy

Recommended Search Terms

- Hydrotherapy
- Water therapy

Important Sites

The Colon Therapists Network: Colon Hydrotherapy: <http://colonhealth.net/colon_hydrotherapy/chthrapy.htm#>

Holistic-Online: Hydrotherapy: <http://www.holistic-online.com/hydrotherapy.htm>

Spine-Health: Water Therapy Exercise Program: <http://www.spine-health.com/topics/conserv/water/water01.html>

79. Smell/Aromatherapy

Recommended Search Terms

- "Alternative medicine" smell
- Aromatherapy
- "Essential oils"
- "Essential oils" "therapeutic use"

Important Sites

American Cancer Society: Making Treatment Decisions: Aromatherapy: <http://www.cancer.org/docroot/eto/content/eto_5_3x_aromatherapy.asp?sitearea=eto>

Gems4Friends: Aromatherapy Information: <http://www.gems4friends.com/oils.html>

Holistic Online: Aromatherapy: <http://www.holistic-online.com/Aromatherapy/hol_aroma.htm>

New York Online Access to Health (NOAH): Ask NOAH About: Aromatherapy: <http://www.noah-health.org/english/alternative/alternative.html#Aromatherapy>

80. Movement/Exercises

NOTE: This topic refers to therapies that focus on movement to gain health.

Recommended Search Terms

- "Dance therapy"
- "Alexander technique"
- "Alternative healing" movement
- "Complementary therapies" exercise
- Feldenkrais
- Naprapathy
- "Physical therapy"
- "Tai chi"

Important Sites

American Dance Therapy Association <http://www.adta.org/>

BoMi (Body and Mind): Massage, Manipulation, Movement, Energy Work and Body Psychotherapies: <http://homepage.tinet.ie/~bomi/bodywork/>

EarthSpirit Therapies: Definitions of Bodywork and Alternative Health Modality Terms: <http://www.earthspirittx.com/definitions_m-n.html>

Holistic Online: Arthritis: Flexibility and Strengthening Exercises: <http://www.holistic-online.com/Remedies/Arthritis/arth_whole-body-exercises.htm>

Holistic Online: Meditation: Meditation Techniques: <http://1stholistic.com/Meditation/hol_meditation_movement.htm>

Nicholas Institute of Sports Medicine and Athletic Trauma (NISMAT): Physical Therapy Corner: Complementary Therapies: <http://www.nismat.org/ptcor/comp_ther/>

Rebecca and John Moores University of California San Diego (UCSD) Cancer Center: Complementary and Alternative Therapies for Cancer Patients: <http://cancer.ucsd.edu/outreach/CAMs/taichi.asp>

What Is Naprapathy?: <http://personal.inet.fi/palvelu/ergo/frmain01.htm>

HOTLINES

National Institutes of Health (NIH): National Center for Complementary and Alternative Medicine:
1-888-644-6226; (301) 519-3153 (International callers)
Food and Drug Administration (FDA):
1-888-463-6332

FAQs

National Center for Complementary and Alternative Medicine (NCCAM): <http://nccam.nih.gov/>
New York Online Access to Health (NOAH): Ask NOAH About: Alternative Health: <http://www.noah-health .org/english/alternative/alternative.html#basics>

ALTERNATIVE/COMPLEMENTARY HEALTH PUBLICATIONS ON THE INTERNET

Alternative Health News Online: <http://www.alt medicine.com/>
Homeopathy Online: <http://www.lyghtforce.com/ HomeopathyOnline/>
Journal of Naturopathic Medicine: <http://www.healthy .net/library/journals/naturopathic/>

PROFESSIONAL ORGANIZATIONS

Acupuncture and Oriental Medicine Alliance: <http:// www.aomalliance.org/>
American Association of Naturopathic Physicians: <http:// www.naturopathic.org/>
American Association of Oriental Medicine: <http://www .aaom.org>
American Chiropractic Association: <http://www.amer chiro.org/>
American Herbalists Guild: <http://www.american herbalist.com>
American Holistic Medical Association: <http://www .holisticmedicine.org/>
American Massage Therapy Association: <http://www .amtamassage.org/>
American Society for the Alexander Technique: <http:// www.alexandertech.com>
Feldenkrais Guild of North America: <http://www .feldenkrais.com>
International Association of Reiki Practitioners: <http:// www.iarp.org>
International Institute of Reflexology: <http://reflexology -usa.net>
National Association for Holistic Aromatherapy: <http:// www.naha.org>
Qigong Association of America: <http://www.qi.org/>
Reflexology Association of America: <http://www .reflexology-usa.org>
Trager International: <http://www.trager.com>

PATIENT SUPPORT ORGANIZATIONS/ DISCUSSION GROUPS

Alternatives for Healthy Living: <http://www.alt-med-ed .com/>
Aetna InteliHealth: <http://www.intelihealth.com/IH/ ihtIH/WSIHW000/21302/21302.html>
Holistic Healing Web Page: <http://www.holisticmed .com/www/mail.html>

BEST ONE-STOP SHOPS

Alternative Medicine—Healthcare or Fraud? You Decide: <http://www.wayne-health.org/nf/nf-wcmedinfo3 .html>
Alternative Medicine Page: <http://www.pitt.edu/~cbw/ internet.html>
Barbara's Health and Medical Page: <http://www.gate.net/ ~barbara/med.htm>
National Center for Complementary and Alternative Medicine (NCCAM): <http://nccam.nih.gov/>
New York Online Access to Health (NOAH): Ask NOAH About: Alternative Health: <http://www.noah-health .org/english/alternative/alternative.html>

REFERENCES

1. "Why Patients Use Alternative Medicine: Results of a National Study." *JAMA* (1998, May 20) Retrieved November 10, 2003, from <http://jama.ama-assn .org/cgi/content/short/279/19/1548>.
2. National Council for Complementary and Alternative Medicine (NCCAM). Press Releases 2002: NIH Announces Institute of Medicine Study of Complementary and Alternative Medicine (2001, October 21). Retrieved November 10, 2003, from <http:// nccam.nih.gov/news/2002/102102.htm>.

Part VI: Multicultural Health

Karyn Pomerantz and Kristine Alpi

SPECIAL SEARCHING ISSUES FOR THIS TOPIC

The relationship of health to race, ethnicity, and culture is complex, and many factors must be considered in order to do an effective search on these topics. An important first step in this process is to become familiar with the meaning of terms used to discuss cultural awareness, or the cultural competency as it relates to health and healthcare. In 1994, the Seattle King County Department of

Public Health (now known as Public Health Seattle-King County) defined cultural competency as follows:

> the ability of individuals and systems to respond respectfully and effectively to people of all cultures, classes, races, ethnic backgrounds and religions in a manner that recognizes, affirms, and values the cultural differences and similarities and the worth of individuals, families, and communities and protects and preserves the dignity of each.[1]

This chapter deals with the complexities of finding information on the health of particular cultural, ethnic and racial groups. Please keep in mind that this chapter uses standard terminology dealing with identity as a means of minimizing possible offense. It is important to find out what terms are preferred and used by the cultural, ethnic, and racial groups about which you are searching.

When searching for information on specific population groups defined by race or ethnicity, it is important to consider what these concepts represent. We often think of "race" as categories of people grouped by biological characteristics—such as skin color and genetic predisposition to health conditions. Words used to describe persons of color or of different racial or ethnic heritages vary greatly. Among the many terms are those that that are technically accurate for a given profession, those that are superficially descriptive without intent to offend, and those that are simply offensive. Because the incidence of some illnesses varies according to race or ethnicity, it can be helpful to use such terms in searches for health information, if done with caution. According to the American Anthropological Association, there are more differences in physical characteristics within "racial" groups than between them: "...present-day inequalities between so-called 'racial' groups are not consequences of their biological inheritance but products of historical and contemporary social, economic, educational, and political circumstances."[2]

It is important to keep this perspective in mind as we conduct searches for information about particular groups divided by race or ancestry/historical heritage, such as ethnicity. Health statistics often reveal different patterns of health and disease for people in particular groups. For example, infant mortality rates and cardiovascular disease rates are higher among people identified as African American; Latinos are at high risk for diabetes; and Native Americans have higher rates of alcohol use and suicide compared to Caucasian populations. What factors contribute to the very real differences in the disease incidence, morbidity, mortality rates, and life expectancy between groups divided by "race" and ethnicity? There are many non-biological factors in society that explain these differences. David Williams, a sociologist at the University of Michigan, created a model that helps explain the influence of race on health. He begins by associating race with particular cultural, socioeconomic, discrimination, and political factors.[3] These factors influence health practices, psychological stress, environmental stress, and medical care which contribute to one's physiological status and well-being.

It is important to consider all of these factors when evaluating the quality of health resources on this topic. Pseudoscientific explanations for the relationships between genes, race, and people's behavioral and cognitive characteristics abound in the literature.

What to Ask

Multicultural health is a broad and multifaceted topic that can be searched for many different reasons. Are you looking for the health status of a particular ethnic or racial group? Then you may want to choose sites focused on that particular group or more general sites that include all groups. Are you interested in treatment or prevention options for particular conditions? If so, you may not need to narrow your search to a particular group since a condition-specific site may cover all options. However, if you are looking for culturally appropriate materials and Web pages for specific conditions, you can start by choosing a site based on ethnicity and then search for the particular condition or health characteristic. Are you researching descriptions and explanations for health disparities between groups? In that case, it may be useful to consider the numerous publications on health disparities that cover a range of groups and topics—such as practitioner interactions with patients, differences in utilization of health services, and health statistics on life expectancy, as well as mortality and morbidity rates for particular populations. Many governmental and educational institutions host this type of information.

Where to Start

When searching U.S. government Web sites, it is important to be aware of the terminology used for race and ethnicity. In the United States, the federal government has defined race and ethnicity for data collection on a variety of issues, including health. In October 1997, the Office of Management and Budget (OMB) announced the revised standards for federal data on race and ethnicity.[4] There are five minimum categories for race:

- American Indian or Alaska Native
- Asian
- Black or African American
- Native Hawaiian or Other Pacific Islander
- White

Of course, these categories continue to be open to discussion. The 2000 Census changed how we measure race in the United States by inviting multiracial identification rather than requiring that every person in the country identify with only one racial group. The OMB offers two minimum categories for ethnicity: "Hispanic or Latino" and "Not Hispanic or Latino." Hispanics and Latinos may be of any race. In certain geographic areas, Hispanics or Latinos are broken into various groups due to large numbers of a particular group or political reasons. In New York City, for example, the data on the leading causes of death is presented for those of Puerto Rican ancestry separate from other Hispanics.[5]

Two U.S. government sites supplying statistics are the National Center for Health Statistics (NCHS), which supplies birth, illness, health care utilization, and death statistics, and the Bureau of the Census, which supplies population statistics. Both sources offer these statistics broken down by racial and ethnic categories. However, the Census Bureau relies on self-identification in assigning racial and ethnic categories while in NCHS data these categories may be assigned by an observer. States, cities, counties, and individual health care institutions may also capture race and ethnicity data. Many states, especially those with large populations of immigrants, have offices of multicultural health that provide potentially useful publications and resources.

Government portal sites, such as healthfinder.gov and Medlineplus.gov, cover resources on many different groups. However, they link primarily to governmental and voluntary health agency sites, such as the American Cancer Association or the American Heart Association. While these sites provide useful information, patrons may not find their messages as compelling or culturally relevant as the sites from community-based organizations and advocacy groups. The Black Women's Health Imperative (formerly known as the Black Women's Health Project) and the links from the National Council of La Raza are two examples of sites that expand on the information provided by government organizations.

ADDITIONAL SEARCH STRATEGIES

In addition to understanding the many facets reflected in the topic of multicultural health, the following issues should be kept in mind when conducting Internet searches on this topic.

Source of information. Many organizations address health disparities by race and ethnicity. Some are newly established governmental agencies and research centers that fund grassroots programs and academic projects, long-standing health provider associations representing particular groups, community-based organizations addressing local issues, and advocacy groups pressing for social change. Sites that are sponsored by non-governmental institutions often express the viewpoints of the groups they represent more completely than is possible on a government Web site. Government Web sites on multicultural health may reflect the priorities and politics of the administration in office. The sites selected for this chapter include a wide range of resources.

Scope of the information. The information may span multiple issues and groups, such as the Intercultural Cancer Council, or concentrate on the health of one particular group of people. Content may focus on diseases or conditions more prevalent for a group, adapt the information for a particular culture, offer options for social change, or explain the context of health disparities.

Content. There are large numbers of sites on the topic of multicultural health. Make sure you check the materials hosted on a site before you branch out to links selected by the site creators. While this chapter focuses on U.S. sites, there is also a rich array of international sites providing relevant information on culture and ethnicity.

Terminology. Terms used to describe specific groups vary over time. Black or African American, Latino or Hispanic, American Indian or Native American are terms that different sources may use to represent the same peoples. Some searching vocabularies designations may be considered offensive, such as the anthropological term "Negroid Race" used as a Medical Subject Heading in the Medline database. In some cases, ethnic groups are clearly identified by country of origin such as Mexicans, Lebanese, or Vietnamese, while others are grouped by region or origin, such as Asian Pacific Islanders or Arabs. While certain terms dominate the current idiom, it may be wise to search more inclusively using more than one term.

Bias. Searches for materials on race and ethnicity and health may retrieve biased sites determined to share their political ideology. Look out for sites that claim that biological or social characteristics are determined by one's race. Conditions traditionally associated with a particular group may have been influenced more by geography, environment, or historical context than genes. Be sensitive to health sites that "blame the victim" for conditions or diseases without acknowledging the social context in which people live. Do sites only document the problems groups have, or do they also call attention to their strengths? Beware of sites that appear to stereotype people by health conditions or behaviors.

TOPIC PROFILE

Who

Applies to all racial, ethnic, cultural, and socioeconomic groups.

What

Multicultural health covers all aspects of health and health care, including social, economic, political, and cultural determinants of health.

Where

Applies to all parts of the body (including mental well-being); most resources cover U.S. sites and issues.

When

Applies to all stages of life.

ABBREVIATIONS USED IN THIS SECTION

CDC = Centers for Disease Control and Prevention
HRSA = Health Resources and Services Administration
IOM = Institute of Medicine of the National Academies
NCHS = National Center for Health Statistics
NCI = National Cancer Institute
NIAMS = National Institute of Arthritis and Musculoskeletal Diseases
NIH = National Institutes of Health
NLM = National Library of Medicine

PROCEDURES AND SPECIAL TOPICS

81. RACISM AND HEALTH/HEALTH DISPARITIES

Recommended Search Terms

- "Border health"
- "Ethnic health"
- Ethnicity health
- "Health disparities
- "Immigrant health"
- "Minority health"
- "Multicultural health"
- "People of color" health
- "Populations of color" health
- Race health
- "Racial Disparities" health
- Racism health
- "Refugee Health"
- [Specific racial and ethnic groups—such as Hispanics, Latinos, or Latinas; Blacks, African Americans, or Afro-Americans (see specific examples below)] [terms for health or medicine]

Important Sites

American Anthropological Association (AAA): American Anthropological Association's "Statement on Race": <http://www.aaanet.org/stmts/racepp.htm>
Health Resources and Services (HRSA): Office of Minority Health (OMH): Eliminating Health Disparities in the United States: <http://www.hrsa.gov/OMH/OMH/disparities/default.htm>
Inequality.org: <http://inequality.org>
Kaiser Family Foundation: Minority Health: <http://www.kff.org/sections.cgi?section=minority>
National Academies Press: Institute of Medicine (IOM): *Unequal Treatment: Confronting Racial and Ethnic Disparities in Health Care*: <http://www.nap.edu/catalog/10260.html>
National Academy of Sciences: Office of News and Public Information: Examining Unequal Treatment in American Health Care from the National Academy of Science: <http://www4.nas.edu/onpi/webextra.nsf/Web/minority?OpenDocument>
RaceSci: History of Race in Science: <http://www.racesci.org/index.html>

82. CULTURAL ASPECTS OF HEALTH CARE

Recommended Search Terms

- "Cross-cultural health"
- "Cross-cultural medicine"
- "Cross-cultural nursing"
- "Cross-cultural practice"
- "Cultural competency"
- "Cultural competence"
- "Cultural diversity" health
- "Cultural medicine"
- "Cultural healthcare"
- "Transcultural health"
- "Transcultural medicine"
- "Transcultural nursing"

Important Sites

American Public Health Association: Maternal and Child Health Community Leadership Institute: Understanding the Health Culture of Recent Immigrants to the United States: A Cross-Cultural Maternal Health Information Catalog: <http://www.apha.org/ppp/red/>
Center for Cross Cultural Health: <http://www.crosshealth.com/>
Cross Cultural Health Care Program: <http://www.xculture.org/>
Culture, Race, and Ethnicity: A Supplement to Mental Health: A Report of the Surgeon General: <http://www.surgeongeneral.gov/library/mentalhealth/cre/>
Diversity Rx: <http://www.diversityrx.org/>

Georgetown University Center for Child and Human Development: National Center for Cultural Competence (NCCC): <http://www.georgetown.edu/research/gucdc/nccc/index.html>

Harborview Medical Center: EthnoMed:<http://www.ethnomed.org/>

83. Governmental Organizations

Important Sites

Agency for Healthcare Research and Quality: Minority Health: <http://www.ahrq.gov/research/minorix.htm>

Department of Health and Human Services (DHHS): Indian Health Service: <http://www.ihs.gov/>

National Center on Minority Health and Health Disparities (NCMHD): <http://ncmhd.nih.gov/>

Office of Minority Health Resource Center: <http://www.omhrc.gov/>

Office of Minority Health Resources Center: Closing the Health Gap: <http://www.healthgap.omhrc.gov/>

U.S. House of Representatives: Congressional Black Caucus Health Braintrust: <http://www.house.gov/christian-christensen/cbc_health_braintrust.htm>

84. Non-Governmental, Community, and Advocacy Organizations

Important Sites

NOTE: Advocacy and community-based groups organized around a particular racial or ethnic group are listed under the heading for that particular group.

Asian and Pacific Islander American (APIA) Health Forum: <http://www.apiahf.org/>

Black Young Professionals' Public Health Network, Inc.: <http://www.bypphn.org/>

Black Women for Wellness (BWW): <http://www.bwwla.com/Home.html>

Kaiser Family Foundation: Minority Health: <http://www.kff.org/sections.cgi?section=minority>

National Council of La Raza (NCLR): <http://www.nclr.org/>

Society for the Analysis of African American Public Health Issues (SAAPHI): <http://www.saaphi.org/>

85. Multiracial and Multi-Ethnic Approaches

Important Sites

Association of Multi-Ethnic Americans (AMEA): <http://www.ameasite.org/>

Centers for Disease Control and Prevention (CDC): National Center for Chronic Disease Prevention and Health Promotion: Tobacco Use Among U.S. Racial/Ethnic Minority Groups: <http://www.cdc.gov/tobacco/sgr-1998/index.htm>

Intercultural Cancer Council: <http://iccnetwork.org/>

National Cancer Institute (NCI): Center to Reduce Cancer Health Disparities: <http://crchd.nci.nih.gov/>

National Institute of Arthritis and Musculoskeletal and Skin Diseases (NIAMS): Health Topics: The Many Shades of Lupus: <http://www.niams.nih.gov/hi/topics/lupus/shades/index.htm>

National Minority AIDS Council (NMAC): <http://www.nmac.org/>

National Minority Organ and Tissue Transplant Education Program (MOTTEP): <http://www.nationalmottep.org/>

86. Refugee, Immigrant, and Border Health

Recommended Search Terms

- "Border health"
- "Border health" [search also with specific group or health condition]
- "Immigrant health"
- "Immigrant health" [search also with specific group or health condition]
- "Refugee health"
- "Refugee health" [search also with specific group or health condition]

Important Sites

EthnoMed: <http://ethnomed.org/>

Mexican American Legal Defense and Educational Fund (MALDEF): <http://www.maldef.org/>

Migrant Clinicians Network (MCN): <http://www.migrantclinician.org/>

National Center for Farmworker Health, Inc. (NCFH): <http://www.ncfh.org/>

National Health Law Program (NHeLP): Immigrant Health: <http://www.healthlaw.org/immigrant.shtml>

Refugee Health—Immigrant Health: <http://www3.baylor.edu/~Charles_Kemp/refugees.htm>

United States–Mexico Border Health Commission: <http://www.borderhealth.org/>

87. Health Resources Organized by Racial and Ethnic Groups

Native Americans

Recommended Search Terms

- "Native Americans" health
- "Alaska natives"

- "American Indians" "traditional healing"
- "First Peoples" "traditional medicine"
- "First Nations" health
- "Indigenous people"
- Names of specific tribes [search also with health condition]

Important Sites

healthfinder: Just for You: American Indians and Alaska Natives: <http://healthfinder.gov/

MedlinePlus: Native American Health: <http://www.nlm.nih.gov/medlineplus/nativeamericanhealth.html>

National Library of Medicine (NLM)/University of Alaska Anchorage (UAA): Arctic Health: <http://www.arctichealth.org/>

National Native American AIDS Prevention Center (NNAAPC) Online: <http://www.nnaapc.org/>

National Network of Libraries of Medicine Pacific Northwest Region (NN/LMPNR): American Indian/Alaska Native Health Resource: Sampler: <http://nnlm.gov/pnr/samplers/natamer.html>

Tribal Connections: <http://www.tribalconnections.org/>

North American Indians and Indigenous People (NAIIP) Health and Medical Path: Information and Resources: <http://www.yvwiiusdinvnohii.net/medinfo.html>

African Americans and Caribbean Americans
Recommended Search Terms

- "African-Americans" [name of specific condition]
- "African-Americans" health
- "Afro-Americans" [name of specific condition]
- "Afro-Americans" health
- Blacks [name of specific condition]
- Blacks health
- "Caribbean Americans" health
- [Specific country of origin groups: Jamaican, etc…] [name of specific condition]

Important Sites

BlackHealthCare.com: <http://blackhealthcare.com/BHC/Index.asp>

Black Womens Health: <http://www.blackwomenshealth.com/>

Black Women's Health Imperative (formerly the National Black Women's Health Project): <http://www.blackwomenshealth.org>

Caribbean Women's Health Association, Inc. (CWHA): <http://www.cwha.org>

healthfinder: Just for You: Blacks or African-Americans: <http://healthfinder.gov/justforyou/>

International Society on Hypertension in Blacks (ISHB): <http://www.ishib.org/main/ishib_open.htm>

National Caucus and Center on Black Aged, Inc. (NCBA): <http://www.ncba-aged.org/>

MedlinePlus: African American Health: <http://www.nlm.nih.gov/medlineplus/africanamericanhealth.html>

Pan American Health Organization (PAHO): <http://www.paho.org/>

Sisters Network, Inc.: <http://www.sistersnetworkinc.org/index.htm>

Asians/Pacific Americans
Recommended Search Terms

- "Arab Americans" health [or medicine or name of specific condition]
- "Asian American" health [or medicine or name of specific condition]
- Asian health
- "Chinese Americans" health
- "Japanese Americans" health [or medicine or name of specific condition]
- "Korean Americans" Health
- "Pacific Americans" Health
- "Pacific Islanders" medicine [or name of specific condition]
- [Specific country of origin groups, such as Hmong, Cambodian, etc.] Health
- [Specific country of origin groups: Hmong, Cambodian, etc.] [name of specific condition]

Important Sites

University of Michigan: School of Public Health: Community-Based Public Health (CBPH): Arab-American Health in Michigan Manual and Bibliography: <http://www.sph.umich.edu/cbph/programs/simhim/arab-manual.pdf>

Asian and Pacific Islander American (APIA) Health Forum: <http://www.apiahf.org/>

Asian and Pacific Islander Coalition on HIV/AIDS (APICHA): <http://www.apicha.org/apicha/main.html>

Association of Asian Pacific Community Health Organizations (AAPCHO): <http://www.aapcho.org>

Consumer Health Information for Asians: <http://hhw.library.tmc.edu/CHIA/>

Harborview Medical Center: Ethnomed: See Cambodian, Chinese, Vietnamese links: <http://ethnomed.org>

healthfinder: Just for You: Asian Americans, Native Hawaiians and Other Pacific Islanders: <http://healthfinder.gov/justforyou/>

New York University School of Medicine: Health Information in Chinese Uniting Patients, Physicians and the Public (HICUP): <http://library.med.nyu.edu/patient/hicup/>

Hmong Health Website: <http://www.hmonghealth.org/>

Islamic Global Health Network (IGHNet): <http://islamicprevention.homestead.com/>

National Asian Pacific Center on Aging (NAPCA): <http://www.napca.org/>

National Asian Women's Health Organization (NAWHO): <http://www.nawho.org/>

MedlinePlus: Asian American Health: <http://www.nlm.nih.gov/medlineplus/asianamericanhealth.html>

University of California, San Francisco: Vietnamese Community Health Promotion Project: <http://www.suckhoelavang.org/>

Hispanics/Latinos

NOTE: Boricua is a term used to represent Puerto Ricans.

Recommended Search Terms

- Boricua health
- Boricua [name of specific condition]
- Chicanas health
- Chicanos [name of specific condition]
- "Hispanic American" health (or specific condition)
- "Hispanic Americans" [name of specific condition]
- Hispanics health
- Latinas health
- Latinos [name specific condition]
- Puerto Rican health
- Puerto Rican [name specific condition]
- [Specific country of origin groups: Puerto Ricans, Dominicans, Mexican Americans, Cuban Americans, etc.] health
- [Specific country of origin groups: Puerto Ricans, Dominicans, Mexican Americans, Cuban Americans etc.] [name of specific condition]

Important Sites

Centers for Disease Control and Prevention (CDC): Office of Minority Health: Hispanic or Latino Populations: <http://www.cdc.gov/omh/Populations/HL/HL.htm>

healthfinder: Just for You: Hispanics: <http://healthfinder.gov/justforyou/>

Latina Salud—WHYY's Latina Health Project: <http://www.latinasalud.org/index.html>

MedlinePlus: Hispanic American Health: <http://www.nlm.nih.gov/medlineplus/hispanicamericanhealth.html>

National Academies Press: Emerging Issues in Hispanic Health: Summary of a Workshop: <http://www.nap.edu/catalog/10485.html>

National Alliance for Hispanic Health: hispanichealth.org: <http://www.hispanichealth.org/>

National Council of La Raza (NCLR): <http://www.nclr.org/>

National Hispanic Leadership on Cancer (NHLIC): En Acción: <http://enaccion.bcm.tmc.edu/>

National Hispanic Council on Aging (NHCoA): <http://www.nhcoa.org/>

National Latina/o Lesbian, Gay, Bisexual, and Transgender Organization (LLEGÓ): <http://www.llego.org/>

National Latino Council on Alcohol and Tobacco Prevention (NLCATP): <http://www.nlcatp.org/>

Hotlines

2003 Toll-Free Numbers for Health Information: <http://www.health.gov/NHIC/Pubs/tollfree.htm>

United States AIDS Hotlines (State by state): <http://www.thebody.com/hotlines/state.html>

HIV Prevention and Education Contact for American Indians and Alaskan Natives: <http://www.thebody.com/hotlines/amerindian.html>

National Hispanic Indoor Air Quality Helpline: 1-800-SALUD-12

National Hispanic Prenatal Helpline (NHPH): 1-800-504-7081

New York Asian Women's Services: 1-888-888-7702

Office of Minority Health Resource Center: 1-800-444-6472

Su Familia: 1-866-Su-Familia/1-866-783-2645

FAQs

Department of Health and Human Services (DHHS): Office for Civil Rights: Frequently Asked Questions with Answers: <http://www.hhs.gov/ocr/newfaq.html>

Office of Minority Health Resource Center: Frequently Asked Questions: <http://www.omhrc.gov/OMHRC/sbfaq.htm>

U.S. Citizenship and Immigration Service: How Do I?: Frequently Asked Questions: <http://uscis.gov/graphics/faqs.htm>

MULTICULTURAL HEALTH PUBLICATIONS ON THE INTERNET

Cross Cultural Health Care Program (CCHCP): Books and Resources: <http://www.xculture.org/resource/index.html>

International Journal for Equity in Health: International Journal for Equity in Health: <http://www.equityhealthj.com/home/>

Office of Minority Health: Publications: Closing the Gap Newsletter: <http://www.omhrc.gov/OMH/sidebar/omh-publications.htm>

Physicians for Human Rights: The Right to Equal Treatment: An Annotated Bibliography of Studies on Racial and Ethnic Disparities in Healthcare, Their Causes, and Related Issues: <http://www.phrusa.org/research/domestic/race/race_report/bibliography.html>

PROFESSIONAL ORGANIZATIONS

American Lebanese Medication Association (ALMA): <http://www.almamater.org/ALMA/Default.html>

Asian Pacific American Medical Student Association (APAMSA): <http://www.apamsa.org/>

Association of American Indian Physicians (AAIP): <http://www.aaip.com/>

Association of Black Social Workers: HARAMBEE: <http://www.nabsw.org>

Association of Clinicians for the Underserved (ACU): <http://www.clinicians.org/>

Black Congress on Health, Law, and Economics (BCHLE): <http://www.bchle.org/main.htm>

Hispanic Dental Association (HAD): <http://www.hdassoc.org/>

Islamic Medical Association of North America (IMANA): <http://www.imana.org/>

National Arab American Medical Association (NAAMA): <http://www.naama.com/>

National Black Nurses Association (NBNA): <http://www.nbna.org/>

National Hispanic Medical Association (NHMA): <http://home.earthlink.net/~nhma/>

National Medical Association (NMA): <http://www.nmanet.org/>

Student National Medical Association (SNMA): <http://www.snma.org/>

PATIENT SUPPORT ORGANIZATIONS/ DISCUSSION GROUPS

American Self-Help Group Clearinghouse: <http://mentalhelp.net/selfhelp/>

DiversityRx: Networking: <http://www.diversityrx.org/HTML/NETWRK.htm>

Dr. John Grohol's PsychCentral: Mental Health and Psychology Resources Online: <http://psychcentral.com/resources>

BEST ONE-STOP SHOPS

Cross Cultural Health Care Program (CCHCP): <http://www.xculture.org>

Harborview Medical Center: EthnoMed: <http://ethnomed.org/>

healthfinder: Just For You: <http://healthfinder.gov/justforyou/>

MedlinePlus: Population Groups Topics: <http://www.nlm.nih.gov/medlineplus/populationgroups.html>

REFERENCES

1. Cross Cultural Health Care Program. Training Programs: What Is Cultural Competence? Retrieved November 10, 2003, from <http://www.xculture.org/training/overview/cultural/>.

2. American Anthropological Association. Statement on Race. Retrieved November 10, 2003 from <http://www.aaanet.org/stmts/racepp.htm>.

3. King, G; and D. Williams. "Race and Health: A Multidimensional Approach to African-American Health" In B. C. Amick, S. Levine, A. R/ Tarlov, and D. C. Walsh, eds. *Society and Health*. New York: Oxford University Press, 1995.

4. U.S. Census Bureau. Racial and Ethnic Classifications Used in Census 2000 and Beyond. (2000, April 12) Retrieved November 10, 2003, from <http://www.census.gov/population/www/socdemo/race/racefactcb.html>.

5. Summary of Vital Statistics 2000. New York: City of New York: Department of Health, 2002. Retrieved November 10, 2003, from <http://www.nyc.gov/html/doh/pdf/vs/2000sum.pdf>.

Part VII: Lesbian, Gay, Bisexual and Transgendered Health Issues

Christopher J. Shaffer and Bryan S. Vogh

SPECIAL SEARCHING ISSUES FOR THIS TOPIC

Because this topic involves issues related to and directly concerning sexuality, searching the Internet for health or disease information on this topic may retrieve inappropriate or potentially offensive information that may not be relevant to health concerns. For this reason, searching in general search engines carries risks and should be undertaken with caution.

Lesbian, gay, bisexual, and transgendered (LGBT) health encompasses a wide variety of people who are members of sexual minorities. There is considerable debate regarding the definitions of the terms used to classify people according to their membership in sexual minority groups. In addition, LGBT people have reclaimed some derogatory words that are still offensive to some people or in certain situations. It is important to be flexible in the selection of terms and use of synonyms when searching for LGBT health information.

Members of sexual minorities must overcome many challenges in their search for health information. As recently as 1973, the American Psychological Association classified homosexuality as a mental disorder. Discrimination is still a daily event in the lives of many LGBT people, who are often reluctant to "come out" when seeking health information or health care. Unfortunately, this discrimination extends to the Internet, and people seeking LGBT health information must be aware that some sites discriminate against LGBT people by providing inaccurate, biased, or offensive information.

TOPIC PROFILE

The standard disease profile (who, what, where, and when) does not apply to this topic. LGBT people are of all ages, races, ethnicities, and cultural backgrounds, and the "alphabet soup" of LGBT continues to be expanded to include new populations. The topic includes physical diseases such as AIDS and breast cancer; mental health problems, such as depression and suicide; and social issues, such as health access and domestic violence.

ABBREVIATIONS USED IN THIS SECTION

LGBT/GLBT = Lesbian, gay, bisexual and transgender (ed): An umbrella term to indicate members of sexual minority groups
LGBTQQIA = Lesbian, gay, bisexual, transgender (ed), queer, questioning, intersex, and allies
MSM = Men who have sex with men
WSW = Women who have sex with women

TERMS USED IN THIS SECTION

Bisexual = A person who is sexually or romantically attracted to both men and women.
Coming out = A revelation or acknowledgment that one is a member of a sexual minority group.

Gay = Sometimes used as an inclusive term encompassing homosexual men and women, but more often used to indicate homosexual men.
Gay men = Men who are attracted sexually or romantically to other men, but not to women.
Gender = Behavioral, social, and psychological characteristics of men and women.
Gender identity = A person's sense of self as male, female, both, or neither.
Heterosexual = A person who is attracted sexually or romantically to members of the opposite sex, but not to members of the same sex.
Homosexual = A person who is attracted sexually or romantically to members of the same sex, but not to members of the opposite sex.
Intersex(ed) person = A person who is born with sex chromosomes, external genitalia, or an internal reproductive system that is not considered "standard" for either male or female.
Lesbians = Women who are attracted sexually or romantically to other women, but not to men.
Queer = An umbrella term used to indicate sexual minority groups. "Queer" is a reclaimed word that is offensive to some people.
Sex = Biological aspects of being male and female.
Sexual identity = A person's sense of self as male, female, both, or neither.
Sexual orientation = Indication of whom a person is attracted to or relates to sexually.
Transgender(ed) person = An umbrella term including just about anyone who acts or thinks in a manner not socially approved for the gender assigned him or her at birth.
Transition = The process of undergoing hormone treatments, behavior modification, and surgery to change the body to match gender identity.
Tranz = Slang term for transgender.
NOTE: *See also* Family Pride Canada: Glossary of LGBT Terms: <http://familypride.uwo.ca/glossary/>.

PROCEDURES AND SPECIAL TOPICS

88. SEXUAL ORIENTATION AND IDENTITY

[*See also* "Adolescents' Health Issues and the Internet: Sexual Behaviors and Choices," p. 128.]

Recommended Search Terms

- "Coming out"
- "Gender identity"
- "Sexual attraction" "same sex"
- "Sexual identity"
- "Sexual orientation"

Important Sites

American Psychological Association (APA) Online: Public Affairs: Answers to Your Questions about Sexual Orientation and Homosexuality: <http://www.apa.org/pubinfo/answers.html>

Basic TG/TS/IS [Transgender/Transexual/Intersexual] Information: <http://ai.eecs.umich.edu/people/conway/TS/TS.html>

Seattle and King County Public Health: Gay Lesbian Bisexual Transgendered (GLBT) Health Webpage: Definitions: <http://www.metrokc.gov/health/glbt/definitions.htm>

Human Rights Campaign Foundation: National Coming Out Project: <http://www.hrc.org/ncop/>

Palo Alto Medical Foundation: Teen Health: Sexual Health and Experience: Sexual Orientation: <http://www.pamf.org/teen/sex/orientation.html>

Sexual Orientation: Science, Education, and Policy: <http://psychology.ucdavis.edu/rainbow/>

89. MEN WHO HAVE SEX WITH MEN

Recommended Search Terms

- Bisexual men health
- Gay hepatitis
- Gay HIV
- Gay "men's health"
- Gay "sexually transmitted diseases"
- "Men who have sex with men"

Important Sites

AIDS.org: <http://www.aids.org/>

GayHealth: General Health: Men: Diseases and Conditions Male Issues: <http://www.gayhealth.com/templates/10684885097855431301400002/general/men>

HepClinics: <http://www.hepclinics.com/>

LgbthealthChannel: Safer Sex (MSM) for Men Who Have Sex with Men: <http://www.gayhealthchannel.com/stdmsm/>

Sexually Transmitted Infections: A Guide for Gay and Bisexual Men: <http://www.gmhp.demon.co.uk/guides/std/>

Gay and Lesbian Medical Association (GLMA): News Releases: Ten Things Gay Men Should Discuss with Their Health Care Providers: <http://www.glma.org/news/releases/n02071710gaythings.html>

90. WOMEN WHO HAVE SEX WITH WOMEN

[*See also* "Breast, Cervical and Other Reproductive Cancers (Women)," p. 15, vol. 2; "Sexuality" (Cancer Issues), p. 26, vol.II; "Sexually Transmitted Diseases," p. 145; "Part XI: Sexual Health Issues," p. 178.]

Recommended Search Terms

- Gay "women's health"
- Lesbian cancer
- Lesbian depression
- Lesbian health
- "Women who have sex with women"

Important Sites

Gay and Lesbian Medical Association (GLMA): News Release: Ten Things Lesbians Should Discuss with Their Health Care Providers: <http://www.glma.org/news/releases/n02071710lesbianthings.html>

GayHealth: General Health: Women: <http://www.gayhealth.com/templates/10684885814142914381800002/general/women>

Human Rights: Background Information on Lesbian Health: <http://www.hrc.org/issues/lesbianh/background/index.asp>

Lesbian.com: Health: <http://www.lesbian.com/health/health_intro.html>

The Mautner Project: <http://www.mautnerproject.org/>

National Women's Health Information Center: 4woman.gov: Lesbian Health: <http://www.4woman.gov/faq/Lesbian.htm>

Safersex.org: The Lesbian Safer Sex Page: <http://www.safersex.org/women/lesbianss.html>

University of California San Francisco: Lesbian Health Research Center (LHRC): <http://www.lesbianhealthinfo.org/>

University of Washington: LesbianSTD: <http://depts.washington.edu/wswstd/>

91. TRANSGENDERED PEOPLE

[*See also* "Part XI: Sexual Health Issues," p. 178.]

Recommended Search Terms

- Female to male health
- FTM health
- Intersex health
- male to female health
- M>F health
- Sex change
- Tranz health

- Transgender hormones
- Transsexual

Important Sites

GayHealth: General Health: Transgender: <http://www.gayhealth.com/templates/1068488581414291438 18000002/general/transgender>

Intersex Society of North America (ISNA): <http://www.isna.org/>

Kenyon College: Women's and Gender Studies Program: Trans 2000: Terms To Know That May Help You Grow: <http://www2.kenyon.edu/Depts/WMNS/Projects/Trans2000/terms.htm>

LgbthealthChannel: Transgender Health: <http://www.lgbthealthchannel.com/transgender/>

Open Directory Project (DMOZ): Society: Transgendered: Health and Wellness: <http://dmoz.org/Society/Transgendered/Health_and_Wellness/>

Open Directory Project (DMOZ): Society: Transgendered: Intersexed: Health and Wellness: <http://dmoz.org/Society/Transgendered/Intersexed/Health_and_Wellness/>

Seattle and King County Public Health: Transgender Health: <http://www.metrokc.gov/health/glbt/transgender.htm>

TransGender Care: Guidance and Transition: Library: What Is Gender and Who Is Transgendered?: <http://www.transgendercare.com/guidance/what_is_gender.htm>

Wellness: Health Care Information Resources: Transgender Issue Links: <http://hsl.mcmaster.ca/tomflem/transgender.html>

Wikipedia: Sexual Reassignment Surgery: <http://wikipedia.org/wiki/Sexual_reassignment_surgery>

92. INTERSEXUALITY

[*See also* "Part XI: Sexual Health Issues," p. 178.]

Recommended Search Terms

- "Congenital adrenal hyperplasia"
- "Genital surgery" intersex
- Hermaphroditism
- Hypospadias
- Intersexuality glossary
- Intersexuality surgery
- Intersexual writings
- Intersexuality "hormone replacement therapy"
- "Klinefelter syndrome"
- "Medicalized intersexuals"
- XYY male

Important Sites

eMedicine: Specialties: Pediatrics: Genetics and Metabolic Disease: Klinefelter Syndrome: <http://www.emedicine.com/PED/topic1252.htm>

Endocrine Society/Hormone Foundation: Patient Fact Sheet: Endocrinology and Congenital Adrenal Hyperplasia (CAH): <http://www.endo-society.org/pubrelations/patientInfo/cah.cfm>

Gene Tests: Gene Reviews: Androgen Insensitivity Syndrome: <http://www.geneclinics.org/profiles/androgen/>

Intersex Association (UK): Management of Intersexuality: Guidelines for Dealing with Individuals with Ambiguous Genitalia: <http://www.ukia.co.uk/diamond/diaguide.htm>

Intersex Society of North America (ISNA): <http://www.isna.org/>

Open Directory Project (DMOZ): Society: Transgendered: Intersexed: Health and Wellness: http://dmoz.org/Society/Transgendered/Intersexed/Health_and_Wellness/>

93. HEALTH ACCESS

[*See also* "Finding and Choosing a Therapist," p. 218, vol. 2.]

Recommended Search Terms

- LGBT health access
- Lesbian gay doctor referral
- "Culturally competent health care"
- "Domestic partner" rights

Important Sites

Federal Globe: Workplace Issues: Long Term Health Care and Domestic Partner Benefits: <http://www.fedglobe.org/issues/issueshome.htm#lthc>

Gay and Lesbian Medical Association: Programs: Online Health Care Referrals: <http://www.glma.org/programs/prp/>

The Gay, Lesbian, Bisexual, and Transgender Health Access Project: <http://www.glbthealth.org/>

Lambda Legal: Resources: Hospital Visitation—A Right for All Families: <http://www.lambdalegal.org/cgi-bin/iowa/documents/record?record=1013>

LgbthealthChannel: Getting Good Health Care: <http://www.lgbthealthchannel.com/healthcare.shtml>

Seattle and King County Public Health: Discrimination in Health Care: Recent Studies: <http://www.metrokc.gov/health/glbt/providers.htm#discrimination>

94. MENTAL HEALTH

[*See also* Living with a Disability: Sexuality," p. 93; "Finding and Choosing a Therapist," p. 218, vol. 2; "Underserved Communities and Populations, Suicide," p. 235, vol. 2.]

Recommended Search Terms

- Homosexual mental health
- Gay psychology
- Lesbian counseling
- LGBT depression

Important Sites

American Psychoanalytic Association: Committee on Gay and Lesbian Issues: <http://www.apsa-co.org/ctf/cgli/>

American Psychological Association (APA) Online: Lesbian, Gay, and Bisexual Concerns: <http://www.apa.org/pi/lgbc/>

National Coalition for LGBT Health: Mental Health and the LGBT Community: <http://www.lgbthealth.net/mental_health.html>

Sexual Orientation: Science, Education, and Policy: Facts about Homosexuality and Mental Health: <http://psychology.ucdavis.edu/rainbow/html/facts_mental_health.html>

95. LIFE STAGES

Youth

[*See also* "Adolescents' Health Issues: Sexual Behaviors and Choices," p. 128; "Suicide," p. 317, vol. 2.]

Recommended Search Terms

- Bisexual youth health
- Gay youth depression
- LGBT youth
- Young queer health

Important Sites

Advocates for Youth: Gay, Lesbian, Bisexual, Transgender, and Questioning (GLBTQ) Youth: <http://www.advocatesforyouth.org/glbtq.htm>

Advocates for Youth: Issues at a Glance: HIV/STD Prevention and Young Men Who Have Sex with Men: <http://www.advocatesforyouth.org/publications/iag/ymsm.htm>

Advocates for Youth: Issues at a Glance: Young Women Who Have Sex with Women: Falling through Cracks

for Sexual Health Care: <http://www.advocatesforyouth.org/publications/iag/ywsw.htm

American Academy of Child and Adolescent Psychiatry (AACAP): Publications: Facts for Families: Gay and Lesbian Adolescents: <http://www.aacap.org/publications/factsfam/63.htm>

American Psychological Association (APA) Online: Healthy Lesbian, Gay, and Bisexual Students Project: <http://www.apa.org/ed/hlgb/>

Children's Hospital Boston: Center for Young Women's Health: Information for Teens: Lesbian Health: A Guide for Teens: <http://www.youngwomenshealth.org/lesbianhealth.html>

Health Canada: The Journey Begins: Who Am I?: <http://www.hc-sc.gc.ca/hppb/hiv_aids/youth/journey/index.html>

Hetrick-Martin Institute: For the Community: Lesbian, Gay, Bisexual and Transgender (LGBTQ) Youth Statistics: <http://www.hmi.org/Community/LGBTQYouthStatistics/default.aspx>

Parents, Families, and Friends of Lesbians and Gays (PFLAG) Transgender Network: Our Trans Children: <http://www.youth-guard.org/pflag-tnet/>

Sexuality Information and Education Council of the United States (SIECUS): Lesbian, Gay, Bisexual and Transgender Youth Issues: <http://www.siecus.org/pubs/fact/fact0013.html>

Youth.org: I Think I Might Be Gay...Now What Do I Do?: <http://www.youth.org/yao/docs/i-think-article-gay.html>

Youth.org: I Think I Might Be a Lesbian...Now What Do I Do?: <http://www.youth.org/yao/docs/i-think-article-lesbian.html>

Aging

[*See also* "Sexuality and Aging," p. 152.]

Recommended Search Terms

- Aging gay health
- LGBT gerontology
- Older lesbian health

Important Sites

American Society on Aging (ASA): Lesbian and Gay Issues Aging Network: <http://www.asaging.org/networks/lgain/>

Classic Dykes Online: <http://www.classicdykes.com/>

For Ourselves: Reworking Gender Expression (FORGE): Transgender Aging Network (TAN): <http://www.forge-forward.org/TAN>

Human Rights Campaign: FamilyNet: Aging: Senior Health: <http://www.hrc.org/familynet/chapter.asp?article=385>

Senior Action in a Gay Environment (SAGE): Links: <http://www.sageusa.org/links.htm>

HOTLINES

Gay and Lesbian National Hotline: 1-888-THE-GLNH/1-888-843-4564, or e-mail: <glnh@glnh.org>

Transgender Health Action Coalition (THAC) Hotline: (215) 732-1207

Trevor Project: Youth Support Hotline: 1-800-850-8078, or email: <Support@TheTrevorProject.org>

FAQs

American Medical Student Association: Health Concerns of the LGBT Community: <http://www.amsa.org/adv/lgbtpm/concerns.cfm>

Substance Abuse and Mental Health Services Administration (SAMHSA): National Clearinghouse for Alcohol and Drug Information (NCADI): Celebrating the Pride and Diversity among and within the Lesbian, Gay, Bisexual, and Transgender Populations: <http://www.health.org/features/lgbt/>

PUBLICATIONS ON THE INTERNET:

American Journal of Public Health: Lesbian/Gay/Bisexual/Transgender Persons: <http://www.ajph.org/cgi/collection/lesbian_gay_bisexual_transgender_persons>

Gay and Lesbian Medical Association (GLMA): GLMA Public Policy: Healthy People 2010 Companion Document for LGBT Health: <http://www.glma.org/policy/hp2010/>

Gay and Lesbian Medical Association (GLMA): GLMA Public Policy: The GMLA-Columbia University White Paper on LGBT Health: <http://www.glma.org/policy/whitepaper/>

Journal of the Gay and Lesbian Medical Association: <http://www.kluweronline.com/issn/1090-7173/contents>

Sexuality Information and Education Council of the United States (SIECUS): Lesbian, Gay, Bisexual, and Transgender Sexuality and Related Issues Annotated Bibliography: <http://www.siecus.org/pubs/biblio/bibs0005.html>

PROFESSIONAL ORGANIZATIONS

Association for Gay, Lesbian and Bisexual Issues in Counseling (AGLBIC): <http://www.aglbic.org/>

Association of Gay and Lesbian Psychiatrists (ALGP): <http://www.aglp.org/>

American Medical Student Association (AMSA): Lesbian, Gay, Bisexual and Transgender People in Medicine (LGBTPM): <http://www.amsa.org/adv/lgbtpm/>

Gay and Lesbian Medical Association (GLMA): <http://www.glma.org/>

Lesbian, Gay, Bisexual and Transgendered Health Science Librarians: Special Interest Group (SIG) of the Medical Library Association (MLA): <http://www.lgbtsig.org/>

National Association of Lesbian and Gay Addiction Professionals (NALGAP): <http://www.nalgap.org/>

The Sexuality Information and Education Council of the United States (SIECUS): <http://www.siecus.org/>

Women in Medicine: <http://www.wimretreat.org/>

BEST ONE-STOP SHOPS

Gay and Lesbian Health Services (GLHS) of Saskatoon (Canada): Issues in the Gay and Lesbian Community Fact Sheet: <http://www.glhs.ca/html/fact.html>

GayHealth.com: <http://www.gayhealth.com/>

Illness: Health Care Information Resources: Gay and Lesbian Health Problems Links: <http://hsl.mcmaster.ca/tomflem/gayprob.html>

LgbthealthChannel: <http://www.lgbthealthchannel.com/>

MedlinePlus: Gay/Lesbian Health: <http://www.nlm.nih.gov/medlineplus/gaylesbianhealth.html>

National Latina/o Lesbian, Gay, Bisexual and Transgender Organization (LLEGO) Resources (English): <http://www.llego.org/main_pages/links.html>

National Latina/o Lesbian, Gay, Bisexual and Transgender Organization (LLEGO) Resources (Spanish): <http://www.llego.org/main_pages/linkssp.htm>

National Women's Health Information: 4woman.gov: Office of Women's Health: Lesbian Health Fact Sheet: <http://www.4woman.gov/owh/pub/factsheets/Lesbian.htm>

New York Online Access to Health (NOAH): Ask NOAH About: Gay, Lesbian, Bisexual and Transgender (GLBT) Personal Health: <http://www.noah-health.org/english/wellness/healthyliving/gaylesbian.html>

Open Directory Project (DMOZ): Society: Gay, Lesbian, and Bisexual: Health and Wellness: <http://dmoz.org/Society/Gay,_Lesbian,_and_Bisexual/Health_and_Wellness/>

Seattle and King County Public Health: Gay Lesbian Bisexual Transgender Health Pages: <http://www.metrokc.gov/health/glbt/>

Wellness: Health Care Information Resources: Gay, Lesbian and Bisexual Health Links: <http://hsl.mcmaster.ca/tomflem/gay.html>

Part VIII: Living with a Chronic Illness

P. F. Anderson

[*See also* "Internet Access for Persons with Disabilities," vol. 1, p. 12; "Tools and Support," p. 133, vol. 1;" Seniors' Health Issues," p. 148; "Living with a Disability," p. 77; "Pain and Pain Management," p. 99.]

SPECIAL SEARCHING ISSUES FOR THIS TOPIC

A great majority of the special disease topics discussed later in this book are chronic diseases or have an aspect of the disease that involves making some sort of long standing modification to your lifestyle. The essence of the concept "chronic" is something that will last for a long time. Most medical definitions use a time frame of a year or longer. Another way to think of this may be that, while a quick cure may not be expected, it is usually reasonable to assume a long and satisfying life. "I have survived and, in many ways, flourished for almost 10 years," said Howard Harrod of his life following prostate cancer treatments.[1] The take-home message here is much the same as throughout this book: you are in charge. The decisions you make—the changes you choose to make or not to make—will have a direct and long-lasting impact on your quality of, and your satisfaction with, life.

Many of the concepts in this chapter are also discussed under specific disease topics, and you are encouraged to explore those topics as well as these. The reverse is also true—try these search examples with the names of a specific health concern or diagnosis. For most topics in this chapter, the sites selected will include both a few general sites as well as a few examples of that issue or coping strategy from sites on a specific disorder. One of the major advocacy organizations for chronic illness, Partnership for Solutions, has a Web page named "Different Conditions, Common Problems." The message is that there are many overarching issues of concern not unique to just one diagnosis—a Web page on cancer fatigue may have tips and strategies helpful to a patient with chronic fatigue syndrome; some of the ideas for coping with arthritis pain may work for persons with migraines or back pain. Be open-minded—the answer to your question may come from an unexpected source.

In searching, since so many of the disorders people are most aware of are chronic, searching with any of the groups of terms about chronic conditions or illness may actually be self-defeating. Often you may get better results by focusing just on the health issue —fatigue, pain, impact

of medications on your body, impact of caregiving on your family, and support. In most discussions in this book, the emphasis is on being more specific and precise in your search. Here the reverse, an oblique approach, is sometimes better. Explore concepts and search strategies mentioned elsewhere in the book, and try being especially creative in your use of language and terms to get the most useful results.

ABBREVIATIONS USED IN THIS SECTION

AAFP = American Academy of Family Physicians
AAP = American Academy of Pediatrics
CDC = Centers for Disease Control and Prevention
DHHS = Department of Health and Human Services
NAP = National Academies Press
NCCDPHP = National Center for Chronic Disease Prevention and Health Promotion
NIH = National Institutes of Health

PROCEDURES AND SPECIAL TOPICS

96. GENERAL

Recommended Search Terms

- "Chronic illness"
- "Chronic disease"
- "Chronic disorders"
- "Chronic conditions"
- "Chronic care"
- "Long term illness"

Important Sites

American Geriatrics Society (AGS) Foundation for Health in Aging: <http://www.healthinaging.org/>
California Department of Health Services: Chronic Disease and Injury Control (CDIC): <http://www.dhs.cahwnet.gov/ps/cdic/cdicindex.htm>
Centers for Disease Control and Prevention (CDC): National Center for Chronic Disease Prevention and Health Promotion: <http://www.cdc.gov/nccdphp/>
Chronic Conditions Information Network (CCIN): <http://www.cc-info.net/>
Chronic Ill Net: <http://www.chronicillnet.org/>
Chronic Illness Resource Center: Chronic Illness: <http://www.chronicillness.com/>
Department of Health and Ageing (Australia): Chronic Disease Prevention and Management: <http://www.chronicdisease.health.gov.au/>

ElderCare Advocates: Eldercare Resource Center: <http://www.eldercareadvocates.com/pages/recenter.htm>

Harvard School of Public Health: Burden of Disease: Avoidable Causes of Adult Chronic Disease and Death: <http://www.hsph.harvard.edu/burdenofdisease/AvoidableChronic.htm>

Health Disparities Collaboratives: Chronic Care Model: <http://www.healthdisparities.net/about_chronic.html>

Improving Chronic Illness Care (ICIC): <http://www.improvingchroniccare.org/>

Improving Chronic Illness Care (ICIC): The Chronic Care Model: Model Components: <http://www.improvingchroniccare.org/change/model/components.html>

Invisible Disabilities Advocate: Chronic Illness: <http://www.invisibledisabilities.com/>

Iron Disorders Institute: Disorders: Anemia of Chronic Disease (ACD): <http://www.irondisorders.org/disorders/acd/>

Johns Hopkins University: Bloomberg School of Public Health: <http://www.jhsph.edu/>

Massachusetts Chronic Disease Improvement Network (MCDIN): <http://www.mcdin.org/>

MedlinePlus Medical Encyclopedia: Acute vs. Chronic Conditions: <http://www.nlm.nih.gov/medlineplus/ency/imagepages/18126.htm>

National Center for Health Statistics (NCHS): Prevalence of Selected Chronic Conditions: United States, 1990-92: <http://www.cdc.gov/nchs/products/pubs/pubd/series/sr10/199-190/se10_194.htm>

Partnership for Solutions: The Problem: About Chronic Conditions: Definition: <http://www.partnershipforsolutions.org/problem/chronic_conditions.cfm>

Public Broadcasting Service (PBS): Fred Friendly: Who Cares: Chronic Illness in America: <http://www.pbs.org/fredfriendly/whocares/>

Trust for America's Health (TFAH): Nationwide Health Tracking Network: <http://healthyamericans.org/campaigns/tracking/>

Washington Post: From Killer to Chronic Disease: Drugs Redefine Cancer for Many: <http://www.washingtonpost.com/wp-dyn/articles/A57393-2003Jan28.html>

World Health Organization (WHO): Best Practices in Health Care for Chronic Conditions: <http://www.who.int/entity/chronic_conditions/best_practices/en/>

97. ADJUSTMENT

- Chronic adjustment "my diagnosis"
- Diagnosis coping
- Diagnosis "now what"
- Diagnosis "what now"
- Diagnosis "what next"
- "Have a diagnosis" start where
- "Have a diagnosis" coping
- "Psychosocial adjustment" disease
- "Psychosocial adjustment" illness

Important Sites

Agency for Healthcare Research and Quality (AHRQ): Now You Have a Diagnosis: What's Next?: <http://www.ahcpr.gov/consumer/diaginfo.htm>

Contact a Family: Factsheet: Living without a Diagnosis: <http://www.cafamily.org.uk/undiagno.html>

Diary of an Illness (Dennis W. Pyritz, RN): <http://www.ons.org/xp6/ONS/Library.xml/ONS_Publications.xml/Diary/Main.xml>

From Diagnosis to Acceptance: One Woman's Journey: <http://www.makinglifeeasier.com/articles/article6.html>

I Have Alzheimer's: Helping Your Family and Friends: <http://www.alz.org/IHaveAD/Helping.htm>

Med Help International: Getting Started: <http://www.medhelp.org/GettingStarted.htm>

Royal National Institute of the Blind: Parent's Place: <http://www.rnib.org.uk/parents/where.htm>

Taking the Fear Out of Cancer: Don't Panic!: <http://www.takingthefearoutofcancer.com/dontpanic.htm>

TumorFree: Diagnosis: <http://www.tumorfree.com/diagnosis.htm>

98. ADVOCACY AND AWARENESS

- "Chronic condition" awareness
- "Chronic disease" advocate
- "Chronic illness" advocacy

Important Sites

American Pain Foundation: <http://www.painfoundation.org/>

Center for Health Care Strategies (CHCS): <http://www.chcs.org/>

Center for the Advancement of Health (CFAH): <http://www.cfah.org/>

Chronic Disease Directors (CDD): <http://www.chronicdisease.org/>

Chronic Illness Alliance (Australia): <http://www.chronicillness.org.au/>

Homebound'ers XChange (Canada): Chronic Illness Advocacy and Projects: <http://members.shaw.ca/zonaszone/hx/projects.html>

Improving Chronic Illness Care: <http://www.improving chroniccare.org/>

Invisible Disabilities Advocate: <http://www.invisible disabilities.com/>

National Invisible Chronic Illness Awareness Week: <http://www.mychronicillness.com/invisibleillness/ home.htm>

National Chronic Care Consortium (NCCC): <http:// www.nccconline.org/>

National Conference of State Legislatures (NCSL): Health: Chronic Disease Prevention: <http://www .ncsl.org/programs/health/chronic.htm>

National Health Council: <http://www.nhcouncil.org/>

National Organization for Rare Disorders (NORD): <http://www.rarediseases.org/>

Partnership for Solutions: <http://www.partnershipfor solutions.org/>

Physician, Public, and Policymaker Perspectives on Chronic Conditions (Gerard F. Anderson): <http:// archinte.ama-assn.org/cgi/content/abstract/163/4/ 437>

World Health Organization (WHO): Observatory on Health Care for Chronic Conditions: <http://www .who.int/entity/chronic_conditions/en/>

99. CHILDREN AND ADOLESCENTS

[*See also* "Children's Health Issues," p. 119; "Adolescents' Health Issues," p. 125.]

Recommended Search Terms

- Adolescent "chronically ill"
- Adolescents "chronic conditions"
- Boys "chronic illness"
- Child "special needs"
- Children chronic conditions
- Girls "chronic disease"
- Kids "chronic disorders"
- Teens "chronic illness"

Important Sites

4Girls.gov: Disabilities and Chronic Illness in Girls: <http://www.4girls.gov/chronic/>

American Academy of Pediatrics (AAP): Committee on Children with Disabilities and Committee on Psychosocial Aspects of Child and Family Health: *Pediatrics* 92 (6) 1993: 876-878, Policy Statement: Psychosocial Risks of Chronic Health Conditions in Childhood and Adolescence (RE9338): <http://www .aap.org/policy/05127.html>

American Academy of Pediatrics (AAP): General Principles in the Care of Children and Adolescents with

Genetic Disorders and Other Chronic Health Conditions (RE9717): <http://www.aap.org/policy/re9717 .html>

All Kids Count: <http://www.allkidscount.org/>

Brave Kids: <http://www.bravekids.org/>

Canadian Paediatric Society (CPS): Adolescent Medicine Committee: Care of the Chronically Ill Adolescent: <http://www.cps.ca/english/statements/AM/am94-05 .htm>

Canadian Paediatric Society (CPS): Adolescent Medicine Committee: Sexual Abuse of Adolescents with Chronic Conditions: <http://www.cps.ca/english/ statements/AM/am96-01.htm>

Band-Aides and Blackboards: <http://www.faculty.fairfield .edu/fleitas/contents.html>

Contact a Family (UK): Factsheet: Living without a Diagnosis: <http://www.cafamily.org.uk/undiagno.html>

Dartmouth Medical College: The C. Everett Koop Institute: Chronic Illness Resources for Teens: <http:// www.dartmouth.edu/dms/koop/resources/chronic_ illness/chronic.shtml>

Children's Hospitals and Clinics: Encourage Online: <http://www.encourageonline.org/>

Head Start Information and Publication Center (HSIPC): Head Start: Caring for Children with Chronic Conditions: <http://www.headstartinfo.org/publications/ children_cc/ccccont.htm>

KidsHealth: Dealing with a Chronic Illness: <http:// kidshealth.org/teen/your_mind/problems/deal_chroni c_illness.html>

KidsHealth: When Someone You Know Has a Chronic Illness: <http://kidshealth.org/kid/feeling/thought/ someone_chronic.html>

National Academies Press (NAP): America's Children: Health Insurance and Access to Care: <http:// www.nap.edu/catalog/6168.html>

National Association of School Nurses (NASN): <http:// www.nasn.org/>

American Academy of Pediatrics (AAP): National Center for Medical Home Initiatives For Children with Special Needs: Resources/State Pages: Transitions Resources: <http://www.medicalhomeinfo.org/ resources/trans.html>

University of Michigan Health System (UMHS): Your Child: Development and Behavior Resources: Children with Chronic Conditions: <http://www.med .umich.edu/1libr/yourchild/chronic.htm>

100. COPING AND STRESS

Recommended Search Terms

- "Chronic illness" "stress management"
- Chronic coping "self-management"

- Chronic health stress coping
- "Living with" [name of diagnosis]
- "Psychosocial adjustment" "chronic illness"

Important Sites

All of a Piece: A Life with Multiple Sclerosis: After the Diagnosis: <http://www.lifewithms.com/after~1.htm>

All of a Piece: A Life with Multiple Sclerosis: Beyond Acceptance: <http://www.lifewithms.com/beyacc.htm>

Alpine Guild: Coping with Chronic Illness (JoAnn LeMaistre): <http://www.alpineguild.com/COPING%20WITH%20CHRONIC%20ILLNESS.html>

Autoimmune Disease Support Organization: Living with Chronic Illness: Thriving in the Face of Adversity!: <http://members.tripod.com/lvngwell/>

Center for the Advancement of Health (CFAH): Social-Emotional Competence and Physical Health: <http://www.cfah.org/pdfs/social_emotional.pdf>

Chronic Fatigue Support: Dealing with Personal Losses: <http://www.chronicfatiguesupport.com/library/show article.cfm/ID/3161/e/1/T/CFIDS_FM/>

Committment: Coping with Fibromyalgia: <http://www.committment.com/barrett.html>

Coping with Personal Memory Loss (CWPML): <http://www.ycsi.net/users/laura/coping.html>

ElderCare Advocates: Eldercare Resource Center: Coping with a Chronic Illness in Your Family: <http://www.eldercareadvocates.com/pages/art22.htm>

Food and Drug Administration (FDA): FDA Consumer: Coping with Arthritis in Its Many Forms: <http://www.fda.gov/fdac/features/296_art.html>

National Fibromyalgia Association: Fibromyalgia: After the Diagnosis: <http://fmaware.org/patient/coping/after thedx.htm>

HealingWell: Conditions: Coping with the Stress of Chronic Illness: <http://www.healingwell.com/library/health/malik1.asp>

HealingWell: Conditions: Living with Chronic Illness Builds Courage: <http://www.healingwell.com/library/health/article.asp?author=salvucci&id=4>

National Mental Health Association (NMHA): Mental Health Information Fact Sheets: Stress: Coping with Everyday Problems: <http://www.nmha.org/infoctr/factsheets/41.cfm>

SelfHelp Magazine: Chronic Illness: <http://www.selfhelp magazine.com/articles/chronic/index.shtml>

Virtual Health Care Team: Systemic Lupus Erythematosus (SLE): Self-Management Skills: Coping Strategies and Stress Reduction: <http://www.vhct.org/case 2700/coping.shtml>

National Academies Press: The End of Stress As We Know It: <http://www.nap.edu/catalog/10247.html>

101. DECISION MAKING AND TREATMENT PLANNING

Recommended Search Terms

- Chronic patient "decision making"
- Chronic shared decisionmaking
- "Chronic condition" "informed consent"
- Collaborative "decision making"
- Informed health "decision making"
- Informed medical decisionmaking
- Patient choice "treatment planning"
- Patient involvement "treatment planning"

Important Sites

CJNR (Canadian Journal of Nursing Research): Disease-Specific Influences on Meaning and Significance in Self-Care Decision-Making in Chronic Illness: <http://www.cjnr.nursing.mcgill.ca/archive/34/abst34_3_paterson.html>

Chronic Illness Resource Center: <http://www.chronic illness.com/SUPPORT2.htm>

Dartmouth Atlas of Health Care: <http://www.dart-mouthatlas.org/>

Dartmouth Atlas of Health Care: Major Topics: Shared Decision Making Overview: <http://www.dartmouth atlas.org/shareddecisionmaking/sdm_1.php>

Foundation for Informed Medical Decision Making (FIMDM): <http://www.fimdm.org/>

Foundation for Informed Medical Decision Making (FIMDM): Common Questions: <http://www.fimdm.org/faq.phpl>

HealingWell.com: Is a Clinical Trial Right for Me?: <http://www.healingwell.com/library/health/thomas1.asp>

Kaiser Permanente: The Permanente Journal: Strengthening Self-Care, Self-Management, and Shared Decision-Making: <http://www.kaiserpermanente.org/medicine/permjournal/spring02/practices.html>

Milbank Memorial Fund: Center for the Advancement of Health (CFAH): Patients as Effective Collaborators in Managing Chronic Conditions: <http://www.Milbank.org/reports/990811chronic.html>

National Guideline Clearinghouse: <http://www.guideline.gov/>

National Vaccine Information Center (NVIC): Chronic Illness and Vaccines: <http://www.909shot.com/Diseases/Chronic_Illness.htm>

New York State Department of Health: Info for Consumers: Chronic Disease Teaching Tools: <http://www.health.state.ny.us/nysdoh/chronic/>

Ottawa Health Research Institute (OHRI): Patient Decision Aids: <http://www.ohri.ca/programs/clinical_epidemiology/OPDSL/a_to_z.asp>

102. Family Life and Caregiving

Recommended Search Terms

- "Chronic conditions" family
- "Chronic diseases" families
- "Chronic illness" spouse
- "Chronic illness" partner home
- "Chronic illness" effect "significant other"
- Family caregivers

Important Sites

American Association for Marriage and Family Therapy (AAMFT): Updates on Family Problems: Families and Health: Chronic Illness: <http://www.aamft.org/families/Consumer_Updates/ChronicIllness.asp>

Empowering Caregivers: <http://www.care-givers.com/>

Family Caregiver Alliance/National Center on Caregiving: <http://www.caregiver.org/>

Family Voices: <http://www.familyvoices.org/>

National Family Caregivers Association (NFCA): <http://www.nfcacares.org/>

National Organization for Empowering Caregivers: <http://www.nofec.org/>

University of Minnesota, Extension Office: Chronic Conditions Affect Families: <http://www.extension.umn.edu/info-u/families/BE803.html>

103. Fatigue

Recommended Search Terms

- Fatigue coping
- Fighting fatigue

Important Sites

CancerBACUP: Coping with Fatigue: Coping at Home: <http://www.cancerbacup.org.uk/info/fatig/fatig5.htm>

Coping with Fatigue of Post-Polio Syndrome: <http://www.skally.net/ppsc/ftg.html>

International Psycho-Oncology Society (IPOS): Research Update: The Fatigue Symptom Inventory (FSI) and the Multidimensional Fatigue Symptom Inventory (MFSI): <http://www.ipos-society.org/news/fsi.htm>

Multiple Sclerosis International Federation (MSIF) (Multilingual): World of MS: Symptoms and Treatments: Coping with Fatigue: <http://www.msif.org/en/symptoms_treatments/relationships_intimacy_sexuality/indirect_factors/fatigue.html>

Multiple Sclerosis Society (UK): Coping with Fatigue in MS Takes Understanding and Planning (Alexander Burnfield): <http://www.infosci.org/MS-UK-MSSoc/coping.html>

New Hope: Functional Foods and Nutraceuticals (February 2002): Fighting Fatigue: Iron Overload vs. Anaemia: <http://www.newhope.com/ffn/ffn_backs/Feb_02/fatigue.cfm>

Schering Hepatitis Innovations: Coping with Fatigue: <http://www.hepatitisinnovations.com/about/managing/fatigue.html>

University of Virginia: Cancer Center: Dog Tired: Coping with Fatigue: <http://www.healthsystem.virginia.edu/internet/cancer/fatigue.cfm>

University of Washington: Orthopaedics and Sports Medicine: Fatigue: Coping: <http://www.orthop.washington.edu/arthritis/living/fatigue/04/>

Yale University Press: Facing and Fighting Fatigue (Benjamin H. Natelson): <http://www.yale.edu/yup/chapters/068484chap.htm>

104. Financial Planning and Resources

Recommended Search Terms

- "Chronic care" "assistance programs"
- "Chronic care" medication costs -".com"
- "Chronic disease" financial planning -".com"
- "Chronic illness" financial services -".com"
- "Long term illness" "financial assistance" -".com"
- "Long-term illness" "what will it cost" -".com"

Important Sites

All of a Piece: Chronically Ill in America: <http://www.lifewithms.com/chron.htm>

American Association of Health Plans (AAHP)/Health Insurance Association of America (HIAA): <http://www.hiaa.org/>

Angel Care Community—Long Term Illness: <http://www.angelcare.net/>

Arthritis Foundation: Financial Planning: An Introduction: <http://www.arthritis.org/resources/Financial_Planning/Introduction/financial_intro.asp>

Carers Association ACT (Australia): Financial Assistance: <http://www.carersact.asn.au/Financial_assist.htm>

Centers for Disease Control and Prevention (CDC): National Center for Chronic Disease Prevention and Health Promotion (NCCDPHP): *The Burden of Chronic Diseases and Their Risk Factors* (2002): <http://www.cdc.gov/nccdphp/burdenbook2002/>

CareGiving Resource Center: Chronic Conditions Consume Half of Health Care Spending: <http://atsh.org/news/chartbook.html>

Chronic Conditions Information Network (CCIN): Benefits and Disability Information: <http://www.cc-info.net/hiv/benefits.html>

Chronic Conditions Information Network (CCIN): Legal and Financial Planning: <http://www.cc-info.net/legfin.html>

Chronic Fatigue Support: <http://www.chronicfatiguesupport.com/>

Citizens for Long Term Care: Long Term Care Financing: Let's Find a Better Way!: <http://www.citizensforltc.org/>

Jewish Family and Children's Services (JFCS): Services for People with Disabilities: <http://www.jfcsboston.org/fcs/svcs_people_disabilities.cfm>

National Academies Press (NAP): *Coverage Matters: Insurance and Health Care*: <http://www.nap.edu/html/coverage_matters/>

National Academy of Social Insurance: <http://www.nasi.org/>

National PACE Association (NPA): Programs of All-Inclusive Care for the Elderly (PACE): <http://www.natlpaceassn.org/>

Ontario Ministry of Health and Long-Term Care: Ontario Hepatitis C Assistance Plan: Questions and Answers: <http://www.health.gov.on.ca/english/public/project/hepc/hepc.html>

Partnership for Solutions: *Chronic Conditions: Making the Case for Ongoing Care*, December 2002: <http://www.partnershipforsolutions.org/DMS/files/chronicbook2002.pdf>

Rest Ministries: Finances: Life Finances: Living with Illness Financial Resources and Emergency Help: <http://www.restministries.org/life-finances.htm>

Long Term Care Link: <http://www.ltclink.net/>

105. LIFESTYLE CHANGE, HEALTH LIVING, AND SELF-MANAGEMENT

Recommended Search Terms

- "Behavior modification" [name of specific diagnosis]
- "Behaviour modification" "chronic conditions"
- "Goal setting" [name of specific diagnosis]
- "Healthy living" [name of specific diagnosis]
- "Lifestyle change" "goal setting"
- "Lifestyle issues" "chronic disorders"
- "Lifestyle management" [name of specific diagnosis]
- Personal "behavior modification" [name of specific diagnosis]

- Personal "goal setting" [name of specific diagnosis]
- "Risk management" "chronic illness"
- "Self-management" chronic

Important Sites

American Academy of Family Physicians (AAFP): Clinical Care and Research: Role of Nutrition in Chronic Disease Care: <http://www.aafp.org/x16154.xml>

CareGuide: Health and Well-Being: Chronic Conditions: <http://www.careguide.com/Careguide/healthwellbeingcontentview.jsp?ContentKey=959>

City of Fort Worth Public Health Department: Chronic Disease Self-Management: <http://www.fortworthgov.org/health/OR/self_man2001.asp>

Hints and Tips for Surviving the Daily Struggles of Living with Chronic Illness: <http://www.netins.net/showcase/fmd/chronic/>

Health Disparities Collaboratives: Cardiovascular Self-Management Tool: <http://www.healthdisparities.net/CVSelf-ManagementEngSpan.pdf>

Health Disparities Collaboratives: Diabetes Goal [Setting] Contract: <http://www.healthdisparities.net/PatientGoalSetting.pdf>

Health Disparities Collaboratives: Diabetes Self-Management Tool: <http://www.healthdisparities.net/selfmgtform[1]hupke.pdf>

HealthTalk: Multiple Sclerosis Education Network (MSEN): Managing Your MS Medications: <http://www.htinet.com/msen/helpserv.cfm?link=/msen/110602/>

Kaiser Permanente: *The Permanente Journal*: Vohs Award Winner: Chronic Disease Self-Management Program: <http://www.kaiserpermanente.org/medicine/permjournal/spring02/selfmanage.html>

Living a Healthy Life with Chronic Conditions: Chronic Disease Self-Management Program: <http://www.coag.uvic.ca/healthyliving/>

Partnership for Solutions: Different Conditions, Common Problems: <http://www.partnershipforsolutions.org/problem/common_problems.cfm>

Stanford University: Patient Education Resource Center (PERC): Chronic Disease Self-Management Program: <http://patienteducation.stanford.edu/programs/>

Virtual Health Care Team: Lifestyle Issues in Cardiac Health: <http://www.vhct.org/case2800/index.shtml>

Virtual Health Care Team: Lifestyle Management of Adult Obesity: <http://www.vhct.org/case2500/index.shtml>

Virtual Health Care Team: Systemic Lupus Erythematosus (SLE): Self-Management Skills: Benefits and Evidence for Self-Management in Chronic Illness: <http://www.vhct.org/case2700/bene_self_mgmt.shtml>

106. Pain Management

Recommended Search Terms

- Chronic "pain management"
- Coping pain [name of specific diagnosis]
- "Pain management" [name of specific diagnosis]
- "Self-management" pain

Important Sites

American Chronic Pain Association (ACPA) <http://www.theacpa.org/>

American Pain Foundation: <http://www.painfoundation.org/>

Arthritis Foundation: <http://www.arthritis.org/>

Cancer Supportive Care: Post Breast Therapy Pain Syndrome Information Handout: <http://www.cancersupportivecare.com/pbtpsinfo.html>

Chronic Illness Alliance Inc. (Australia): <http://www.chronicillness.org.au/>

Chronic Pain Network: <http://kimberlygraves.tripod.com/chronicpainnetwork/>

Facial Neuralgia Resources: Coping with Pain: <http://facial-neuralgia.org/coping/pain/pain.html>

MedicineNet: Focus on Chronic Pain: <http://www.focusonchronicpain.com/>

National Chronic Pain Outreach Association: <http://neurosurgery.mgh.harvard.edu/ncpainoa.htm>

National Foundation for the Treatment of Pain: <http://www.paincare.org/>

National Institute of Neurological Disorders and Stroke (NINDS): <http://www.ninds.nih.gov/>

National Institute of Neurological Disorders and Stroke (NINDS): Central Pain Syndrome: <http://www.ninds.nih.gov/health_and_medical/disorders/centpain_doc.htm>

National Institute of Neurological Disorders and Stroke (NINDS): Cephalic Disorders: <http://www.ninds.nih.gov/health_and_medical/disorders/cephalic_disorders.htm>

National Institute of Neurological Disorders and Stroke (NINDS): Pain—Hope through Research: <http://www.ninds.nih.gov/health_and_medical/pubs/pain.htm>

National Institute of Neurological Disorders and Stroke (NINDS): Complex Regional Pain Syndrome (also called Reflex Sympathetic Dystrophy Syndrome): <http://www.ninds.nih.gov/health_and_medical/pubs/rsds_fact_sheet.htm>

Pain Online: <http://www.painonline.org/>

107. Research

Recommended Search Terms

- "Chronic disease" research
- "Chronic illness" research
- "Patient-centered care"

Important Sites

Agency for Healthcare Research and Quality (AHRQ): Fact Sheet: Outcomes Research: <http://www.healthlegacy.org/resources/outcomes.htm>

Agency for Healthcare Research and Quality (AHRQ): Focus on Research: Chronic Disease in Adults: <http://www.ahcpr.gov/news/focus/chadult.htm>

Agency for Healthcare Research and Quality (AHRQ): Research in Action, Issue 3: Preventing Disability in the Elderly with Chronic Disease: <http://www.ahcpr.gov/research/elderdis.htm>

Baylor College of Medicine (BCM): Chronic Disease Research Center: <http://cccr.bcm.tmc.edu/>

National Institute of Neurological Disorders and Stroke (NINDS): Pain—Hope through Research: <http://www.ninds.nih.gov/health_and_medical/pubs/pain.htm>

University of Calgary: Faculty of Nursing: Research in Continuing/Chronic Care: <http://www.ucalgary.ca/NU/research/rccc.htm>

University of North Carolina: Carolina School of Nursing: Center for Research on Chronic Illness (CRCI): <http://nursing.unc.edu/crci/>

Yale University: Chronic Disease Epidemiology Research: <http://info.med.yale.edu/eph/html/divisions/cde/cde_research.html>

108. Seniors

[*See also* "Seniors Health Issues," p. 148.]

Recommended Search Terms

- "Chronic conditions" aging
- "Chronic disease" seniors
- "Chronic disease" elderly
- Chronic medication aged
- "Chronic illness" geriatrics

Important Sites

American Geriatrics Society (AGS): <http://www.americangeriatrics.org/>

American Geriatrics Society (AGS): Foundation for Health in Aging: <http://www.healthinaging.org/>

Agency for Healthcare Research and Quality (AHRQ): Research in Action, Issue 3: Preventing Disability in the Elderly with Chronic Disease: <http://www.ahcpr.gov/research/elderdis.htm>

Coping with Personal Memory Loss (CWPML): <http://www.ycsi.net/users/laura/coping.html>

ElderCare Advocates: Eldercare Resource Center: <http://www.eldercareadvocates.com/pages/recenter.htm>

ElderCare Advocates: Eldercare Resource Center: Coping with a Chronic Illness in Your Family: <http://www.eldercareadvocates.com/pages/art22.htm>

National Academies Press (NAP): *The Role of Nutrition in Maintaining Health in the Nation's Elderly: Evaluating Coverage of Nutrition Services for the Medicare Population*: <http://www.nap.edu/catalog/9741.html>

National Council On the Aging (NCOA): <http://www.ncoa.org/>

National PACE Association (NPA): Programs of All-Inclusive Care for the Elderly (PACE): <http://www.natlpaceassn.org/>

109. SEXUALITY AND INTIMACY

[*See also* "Sexual Health Issues," p. 178.]

Recommended Search Terms

- "Chronic conditions" sexuality
- "Chronic disease" intimacy
- Chronic medication sexuality
- "Chronic illness" "sexual response"

Important Sites

Canadian Paediatric Society (CPS): Adolescent Medicine Committee: Sexual Abuse of Adolescents with Chronic Conditions: <http://www.cps.ca/english/statements/AM/am96-01.htm>

Chronic Conditions Information Network (CCIN): Sexuality: <http://www.cc-info.net/sexuality/sexuality.html>

EngenderHealth: Sexual Response and Sexual Practices 4: The Effect of Diseases and Drugs on Sexual Response: <http://www.engenderhealth.org/res/onc/sexuality/response/pg5.html>

Family Health International (FHI): *FHI's Quarterly Health Bulletin, Network*: Contraception and Chronic Conditions Winter 1999, Volume 19, Number 2: <http://www.reproline.jhu.edu/english/6read/6issues/6network/v19-2/v19-2.htm>

SelfHelp Magazine: When the Answer Is "Not Tonight" (Marlene M. Maheu): <http://www.shpm.com/articles/sex/sex.html>

Sexuality and Disability Webliography: Chronic Illness: <http://www.bccpd.bc.ca/wdi/sex_dis_webliog/chronicill.html>

110. SOCIAL SUPPORT AND STORIES

Recommended Search Terms

- "Life with" [name of a specific disease or disorder]
- "My journey" diagnosis
- "My story" illness
- Patient advocacy support
- Patient "support groups" ".gov"
- Patient "support groups" ".org"
- "Patient-to-patient"

Important Sites

All of a Piece: A Life with Multiple Sclerosis (Barbara D. Webster): <http://www.lifewithms.com/>

American Chronic Pain Association (ACPA): <http://www.theacpa.org/>

Center for the Advancement of Health (CFAH): Writing Your Feelings: Good Medicine for Chronic Conditions: <http://www.cfah.org/hbns/newsrelease/990413.cfm>

Diary of an Illness (Dennis W. Pyritz, RN): <http://www.ons.org/xp6/ONS/Library.xml/ONS_Publications.xml/Diary/Main.xml>

From Diagnosis to Acceptance: One Woman's Journey: <http://www.makinglifeeasier.com/articles/article6.html>

From Patient to Patient: A Survival Guide (Patty Cyr): <http://www.geocities.com/bhchcactus/patient.htm>

Guardian Unlimited Observer: Physician, Heal Thyself: <http://www.observer.co.uk/review/story/0,6903,668604,00.html>

111. UNDERSERVED COMMUNITIES AND POPULATIONS

[*See also* "Multicultural Health Issues," p. 54.]

Recommended Search Terms

- "African American" chronic health
- "Health disparities" "chronic diseases"
- Hispanic diabetes
- Immigrant "health care"
- Migrant "access to care" health
- Minorities "chronic illness"
- Rural "access to care" clinics
- Underserved "chronic conditions"

Important Sites

Centers for Disease Control and Prevention (CDC): National Center for Chronic Disease Prevention and

Health Promotion (NCCDPHP): Behavioral Risk Factor Surveillance System (BRFSS): <http://www.cdc.gov/brfss/>

Center for Health Care Strategies (CHCS): <http://www.chcs.org/>

Global Health Council: <http://www.ncih.org/>

Health Disparities Collaboratives: <http://www.healthdisparities.net/>

Migrant Clinicians Network: <http://www.migrantclinician.org/>

National Academies Press (NAP): From Generation to Generation: The Health and Well-Being of Children in Immigrant Families: <http://www.nap.edu/catalog/6164.html>

National Health Care for the Homeless Council: <http://www.nhchc.org/>

National PACE Association (NPA): Programs of All-Inclusive Care for the Elderly (PACE): <http://www.natlpaceassn.org/>

Kaiser Family Foundation: State Health Facts Online: <http://www.statehealthfacts.kff.org/>

112. WOMEN

[*See also* "Women's Health Issues," p. 136.]

Recommended Search Terms

* "Chronic conditions" women
* "Chronic disease" woman
* "Chronic illness" girls

Important Sites

4Girls.gov: Disabilities and Chronic Illness in Girls: <http://www.4girls.gov/chronic/>

American Medical Women's Association (AMWA): <http://www.amwa-doc.org/>

Baylor College of Medicine: Center for Research on Women with Disabilities: National Study of Women with Disabilities: Chronic Conditions: <http://www.bcm.tmc.edu/crowd/national_study/CHRONCON.htm>

National Older Women's League (OWL): <http://www.owl-national.org/>

Womenfolk: Transcending Chronic Illness: Creative Living within Physical Limitations: <http://www.womenfolk.com/transcend/>

HOTLINES

American Cancer Society (ACS):
1-800-227-2345
American Chronic Pain Association:
1-800-533-3231, or e-mail: <ACPA@pacbell.net>

American Diabetes Association (ADA):
1-800-342-2383
American Heart Association (AHA):
1-800-242-8721
American Lung Association (ALA):
1-800-586-4872
American Pain Foundation:
1-888-615-PAIN/1-888-615-7246, or e-mail: <info@painfoundation.org>
Arthritis Foundation: 1-800-283-7800
National Institute of Neurological Disorders and Stroke (NINDS): 1-800-352-9424
National Organization for Rare Disorders (NORD): 1-800-999-6673
Pain Advocacy: 1-800-846-7444
Pain Advocate Foundation: 1-800-532-5274

FAQs

American Academy of Pain Management (AAPM): Patients: We Know You Are Hurting: <http://www.aapainmanage.org/info/Patients.php>

American Chronic Pain Association: Frequently Asked Questions: <http://www.theacpa.org/faqs.htm>

American Lyme Disease Foundation (ALDF): Frequently Asked Questions: <http://www.aldf.com/FAQ.asp>

Chronic Fatigue Syndrome (CFS) FAQ: <http://www.cfs-news.org/faq.htm>

National Women's Health Information Center: 4Woman.gov: Frequently Asked Questions about Women's Health: <http://www.4woman.gov/faq/>

National Information Center for Children and Youth with Disabilities (NICHCY): Frequently Asked Questions: <http://www.nichcy.org/faqs.htm>

Pain Management and Rehabilitation Medical Services of New York: Frequently Asked Questions (FAQs) about Chronic Pain and Pain Management: <http://www.painmanagementny.com/educ_faqs.html>

Pain-Pal: Chronic Pain FAQ: <http://www.pain-pal.com/faq.html>

Patient UK: <http://www.patient.co.uk/>

U.S. Office of Personnel Management (OPM): Insurance: Federal Long Term Care Insurance Program (FLTCIP): Frequently Asked Questions: Basics FAQ: <http://www.opm.gov/insure/ltc/faq/basics.htm>

Veterans Administration (VA): Health: Frequently Asked Questions: <http://www.appc1.va.gov/health/environ/faq.htm>

CHRONIC ILLNESS PUBLICATIONS ON THE INTERNET

Magazines and Journals

Canadian Abilities Foundation: *Abilities Magazine*: <http://www.abilities.ca/>

Family Health International (FHI): *FHI's Quarterly Health Bulletin: Network*: <http://www.reproline.jhu.edu/english/6read/6issues/6network/>

HealingWell: Chronic Illness Resources Online: <http://www.healingwell.com/pages/>

SelfHelp Magazine: <http://www.selfhelpmagazine.com/>

Books

All of a Piece: A Life with Multiple Sclerosis (Barbara D. Webster): <http://www.lifewithms.com/>

National Academies Press (NAP): *Care without Coverage: Too Little, Too Late*: <http://www.nap.edu/catalog/10367.html>

National Academies Press (NAP): *Changing Health Care Systems and Rheumatic Disease*: <http://www.nap.edu/catalog/5472.html>

National Academies Press (NAP): *Coverage Matters*: <http://www.nap.edu/html/coverage_matters/>

National Academies Press (NAP): *Diet and Health: Implications for Reducing Chronic Disease Risk*: <http://www.nap.edu/catalog/1222.html>

National Academies Press (NAP): *Eat for Life: The Food and Nutrition Board's Guide to Reducing Your Risk of Chronic Disease*: <http://www.nap.edu/catalog/1365.html>

National Academies Press (NAP): *Improving the Quality of Long-Term Care*: <http://www.nap.edu/catalog/9611.html>

National Academies Press (NAP): *Promoting Health: Intervention Strategies from Social and Behavioral Research*: <http://www.nap.edu/catalog/9939.html>

National Academies Press (NAP): *The Role of Nutrition in Maintaining Health in the Nation's Elderly: Evaluating Coverage of Nutrition Services for the Medicare Population*: <http://www.nap.edu/catalog/9741.html>

MEDICAL SPECIALTIES

Family practice; Geriatrics; Internal medicine; Pain management; Pediatrics; Physical therapy

PROFESSIONAL ORGANIZATIONS

Alzheimer's Association: <http://www.alz.org/>

American Academy of Family Physicians (AAFP): <http://www.aafp.org/>

American Academy of Pain Management: <http://www.aapainmanage.org/>

American Academy of Pain Medicine: <http://www.painmed.org/>

American Academy of Pediatrics (AAP): <http://www.aap.org/>

American Association of Health Plans (AAHP): <http://www.aahp.org/>

American Cancer Society: <http://www.cancer.org/>

American College of Physicians (ACP): Internal Medicine/Doctors for Adults: <http://www.acponline.org/>

American Chronic Pain Association (ACPA): <http://www.theacpa.org/>

American Diabetes Association (ADA): <http://www.diabetes.org/>

American Geriatrics Society (AGS): <http://www.americangeriatrics.org/>

American Heart Association: <http://www.americanheart.org/>

American Lung Association: <http://www.lungusa.org/>

American Pain Society: <http://www.ampainsoc.org/>

American Pain Foundation: <http://www.painfoundation.org/>

American Public Health Association (APHA): <http://www.apha.org/>

American Society of Pain Management Nurses (ASPMN): <http://www.aspmn.org/>

Association of American Physicians and Surgeons (AAPS): <http://www.aapsonline.org/>

Canadian Association of Psychosocial Oncology: <http://capo.ca/>

Canadian Pain: <http://www.canadianpain.com/>

Chronic Illness Alliance (Australia): <http://www.chronicillness.org.au/>

Chronic Pain Association of Canada (CPAC): <http://ecn.ab.ca/cpac/>

Disease Management Association of America (DMAA): <http://www.dmaa.org/>

International Association for the Study of Pain (IASP): <http://www.iasp-pain.org/index.html>

National Alliance for the Mentally Ill (NAMI): <http://www.nami.org/>

National Association of School Nurses: <http://www.nasn.org/>

National Association of School Nurses for the Deaf: <http://www.nasnd.org/>

National Council On the Aging (NCOA): <http://www.ncoa.org/>

North American Chronic Pain Association of Canada: <http://www.chronicpaincanada.org/>

Pain Relief Foundation (UK): <http://www.painrelieffoundation.org.uk/>

Pain Society (British Chapter of the International Association for the Study of Pain): <http://www.painsociety.org/>

Pain World (Australia): <http://www.painworld.zip.com.au/>

Society for Pain Practice Management (SPPM): <http://www.sppm.org/>

REFERENCES

1. Harrod, Howard L. "Essay on Desire." *JAMA* (2003, February 19,) 289(7):813-14.

Part IX: Living with a Disability

P. F. Anderson

[*See also* "Internet Access for Persons with Disabilities," vol. 1, p. 12; "Tools and Support," p. 133, vol. 1; " Living with a Chronic Illness," p. 67.]

SPECIAL SEARCHING ISSUES FOR THIS TOPIC

Much of the best information is from nonprofit organizations and private individuals with similar concerns. Because of laws such as the Americans with Disabilities Act, more commonly referred to as ADA, there are many government information sources and legislative issues. There are similar laws in many other countries, as well as international organizations. It is particularly important to take these into account if you want to travel outside the United States, but it can also be useful to compare types of resources, standards, and information across countries. Persons interested in advocacy for the civil rights of persons with disabilities may be particularly interested in these types of resources. To focus a search more towards these types of resources (goverment or nonprofit sources), you may wish to add to your search string either (but not both) of the following two search strings.

- ".gov"
- ".org"

Adding these search strings can also help to avoid offensive or inappropriate Web sites, but it will not entirely exclude them. While there have been recommendations on how to avoid pornography and Web sites that focus on the person as an object with many of the health issues discussed, this issue is of special importance in seeking information about disabilities. One of the issues is how to interact with a person who has a disability in daily encounters, at work, at home, or at school.

That it is even necessary to talk about disability etiquette indicates how often people with disabilities are not treated as persons. Given that persons with disabilities are often treated as children or objects by persons who are well meaning, it should not come as a surprise that they are especially targeted by, or vulnerable to, persons whose intentions are not so honorable. For this reason, it may be a wise choice to include one of the following search strings as additions to your search topics.

- -xxx -porn
- -xxx -porn -pornography
- -xxx -porn -pornography -paid -".com"

The language or words used to search for information about disability can also be a sensitive topic. There is a great quantity of pejorative or offensive language that seems to exist solely for the purpose of verbally insulting or injuring persons with differences. In the case of persons with disabilities, preferred language has evolved over time to avoid offense. A Web site may have excellent resources or information, but use outdated language, such as housing sites that use the term "handicapped" in the name of the organization. To locate those sites, one must sometimes use the outdated language in the search. Some persons with disabilities have claimed the offensive terms as a personal badge of identity and pride, and thus you may also see Web sites in which individuals refer to themselves as "gimps," "crips," "cripples," or "wheelies." Use of the offensive terms in this manner creates passionate discussion and dissention within the community of disabled persons.[1] These discussions may offer excellent information, and some such sites are included in the lists of important sites. At the same time, searching with these terms may also retrieve sites intended to offend, which is a risk of including these terms.

ABBREVIATIONS USED IN THIS SECTION

ADA = Americans with Disabilities Act
AAFP = American Academy of Family Physicians
BBC = British Broadcasting Corporation
DHHS = Department of Health and Human Services
DOE = Department of Education
DOL = Department of Labor
DRM = Disability Resources Monthly
EEOC = Equal Employment Opportunity Commission
HUD = Housing and Urban Development
IRSC = Internet Resources for Special Children
NCDRR = National Center for the Dissemination of Disability Research
NCHS = National Center for Health Statistics
NICHCY = National Information Center for Children and Youth with Disabilities

NIH = National Institutes of Health

NINDS = National Institute of Neurological Disorders and Stroke

RADAR = Royal Association for Disability and Rehabilitation (UK)

SAMHSA = Substance Abuse and Mental Health Services Administration

SSA = U.S. Social Security Administration

TTD = Telecommunication device for the deaf

TTY = Teleprinter, teletype, teletypewriter, or text telephone

PROCEDURES AND SPECIAL TOPICS

113. GENERAL

Recommended Search Terms

- Abilities [use with a more specific term]
- Ability [use with a more specific term]
- Able [use with a more specific term]
- Disabilities
- Disability
- Disabled
- Handicap
- Handicaps
- Handicapped
- "Persons with disabilities"
- "Persons with handicaps"
- "PWDs" disabilities
- Rehabilitation

Important Sites

American Civil Liberties Union (ACLU): Disability Rights: <http://www.aclu.org/DisabilityRights/Disability RightsMain.cfm>

American with Disabilities Act (ADA): <http://www.ada .gov/>

BellaOnline: Education: Special Education: Disability Etiquette: <http://www.bellaonline.com/articles/art7003 .asp>

British Council of Disabled People (BCODP): <http:// www.bcodp.org.uk/>

California State University Northridge (CSUN): CSUN Center on Disabilities: <http://www.csun.edu/cod/>

Commission on Accreditation of Rehabilitation Facilities (CARF): <http://www.carf.org/>

Cornucopia of Disability Information: <http://codi.buffalo .edu/>

Department of Education: Office of Special Education and Rehabilitation Services (OSERS): National Institute on Disability and Rehabilitation Research (NIDRR): <http://www.ed.gov/about/offices/list/osers/nidrr/index .html>

Disabilities Studies and Services Center (DSSC): <http:// www.dssc.org/>

DisabilityInfo.gov: <http://www.disabilityinfo.gov/>

DisabilityInfo.gov: Health: <http://www.disabilityinfo.gov/ Health/>

Disability WebLinks (Canada): <http://www.disabilityweb links.ca/>

National Council on Disability: <http://www.ncd.gov/>

New York State: Office of Advocate for Persons with Disabilities: <http://www.advoc4disabled.state.ny.us/>

Persons with Disabilities Online (Canada): <http://www .pwd-online.ca/en/menu.jsp>

Proyecto Vision: A Bilingual Web Site for Latinos with Disabilities (English/Español): <http://www.proyecto vision.net/>

Queer Theory: Disabilities: <http://www.queertheory.com/ cultures/disabilities/>

United Nations: Persons with Disabilities: <http://www.un .org/esa/socdev/enable/>

University of Washington: Dental Education in Care of Persons with Disabilities (DECOD): Referral Service: <http://www.dental.washington.edu/disability/>

114. COMMON DISABILITIES

NOTE: While specific disorders and disabilities are mentioned in this section, the sites were selected primarily for the information on accommodation and lifestyle for these disabilities rather than for the health aspects. For information about the health issues of the disorder or disability, please refer to the appropriate section in volume 1.

Recommended Search Terms

- "Common disabilities"
- Common disabilities -student
- Disabilities "most common" ".gov"
- "Most frequent disabilities"

Important Sites

Disability.gov: <http://www.disability.gov/>

Human Rights Education Associates: An Annotated Primer for Selecting Democratic and Human Rights Education Teaching Materials: <http://www.hrea.org/ pubs/Primer/>

Job Corps Health and Wellness Program: Accommodating Students with Disabilities, a Tutorial: <http://www.job corpshealth.com/disability/>

Nevada Employment Law: ADA: The 10 Most Common Disabilities and How to Accommodate: <http://www.nevadaemploymentlaw.com/articles/10%20most%20common%20disabilities.pdf>

Physical Education (PE) Central: Common Disabilities Defined/Described: <http://www.pecentral.org/adapted/adapteddisabilities.html>

Social Security Administration (SSA): Social Security Online: Disability Programs: Medical/Professional Relations: Disability Evaluation Under Social Security (Blue Book-January 2003): <http://www.ssa.gov/disability/professionals/bluebook/>

United Nations: Persons with Disabilities: <http://www.un.org/esa/socdev/enable/>

115. Back and Spinal Injury

Recommended Search Terms

- "Back injury"
- "Back injury" prevention workplace
- "Back pain"
- "Back injury" accommodation employment
- "Back pain" ADA accommodation employment
- "Spinal cord injury"
- "Spinal cord injury" accommodation employment
- Wheelchair accommodation employment

Important Sites

American Academy of Family Physicians (AAFP): *American Family Physician* (Nov. 15, 1999): Assessment and Management of Acute Low Back Pain: <http://www.aafp.org/afp/991115ap/2299.html>

American Academy of Family Physicians (AAFP): *American Family Physician* (Nov. 15, 1999): Low Back Pain: What to Expect: <http://www.aafp.org/afp/991115ap/991115a.html>

American Pain Society (APS): *APS Bulletin* November/December 1996: The Pain Facts: Back Pain and Associated Disability: <http://www.ampainsoc.org/pub/bulletin/nov96/facts.htm>

American Spinal Injury Association (ASIA): <http://www.asia-spinalinjury.org/>

Brain Injury Rehabilitation Trust (UK): <http://www.birt.co.uk/>

Chiropractic Resource Organization: Lowback Guidelines: <http://www.chiro.org/LINKS/GUIDELINES/Lowback.shtml>

Christopher and Dana Reeve Paralysis Resource Center: <http://www.paralysis.org/>

Healthy Gimp: <http://www.rexdonald.com/index.html>

Job Accommodation Network (JAN): Accommodating Individuals with Back Impairments: <http://janweb.icdi.wvu.edu/media/Back.html>

Job Accommodation Network (JAN): Work-Site Accommodation Ideas for Office Workers Who Use Wheelchairs: <http://janweb.icdi.wvu.edu/media/wheelchair.html>

Kent Waldrep National Paralysis Foundation: <http://www.spinalvictory.org/>

Miami Project to Cure Paralysis: <http://www.themiamiproject.org/>

Mobility-Disability (UK): <http://www.mobility-disability.co.uk/>

National Rehabilitation Information Center (NARIC): <http://www.naric.com/>

National Spinal Cord Injury Association (NSCIA): <http://www.spinalcord.org/>

National Spinal Cord Injury Association (NSCIA): Resource Center: Back Pain: <http://www.spinalcord.org/html/resources/b.php>

National Spinal Cord Injury Association (NSCIA): Resource Center: Disability: <http://www.spinalcord.org/html/resources/d.php>

New Mobility Magazine: <http://www.newmobility.com/>

National Institute of Neurological Disorders and Stroke (NINDS): Spinal Cord Injury Information Page: <http://www.ninds.nih.gov/health_and_medical/disorders/sci.htm>

Paralyzed Veterans of America (PVA): <http://www.pva.org/>

Prevention of Low Back Pain Disability (Jacksonville Medicine/January, 1997): <http://www.dcmsonline.org/jax-medicine/1997journals/jan97/back-school.htm>

SCI-Info-Pages: <http://www.sci-info-pages.com/>

Spinal Cord Injury Network International (SCINI): <http://www.spinalcordinjury.org/>

Spinal Cord Society: <http://members.aol.com/scsweb/>

Hotlines

Christopher Reeve Paralysis Foundation/Paralysis Resource Center:
1-800-225-0292

Kent Waldrep National Paralysis Foundation:
1-877-SCI-CURE/ 1-877-925-2873

Miami Project to Cure Paralysis/ Buoniconti Fund:
1-800-STANDUP/1-800-782-6387

National Rehabilitation Information Center (NARIC):
1-800-346-2742

National Spinal Cord Injury Association: 1-800-962-9629

Paralyzed Veterans of America (PVA):
1-800-424-8200

116. BLOOD DISORDER

Recommended Search Terms

- ADA employment [name of a specific blood disorder]
- ADA employment anemia
- Disabled "blood disease"
- Disability "blood disorder"
- Disability hematologic

Important Sites

American Civil Liberties Union (ACLU): Genetic Discrimination in the Workplace Fact Sheet: <http://www.aclu.org/news/NewsPrint.cfm?ID=9918andc=34>

DisabilityOnline (Australia): Blood: <http://www.disability.vic.gov.au/dsonline/dsarticles.nsf/pages/hc_blood?OpenDocument>

Job Accommodation Network (JAN): Work-Site Accommodation Ideas for Individuals with AIDS/HIV: <http://janweb.icdi.wvu.edu/media/hiv.html>

Job Accommodation Network (JAN): Work-Site Accommodation Ideas for Individuals with Hepatitis (A, B, and C): <http://janweb.icdi.wvu.edu/media/Hep.html>

117. COGNITIVE IMPAIRMENTS

Recommended Search Terms

- ADA employment [name of a specific blood disorder]
- ADA employment psychiatric
- "Cognitive impairment" ADA
- Disabled "mental disease"
- Disability "mental disorder"
- Disability psychiatric
- "Learning disorder"
- "Learning disorder" ADA accommodation
- "Learning disorder" ADA employment
- "Post traumatic stress disorder" ADA accommodation

Important Sites

American Civil Liberties Union (ACLU): Disability Rights: Mentally Disabled: <http://www.aclu.org/DisabilityRights/DisabilityRightslist.cfm?c=74>

The Arc of the United States: <http://www.thearc.org/>

Autism Today: <http://www.autismtoday.com/>

Job Accommodation Network (JAN): Accommodating Workers with Bipolar Disorder: <http://janweb.icdi.wvu.edu/media/Bipolar.html>

Job Accommodation Network (JAN): Accommodations for People with Mental Retardation or Other Developmental Disabilities: <http://janweb.icdi.wvu.edu/media/MR.html>

Job Accommodation Network (JAN): Accommodations for People with PTSD (Post-Traumatic Stress Disorder): <http://janweb.icdi.wvu.edu/media/ptsd.html>

Job Accommodation Network (JAN): Work-Site Accommodation Ideas for Persons with Psychiatric Disabilities: <http://janweb.icdi.wvu.edu/media/Psychiatric.html>

Job Accommodation Network (JAN): Work-Site Accommodation Ideas for People with Learning Disabilities and/or Attention Deficit Disorder: <http://janweb.icdi.wvu.edu/media/LD.html>

MIND (National Association for Mental Health) (UK): <http://www.mind.org.uk/>

National Center for Post-Traumatic Stress Disorder: Frequently Asked Questions: <http://www.ncptsd.org/faq.html>

Substance Abuse and Mental Health Services Administration (SAMHSA): National Mental Health Information Center: The Center for Mental Health Services: <http://www.samhsa.gov/centers/cmhs/cmhs.html>

118. DIABETES

[*See also* "Diabetes," p. 51, vol. 2.]

Recommended Search Terms

- Accommodation employment diabetes
- ADA accommodation diabetes
- ADA disabilities diabetes
- ADA employment diabetes
- Diabetes "reasonable accommodation"
- Diabetes disability accommodation
- Diabetic "reasonable accommodation"
- Disability diabetes
- Disabled diabetic

Important Sites

American Diabetes Association (ADA): Advocacy: Major Federal Employment Laws Affecting People with Diabetes: <http://www.diabetes.org/main/community/advocacy/worklaw.jsp>

American Diabetes Association (ADA): Government Relations Advocacy: <http://www.diabetes.org/advocacy/>

Independent Living Research Utilization (ILRU): Disability Law Resource Project: Employment Considerations for People Who Have Diabetes: <http://www.dlrp.org/html/publications/employment/onthejob/diabetes.html>

Job Accommodation Network (JAN): Work-Site Accommodation Ideas for Individuals with Diabetes: <http://janweb.icdi.wvu.edu/media/Diabetes.html>

119. EXTREMITIES

Recommended Search Terms

- Amputation
- Amputation accommodation employment
- Amputee
- Amputee ADA accommodation employment
- "Extremity loss" ADA accommodation employment
- Wheelchair ADA accommodation employment
- Wheelchair employment rights

Important Sites

Access Board: Accessibility Guidelines and Standards: <http://www.access-board.gov/indexes/accessindex.htm>

Amputee Coalition of America (ACA): Employment Opportunities: <http://www.amputee-coalition.org/aca_employment.html>

WheelchairNet: Working and Using a Wheelchair: <http://www.wheelchairnet.org/WCN_Living/work.html>

120. HEAD AND BRAIN INJURY

Recommended Search Terms

- "Brain injury"
- "Brain injury" accommodation
- "Head injury"
- "Head injury" accommodation
- "Traumatic brain injury"
- "Traumatic brain injury" accommodation

Important Sites

Brain Injury Resource Center: <http://www.headinjury.com/>

Job Accommodation Network (JAN): Work-Site Accommodation Ideas for Persons with Brain Injury: <http://janweb.icdi.wvu.edu/media/BrainInjury.html>

Missouri Head Injury Guide: "What Everyone Should Know about Brain Injury": <http://www.oa.state.mo.us/gs/hi/tbi/HIGUIDE/>

National Alliance for the Mentally Ill (NAMI): Brain Injury Resource Directory: <http://www.nami.org/multnomah/brain%20injury.html>

National Women's Health Information Center: 4woman.gov: Women with Disabilities: Traumatic Brain Injury: <http://www.4woman.gov/>

121. HEARING IMPAIRMENTS

Recommended Search Terms

- Deaf
- Deafness
- "Hearing impairments"
- "Hearing impairment" ADA accommodation employment

Important Sites

Deaf Magazine: <http://www.deaf-magazine.org/>

DeafNation: <http://www.deafnation.com/>

Deaf Resource Library: <http://www.deaflibrary.org/>

Gallaudet University: <http://www.gallaudet.edu/>

Job Accommodation Network (JAN): Work-Site Accommodation Ideas for Individuals Who Are Deaf or Hard of Hearing: <http://janweb.icdi.wvu.edu/media/Hearing.html>

National Technical Assistance Consortium for Children and Young Adults Who Are Deaf-Blind (NTAC): <http://www.tr.wou.edu/ntac/>

National Captioning Institute (NCI): <http://www.ncicap.org/>

National Technical Institute for the Deaf: <http://www.rit.edu/NTID/>

Royal National Institute for the Deaf (RNID) (UK): <http://www.rnid.org.uk/>

122. HEART IMPAIRMENTS

Recommended Search Terms

- "Cardiac rehabilitation"
- "Heart attack" recovery
- "Heart disability"
- "Heart disease" "reasonable accommodation"
- "Heart impairment" accommodation employment
- "Heart impairments" ADA disability accommodation
- Heart lifestyle accommodation
- Stroke recovery rehabilitation

Important Sites

American Heart Association: <http://www.americanheart.org/>

British Heart Foundation (UK): <http://www.bhf.org.uk/>

Canadian Association of Cardiac Rehabilitation (CACR): <http://www.cacr.ca/>

Disability UK: Heart Index Page: <http://www.disabilityuk.com/health/heart/>

Job Accommodation Network (JAN): Accommodating People with Heart Conditions: <http://www.jan.wvu.edu/media/Heart.html>

123. INVISIBLE DISABILITIES

[*See also* "Living with a Chronic Illness," p. 67.]

Recommended Search Terms

- Invisible disability
- "Invisible disability" ADA accommodation employment
- [Name of a specific disability] ADA accommodation employment

Important Sites

Dolfrog's Helpful (C)APD and Invisible Disability Connections (UK): <http://www.dolfrog.com/>

Federation of Invisible Disabilities (FIDS) (Canada): <http://www.fids.bc.ca/>

Paintracking.com: Fibromyalgia: An "Invisible" Disability: <http://www.paintracking.com/fms03.html>

ID Agora: The Invisible Disabilities Agora: <http://www.tertius.net.au/id/>

Invisible Disabilities Advocate: <http://www.invisibledisabilities.com/>

Invisible Disabilities Association of Canada: <http://www.nsnet.org/idans/>

Invisible Disabilities Page: <http://mysite.verizon.net/vze20h45/invisible_disability.html>

Job Accommodation Network (JAN): Accommodating People with Chronic Fatigue Syndrome: <http://janWeb.icdi.wvu.edu/media/cfs.html>

Job Accommodation Network (JAN): Work-Site Accommodation Ideas for Individuals with Fragrance Sensitivity: <http://janweb.icdi.wvu.edu/media/fragrance.html>

Job Accommodation Network (JAN): Work-Site Accommodation Ideas for Natural Latex Allergies in the Healthcare Environment: <http://janweb.icdi.wvu.edu/media/LATEX.html>

Job Accommodation Network (JAN): Work-Site Accommodation Ideas for Individuals Who Experience Limitations Due to Chemical Sensitivity or Environmental Illness: <http://janweb.icdi.wvu.edu/media/MCS.html>

Job Accommodation Network (JAN): Work-Site Accommodation Ideas: Respiratory Impairment: <http://janWeb.icdi.wvu.edu/media/Respiratory.html>

Living with an Invisible Disability: <http://dolfrog4life.homestead.com/AA_index_ZZ.html>

National Chronic Fatigue Syndrome and Fibromyalgia Association (NCFSFA): The Americans with Disabilities Act: CFS and Employment: <http://www.ncfsfa.org/Patients/ada.htm>

Not Done Yet: Column 1: What's an Invisible Disability?: <http://www.tertius.net.au/id/column/1_what_is_ID.html>

Ragged Edge Magazine: A Hard Look at Invisible Disability (March 2001): <http://www.ragged-edge-mag.com/0301/0301ft1.htm>

124. NEUROLOGICAL IMPAIRMENTS

Recommended Search Terms

- Accommodation employment "attention deficit disorder"
- ADA accommodation employment [Name of a specific neurological impairment]
- ADA accommodation employment epilepsy
- ADA accommodation employment hyperactivity
- "Neurological impairment" ADA accommodation employment

Important Sites

HealthyPlace: ADD Adults in the Workplace: The Americans with Disabilities Act: Facts about the Americans with Disabilities Act: <http://www.healthyplace.com/Communities/ADD/ask/legal/ADA_act.html>

Job Accommodation Network (JAN): Accommodating People with Chronic Pain: <http://janweb.icdi.wvu.edu/media/ChronicPain.html>

Job Accommodation Network (JAN): Accommodating People with Multiple Sclerosis: <http://janweb.icdi.wvu.edu/media/MS.html>

Job Accommodation Network (JAN): Accommodating People with Muscular Dystrophy: <http://janweb.icdi.wvu.edu/media/MD.html>

Job Accommodation Network (JAN): Accommodating People with Myasthenia Gravis: <http://janweb.icdi.wvu.edu/media/MG.html>

Job Accommodation Network (JAN): Accommodating People with Parkinson's Disease: <http://janweb.icdi.wvu.edu/media/PD.html>

Job Accommodation Network (JAN): Accommodation Ideas for Employees with Epilepsy: <http://janweb.icdi.wvu.edu/media/epilepsy.html>

Job Accommodation Network (JAN): Work-Site Accommodation Ideas for Individuals Who Have Migraine Headaches: <http://janweb.icdi.wvu.edu/media/Migraine.html>

Job Accommodation Network (JAN): Work-Site Accommodation Ideas for Individuals Who Have Cerebral Palsy: <http://janweb.icdi.wvu.edu/media/CP.html>

National Multiple Sclerosis Society: Brochures: ADA and People with MS: A Guarantee of Full Participation in Society: <http://www.nationalmssociety.org/Brochures-ADA%20and.asp>

United Cerebral Palsy (UCP) of New York City: Americans with Disabilities Act: <http://www.ucpnyc.org/advoc/disabilitiesact.cfm>

125. Stuttering and Speech Impairment

Recommended Search Terms

- Disfluency
- Disfluency employment
- Dysfluency
- Dysfluency accommodation
- Stammering
- Stammering "civil rights"
- Stuttering
- Stuttering advocacy
- "Speech disorders"
- "Speech impairment"

Important Sites

Allan Tyrer's Stammering Page: Discrimination against People Who Stammer in the UK: <http://www.atyrer.demon.co.uk/stammer/dda/>

Apraxia-Kids: Stuttering or Dysfluency: <http://www.apraxia-kids.org/links/linksstuttering.html>

Association for Research into Stammering in Childhood: <http://www.stammeringcentre.org/>

Canoe (Canada): Stuttering Is Society's Hidden Disability: <http://www.canoe.ca/Health0002/17_stutter_CP.html>

DiSS'01: Disfluency in Spontaneous Speech, 2001 (Scotland): <http://www.ling.ed.ac.uk/DISS-01/>

Human Rights and Equal Opportunity Commission (Australia): Disability Rights: Frequently Asked Questions: Who Is Protected by the DDA?: <http://www.hreoc.gov.au/disability_rights/faq/Who_is_protected_/who_is_protected_.html>

International Stuttering Awareness Day 1999 On-Line Conference: Stuttering and Employment Discrimination: <http://www.mankato.msus.edu/dept/comdis/isad2/papers/parry.html>

International Stuttering Association (ISA): <http://www.stutterisa.org/>

Language Express (Canada): What Is Normal Dysfluency? (Stuttering): <http://www.language-express.ca/comdisorder/dysfluency.htm>

Minnesota State University, Mankato: The Stuttering Homepage: <http://www.mankato.msus.edu/dept/comdis/kuster/stutter.html>

National Center for Stuttering: <http://www.stuttering.com/>

National Center for Stuttering: Stutter No More, Online Book: <http://www.stuttering.com/stutter.htm>

National Organization on Disability: Can Technology Cure Stuttering? (John Williams): <http://www.nod.org/cont/dsp_cont_item_view.cfm?contentId=1188>

National Stuttering Association (NSA): <http://www.nsastutter.org/>

National Stuttering Association (NSA): Letting Go (Newsletter): <http://www.nsastutter.org/lettinggo.html>

National Stuttering Project Advocacy Committee: Stuttering as a Disability under the Americans with Disabilities Act of 1990: <http://members.aol.com/wdparry/ada.htm>

Stuttering Foundation of America: <http://www.stuttersfa.org/> or <http://www.stutteringhelp.org/>

Valsalva-Stuttering Network: <http://www.valsalva.org/>

126. Substance Abuse

Recommended Search Terms

- Addiction accommodation employment
- Alcoholic employee accommodation
- Alcoholism accommodation employment ".gov"
- Disability "substance abuse"
- "Substance abuse" accommodation employment

Important Sites

Department of Health and Human Services: Substance Abuse and Mental Health Services Administration (SAMHSA): Center for Substance Abuse Treatment: <http://www.samhsa.gov/centers/csat2002/csat_frame.html>

Department of Health and Human Services: Substance Abuse and Mental Health Services Administration (SAMHSA): National Clearinghouse for Alcohol and Drug Information (NCADI): <http://www.health.org/>

Job Accommodation Network (JAN): Ideas for Accommodating Persons with Alcoholism: <http://janweb.icdi.wvu.edu/media/alcohol.html>

LawSight.com: Alcoholism Is a Disability under the ADA: <http://www.lawsight.com/jjart2.htm>

National Center for the Dissemination of Disability Research (NCDDR): Guide to Substance Abuse and Disability Resources: <http://www.ncddr.org/du/products/saguide/>

National Institute for Drug Abuse (NIDA): <http://www.nida.nih.gov/>

National Institute of Alcohol Abuse and Alcoholism (NIAAA): <http://www.niaaa.nih.gov/>

127. Vision Impairments

Recommended Search Terms

- Blind accommodation employment
- Blindness ADA
- "Impaired vision"
- "Vision impairment"

Important Sites

American Council for the Blind (ACB): <http://acb.org/>

American Foundation for the Blind (AFB): <http://www.afb.org/>

American Printing House for the Blind (APH): <http://www.aph.org/>

Association for Education and Rehabilitation of the Blind and Visually Impaired (AER) Online: <http://www.aerbvi.org/>

Blindness-Specific Emailing Lists: BLIST: <http://www.hicom.net/~oedipus/blist.html>

Blindness-Related Resources on the Web and Beyond: <http://www.hicom.net/~oedipus/blind.html>

Canadian National Institute for the Blind (CNIB): <http://www.cnib.ca/>

Canadian National Institute for the Blind (CNIB): Workopolis.com: Job Seekers: <http://cnib.workopolis.com/jobseekers.html>

Helen Keller Worldwide: <http://www.hkworld.org/>

International Blind Sports Federation (IBSA): <http://www.ibsa.es/>

Job Accommodation Network (JAN): Work-Site Accommodation Ideas for Individuals with Vision Impairments: <http://janweb.icdi.wvu.edu/media/sight.html>

Library of Congress: National Library Service for the Blind and Physically Handicapped (NLS): <http://lcweb.loc.gov/nls/>

Lighthouse International: <http://www.lighthouse.org/>

Lighthouse International: Guide to Employment Resources for People with Impaired Vision: <http://www.lighthouse.org/download/fact_sheets/emp_res.pdf>

National Braille Press: <http://www.nbp.org/>

National Federation of the Blind (NFB): <http://www.nfb.org/>

Prevent Blindness America: <http://www.preventblindness.org/>

Royal National Institute for the Blind (RNIB) (UK): <http://www.rnib.org.uk/>

Sight Savers International (UK): <http://www.sightsavers.org.uk/>

Vision World Wide: <http://www.visionww.org/>

128. Access and Accommodation

Recommended Search Terms

- Accessibility disability
- Disabilities accommodation
- Disability accommodations
- Disabled "public access"
- Disabled "public accommodations"
- Disabled "reasonable accommodation"

Important Sites

Access-Ability (UK): <http://www.access-ability.co.uk/>

Access Board: <http://www.access-board.gov/>

Access Board: Access Currents: <http://www.access-board.gov/news/Access%20Currents/General.htm>

Access Board: Accessibility Guidelines and Standards: <http://www.access-board.gov/indexes/accessindex.htm>

American Civil Liberties Union (ACLU): Disability Rights: Public Accommodations: <http://www.aclu.org/DisabilityRights/DisabilityRightslist.cfm?c=75>

The Arc: ADA Access Strategies Chart: <http://www.thearc.org/ada/adachart.html>

Department of Health and Human Services (DHHS): Delivering on the Promise: Preliminary Report of Federal Agencies' Actions to Eliminate Barriers and Promote Community Integration: <http://www.hhs.gov/newfreedom/prelim/>

Rocky Mountain Disability and Business Technical Assistance Center: ADA Info Net: *ADA Quiz Book*: <http://www.ada-infonet.org/training/quizbook/>

Department of Health and Human Services (DHHS): Delivering on the Promise: Self-Evaluation to Promote Community Living for People with Disabilities: <http://cms.hhs.gov/newfreedom/hhsselfeval.pdf>

Department of Health and Human Services (DHHS): Fulfilling America's Promise to Americans with Disabilities: New Freedom Initiative: <http://cms.hhs.gov/newfreedom/>

Disabilities Resources Monthly (DRM): Architecture/Home Modification: <http://www.disabilityresources.org/ARCHITECTURE.html>

DisabilityInfo.gov: <http://www.disability.gov/>

Equal Employment Opportunity Commission (EEOC): Enforcement Guidance: Reasonable Accommodation and Undue Hardship Under the Americans with Disabilities Act: <http://www.eeoc.gov/docs/accommodation.html>

Job Accommodation Network (JAN): Searchable Online Accommodation Resource (SOAR): <http://www.jan.wvu.edu/soar/>

Kid Design: <http://pt.creighton.edu/kiddesign/>

RADAR: Access: <http://www.radar.org.uk/RANE/Templates/Article1.asp?lHeaderID=252>

White House: New Freedom Initiative: <http://www.whitehouse.gov/news/freedominitiative/freedominitiative.html>

129. ADVOCACY

Recommended Search Terms

- Disabilities advocacy
- Disability "civil disobedience"
- Disabled activism

Important Sites

ADAPT: <http://www.adapt.org/>

American Civil Liberties Union (ACLU): ACLU Briefing Paper #21 on Disabilities Rights: <http://www.aclu.org/DisabilityRights/DisabilityRights.cfm?ID=9474&c=18>

American Association of People with Disabilities (AAPD): <http://www.aapd.com/>

American Disability Association: <http://www.adanet.org/>

American RehabACTion Network (ARAN): <http://www.americanrehabaction.org/>

Department for Work and Pensions (DWP) (UK): Disability: <http://www.disability.gov.uk/>

Disability Rights Education and Defense Fund (DREDF): <http://www.dredf.org/>

Disabled People's International (DPI) [Multilingual]: <http://www.dpi.org/>

Disabled People's International Europe: <http://www.dpieurope.org/>

National Association of Protection and Advocacy (NAPAS): <http://www.protectionandadvocacy.com/>

Parents Educating Parents and Professionals (PEPP), Inc.: United Parent Syndicate on Disabilities (UPSD): <http://www.peppinc.org/upsdoverview.htm>

Planned Lifetime Advocacy Network (PLAN): <http://www.plan.ca/>

RADAR: Bioethics: <http://www.radar.org.uk/RANE/Templates/Article1.asp?lHeaderID=127>

Red Pepper: Directory: Disability: <http://www.redpepper.org.uk/direct.html#disable>

130. CHILDREN WITH DISABILITIES

NOTE: Information for parents of children with disabilities is included in this section. Information for parents who themselves are disabled is under "Parenting," p. 92.

Recommended Search Terms

- Disabilities children
- Disabilities parenting
- Disabilities parents
- Disability children
- Disability parents
- Parenting [name of a specific disability or diagnosis]
- Parenting "children with disabilities"
- Parent "disabled child"
- Parents "handicapped child"
- "Special needs" parenting
- "Special needs" parents

Important Sites

The Arc: Sibling Support Project: <http://www.thearc.org/siblingsupport/>

The Arc of the United States: <http://www.thearc.org/>

Autism Today: <http://www.autismtoday.com/>

Child Rights Information Network (CRIN) (International): <http://www.crin.org/>

Children with Disabilities: <http://www.childrenwithdisabilities.ncjrs.org/>

Contact a Family (UK): <http://www.cafamily.org.uk/>

Council for Exceptional Children (CEC): <http://www.cec.sped.org/>

Disability Resource Monthly (DRM): The DRM Web-Watcher (Subjects): Just for Kids: <http://www.disabilityresources.org/KIDS.html>

Disability Resource Monthly (DRM): The DRM Web-Watcher (Subjects): Just for Parents (and Service Providers): <http://www.disabilityresources.org/PARENTS-OF.html>

Educational Resources Information Center (ERIC) Clearinghouse on Disabilities and Gifted Education: <http://ericec.org/>

Exceptional Parent (EP) Magazine: <http://www.eparent.com/>

Federal Interagency Coordinating Council: <http://www.fed-icc.org/>

Internet Resources for Special Children (IRSC): <http://www.irsc.org/>

Kid Design: <http://pt.creighton.edu/kiddesign/>

Kids Together, Inc.: <http://www.kidstogether.org/>

Learning Disabilities Association of America (LDA): <http://www.ldanatl.org/>

Learning Disabilities (LD) Online: <http://www.ldonline.org/>

National Association of Councils on Developmental Disabilities (NACDD): <http://www.naddc.org/>

National Center for Learning Disabilities: LD InfoZone: <http://www.ncld.org/LDInfoZone/index.cfm>

National Information Center for Children and Youth with Disabilities (NICHCY) [English/Spanish]: <http://www.nichcy.org/>

National Information Center for Children and Youth with Disabilities (NICHCY): Basics for Parents: <http://www.nichcy.org/basicpar.asp>

National Information Center for Children and Youth with Disabilities (NICHCY): Parent Guides: <http://www.nichcy.org/parents.asp>

National Information Center for Children and Youth with Disabilities (NICHCY): Student Guides: <http://www.nichcy.org/stuguid.asp>

Oklahoma Parent e-Network: <http://pages.ivillage.com/okparentnetwork/>

Parents for Inclusion (Pi) (UK): <http://www.parentsforinclusion.org/pihomepage.htm>

Social Security Online: Benefits for Children with Disabilities: <http://www.ssa.gov/pubs/10026.html>

Special Child: For Parents of Children with Disabilities: <http://www.specialchild.com/>

SpecialLink (National Centre for Child Care Inclusion): <http://www.specialinkcanada.org/>

Social Security Administration (SSA): The Blue Book: Listing of Impairments—Childhood: <http://www.ssa.gov/disability/professionals/bluebook/Childhood Listings.htm>

The Vanier Institute of the Family: Transition Magazine (Spring 2002): A Family PLAN for the Future of People with Disabilities: <http://www.vifamily.ca/library/321/321.html#4>

131. CREATIVE ARTS, ENTERTAINMENT, LEISURE, RECREATION, AND SPORTS

Recommended Search Terms

- Disabilities arts
- Disabilities music
- Disability creativity
- Disability entertainment
- Disabled leisure
- Disabled artists
- Disabled musicians
- Handicap recreation
- Handicapped sports

Important Sites

Activeamp: <http://www.activeamp.org/>

AllAbilities: Arts and Entertainment: <http://www.allabilities.com/arts.html>

AllAbilities: Sports and Recreation: <http://www.allabilities.com/sports.html>

Association of Mouth and Foot Painting Artists (AMFPA): <http://www.amfpa.com/>

British Broadcasting Corporation (BBC): Watchdog: Guides to Disability: Entertainment: <http://www.bbc.co.uk/watchdog/guides_to/disability/index8.shtml>

International Games Archive: British Commonwealth Paraplegic Games: <http://www.internationalgames.net/britishCommParGames.htm>

Special Olympics Canada: <http://www.cso.on.ca/>

Coalition for Disabled Musicians, Inc.: <http://www.disabled-musicians.org/>

Deaf Art: <http://www.deafart.org/>

Disabled Sailing Association of British Columbia: <http://www.reachdisability.org/dsa/>

Disability Resources Monthly (DRM): DRM WebWatcher (Subjects): Sports and Recreation (General): <http://www.disabilityresources.org/SPORTS-GENERAL.html>

International Games Archive: Games for Athletes with Physical Disabilities: <http://www.internationalgames.net/gamesfor.htm>

Google Directory: Society: Disabled: Arts: <http://directory.google.com/Top/Society/Disabled/Arts/>

Google Directory: Society: Disabled: Sports: <http://directory.google.com/Top/Sports/Disabled/>

Handicapped Scuba Association (HSA) International: <http://www.hsascuba.com/>

Institute on Disability Culture: <http://www.dimenet.com/disculture/>

International Paralympic Committee: <http://www.paralympic.org/>

International Disabled Self-Defense Association (IDSA): <http://www.defenseability.com/>

London Disability Arts Forum (UK): <http://www.ldaf.net/>

Michigan State University: Kinesiology: Disability Sports: <http://ed-Web3.educ.msu.edu/kin866/>

National Arts and Disability Center (NADC): <http://nadc.ucla.edu/>

National Disability Arts Forum: <http://www.ndaf.org/>

National Forum on Careers in the Arts for People with Disabilities: <http://artsedge.kennedycenter.org/forum/>

National Theatre Workshop of the Handicapped: <http://www.ntwh.org/>

North American Riding for the Handicapped Association (NARHA): <http://www.narha.org/>

Orpheus Centre (UK): <http://www.orpheus.org.uk/>

International Games Archive: Pan-American Wheelchair Games: <http://www.internationalgames.net/panamwheel.htm>

Project Ability (UK): <http://www.project-ability.co.uk/>

Special Olympics: <http://www.specialolympics.org/>

RADAR: Creative Arts: <http://www.radar.org.uk/RANE/Templates/Article1.asp?lHeaderID=371>

VSA Arts (Very Special Arts) [International]: <http://www.vsarts.org/>

World Leisure: Commission on Access and Inclusion: <http://www.worldleisure.org/Commissions/Access%20and%20Inclusion/main.html>

World Wheelchair Sports: <http://www.efn.org/~wwscoach/>

132. EDUCATION

Recommended Search Terms

- Disability education
- "Disability rights" education
- "Distance learning" disabled
- "Educational technologies" disability
- "Educational technology" disabilities
- Handicapped education

Important Sites

American Civil Libraries Union (ACLU): Disability Rights: Education: <http://www.aclu.org/DisabilityRights/DisabilityRightslist.cfm?c=71>

Centre for Educational Technology Interoperability Standards (CETIS): <http://www.cetis.ac.uk/>

Department for Works and Pensions (DWP) (UK): Disability: Campaigns and Consultations: Policy and Programmes: Special Educational Needs: Special Educational Needs and Disability Act 2001: <http://www.disability.gov.uk/policy/sen/>

Department of Education: ED.gov: Office of Civil Rights: <http://www.ed.gov/ocr/>

Department of Education: Office of Special Education and Rehabilitative Services (OSERS): <http://www.ed.gov/about/offices/list/osers/index.html?src=mr>

Disabilityinfo.gov: Education: <http://www.disabilityinfo.gov/Education/>

Disability Resources Monthly (DRM): DRM WebWatcher (Subjects): Education: <http://www.disabilityresources.org/EDUCATION.html>

Educational Testing Service (ETS): Disabilities and Testing: General Information: <http://www.ets.org/disability/>

George Washington University HEATH Resource Center: The National Clearinghouse on Postsecondary Education for Individuals with Disabilities: <http://www.heath.gwu.edu/>

National Educational Association of Disabled Students (Canada): <http://www.neads.ca/>

Parents for Inclusion (UK): <http://www.parentsforinclusion.org/pihomepage.htm>

RADAR: Education: <http://www.radar.org.uk/RANE/Templates/Article1.asp?lHeaderID=129>

Skill: National Bureau for Students with Disabilities (UK): <http://www.skill.org.uk/>

133. EMERGENCY AND DISASTER PREPAREDNESS

Recommended Search Terms

- Disabilities "disaster preparedness"
- Disabilities "emergency preparedness"
- Disabled "disaster preparedness"
- Disabled "emergency preparedness"
- Disaster emergency preparedness [name of a specific disability]
- Disaster emergency preparedness blindness
- Disaster emergency preparedness disability
- Disaster emergency preparedness wheelchair

Important Sites

American Red Cross: Disaster Services—Be Prepared: Special Needs and Concerns: People with Disabilities: Disaster Preparedness for People with Disabilities: <http://www.redcross.org/services/disaster/beprepared/disability.html>

Department of Health and Human Services: Administration on Developmental Disabilities (ADD): Coping with Disaster: Suggestions for Helping Children with Cognitive Disabilities: <http://www.acf.dhhs.gov/programs/add/Sept11/addcoping.html>

Disabilities: Tips for People with Special Needs and Concerns: <http://www.redcross.org/services/disaster/beprepared/mobileprogs.html>

DisabilityInfo.gov: Emergency Preparedness: <http://www.disabilityinfo.gov/Community/6/>

Disability Resources Monthly (DRM): DRM WebWatcher (Subjects): Disaster Preparedness for People with

Disabilities: <http://www.disabilityresources.org/DISASTER.html>

Earthquake Tips for Persons with Disabilities (English/Spanish): <http://www.jik.com/disaster.html#Earthquakes>

Easter Seals: Resources: s.a.f.e.t.y. first: Evacuation Planning Guide: <http://www.easter-seals.org/site/PageServer?pagename=ntl_safety_first>

Federal Emergency Management Agency (FEMA): Disaster Preparedness for People with Disabilities: <http://www.fema.gov/library/disprepf.shtm>

Independent Living Resource Center San Francisco (ILRCSF): Emergency Preparedness for People with Disabilities: <http://www.ilrcsf.org/Publications/prepared/>

Job Accommodation Network (JAN): Employers' Guide to Including Employees with Disabilities in Emergency Evacuation Plans: <http://www.jan.wvu.edu/media/emergency.html>

National Center on Emergency Preparedness for People with Disabilities (NCEPPD): <http://www.disabilitypreparedness.com/>

National Institute of Standards and Technology: Building and Fire Research Laboratory: Emergency Procedures for Employees with Disabilities in Office Occupancies: <http://fire.nist.gov/bfrlpubs/fire95/art043.html>

National Organization On Disability: Community Involvement: Emergency Preparedness Initiative: Emergency Preparedness Initiative (EPI) Guide for Emergency Managers, Planners and Responders: <http://www.nod.org/cont/dsp_cont_item_view.cfm?viewType=itemView&contentId=1267>

PrepareNow.org: Supporting Special Needs and Vulnerable Populations in Disaster: <http://www.preparenow.org/>

U.S. Fire Administration: Public: Home Fire Safety: Factsheets: Removing the Barriers: A Fire Safety Factsheet for People with Disabilities and their Caregivers: <http://www.usfa.fema.gov/public/factsheets/fswy22.shtm>

134. Employment and Work Place

Recommended Search Terms

- Disabilities employment
- Disabilities professional
- Disabilities [name of a specific profession]
- Disability employment
- Disability jobseekers
- Disability "job seeker"
- Disability job-seeking
- Disability "job seeking"
- Disability workplace accommodation

- Disability "work place" accommodation
- Disabled employment rights
- Disabled unemployment
- Disabled professional
- Disabled [name of a specific profession]
- "Employment rights"
- Employment rights disability
- "Equal opportunity" disabled
- Handicapped employment
- Handicapped jobseekers
- Handicapped [name of a specific profession]
- Workplace accommodation

Important Sites

Abilities for Life—Taking Charge: <http://www.angelfire.com/ok4/abilitiesforlife/>

American Civil Liberties Union (ACLU): Disability Rights: Employment: <http://www.aclu.org/DisabilityRights/DisabilityRightslist.cfm?c=72>

The Arc: ADA and Title III Business Guide: <http://www.thearc.org/ada/adaguide.html>

British Broadcasting Corporation (BBC): Equal Opps: Disability and Work: <http://www.bbc.co.uk/radio1/onelife/work/rights/eq_disability.shtml>

Cornell University: School of Industrial and Labor Relations: Program on Employment and Disability: Disability Employment Policy: <http://www.ilr.cornell.edu/ped/dep/dep.html>

Careers in Vocational Rehabilitation: <http://www.rehabjobs.org/>

Department of Labor (DOL): Office of Disability Employment Policy: <http://www.dol.gov/odep/welcome.html>

Disabilities Concerns (DISC): <http://gbgm-umc.org/DISC/>

Disabilityinfo.gov: Employment: <http://www.disabilityinfo.gov/Employment/>

Disabled Businesspersons Association: <http://www.disabledbusiness.com/>

disABLEDperson.com: RecruitABILITY: <http://www.disabledperson.com/recruitability.asp>

Disability Resources Monthly (DRM): DRM WebWatcher (Subjects): Employment: <http://www.disabilityresources.org/EMPLOYMENT.html>

Equal Employment Opportunity Commission (EEOC): <http://www.eeoc.gov/>

Equal Employment Opportunity Commission (EEOC): The ADA: Questions and Answers: Employment: <http://www.eeoc.gov/facts/adaqa1.html>

Equal Employment Opportunity Commission (EEOC): The ADA: Your Employment Rights as an Individual with a Disability: <http://www.eeoc.gov/facts/ada18.html>

Equip for Equality: Employment Rights: <http://www.equipforequality.org/employment.html>

Exceptional Nurse: <http://www.exceptionalnurse.com/>

Gallaudet University: Deaf, Hard of Hearing, and Hearing Social Workers (DHHHSW): <http://academic.gallaudet.edu/prof/dhhhswweb.nsf>

iCan Online: Employment: For Employers: <http://www.ican.com/channels/employment/for_employers/index.cfm>

Information for Decision Making (IFDM): Welfare Information Network (WIN): <http://www.financeprojectinfo.org/win/>

Job Accommodation Network (JAN): <http://janweb.icdi.wvu.edu/>

National Association of State Work Force Agencies: <http://www.workforceatm.org/>

National Business and Disability Council: <http://www.business-disability.com/>

National Center for Disability Services (NCDS): <http://www.ncds.org/>

National Clearinghouse of Rehabilitation Training Materials (NCRTM): <http://www.nchrtm.okstate.edu/>

National Collaborative on Workforce and Disability for Youth (NCWD): <http://www.ncwd-youth.info/>

Department for Work and Pensions (DWP) (UK): New Deal: <http://www.newdeal.gov.uk/>

Department for Work and Pensions (DWP) (UK): New Deal for Jobseekers: <http://www.newdeal.gov.uk/home_job.asp>

Proyecto Vision: A Bilingual Web Site for Latinos with Disabilities: Bridges to Employment: <http://www.proyectovision.net/english/news/06/>

Protection and Advocacy, Inc.: Employment Rights Under the Americans with Disabilities Act: <http://www.pai-ca.org/pubs/506801.html>

RADAR: Employment: <http://www.radar.org.uk/RANE/Templates/Article1.asp?lHeaderID=121>

Raise-Up.org: Employers' Frequently Asked Questions (FAQ): <http://www.raiseup.org/html/FAQ.php>

Ticket to Work: <http://www.yourtickettowork.com/>

Victoria University of Wellington (New Zealand): Reasonable Accommodations an Introduction: <http://www2.vuw.ac.nz/home/publications/disabilities/>

135. Housing

Recommended Search Terms

- Accessible housing
- "Accessible housing" [with geographic location name, such as state or city]
- Disability housing
- Handicapped housing

Important Sites

ABLEDATA: Informed Consumer's Guide to Accessible Housing: <http://www.abledata.com/Site_2/icg_hous.htm>

ABLEDATA: Resource Center on Accessible Housing and Universal Design: <http://www.abledata.com/Site_2/accessib.htm>

American Civil Liberties Union (ACLU): Disability Rights: Housing: <http://www.aclu.org/DisabilityRights/DisabilityRightslist.cfm?c=73>

Center for Universal Design: <http://www.design.ncsu.edu/cud/>

Department of Housing and Urban Development (HUD): Homes and Commnities: People with Disabilities: <http://www.hud.gov/groups/disabilities.cfm>

Department of Housing and Urban Development (HUD): Informacion en Español: <http://www.hud.gov/directory/800/parainformacion.cfm>

Disabilityinfo.gov: Housing: <http://www.disabilityinfo.gov/Housing/>

HoDis, the National Disabled Persons Housing Services (DPHS) (UK): <http://www.hodis.org.uk/>

Housing and Neighborhood Development Service (HANDS): Housing: <http://www.hands-erie.org/disabilities.htm>

National Accessible Apartment Clearinghouse: <http://www.forrent.com/naac/>

National Housing and Rehabilitation Association (NHandRA): HousingOnline: <http://www.housingonline.com/>

RADAR: Housing: <http://www.radar.org.uk/RANE/Templates/Article1.asp?lHeaderID=33>

136. Independent Living, Community Living, and Home Care

Recommended Search Terms

- Disability "independent living"
- "Independent living"
- "Community living" disabled

Important Sites

Access-Ability (UK): <http://www.access-ability.co.uk/>

Canadian Association for Community Living (CACL): <http://www.cacl.ca/>

Canadian Association of Independent Living Centres (CAILC): <http://www.cailc.ca/>

Center for Independent Living (CIL): <http://www.cilberkeley.org/>

Cornell University: School of Industrial and Labor Relations: Program on Employment and Disability: Independent Living: <http://www.ilr.cornell.edu/ped/il/il.html>

Department of Health and Human Services (DHHS): Independence Plus: <http://cms.hhs.gov/independenceplus/>

Disability: Independent Living: <http://www.ilr.cornell.edu/ped/il/il.html>

Disabled Living Foundation: Solutions for Independent Living: <http://www.dlf.org.uk/>

Digital Federal Credit Union (DFCU): *StreetWise: Resource Guide for Persons with Disabilities*: <http://www.dcu.org/streetwise/ability/>

Disabilityinfo.gov: Community Life: <http://www.disabilityinfo.gov/Community/>

Independent Living Research Utilization (ILRU): <http://www.ilru.org/>

National Organization on Disability: Emergency Preparedness Initiative: EPI Guide for Emergency Managers, Planners and Responders: <http://www.nod.org/cont/dsp_cont_item_view.cfm?viewType=itemView&contentId=1267>

RADAR: Independent Living: <http://www.radar.org.uk/RANE/Templates/Article1.asp?lHeaderID=130>

University of Kansas: Research and Training Center on Independent Living (RTC/IL): <http://rtcil.org/>

137. LEGAL, INSURANCE, SOCIAL SECURITY, AND INCOME SUPPORT

Recommended Search Terms

- "Civil rights" disabled
- Disabilities discrimination
- Disabilities laws
- Disabilities "legal assistance"
- Disabilities rights
- Disability "equal opportunity"
- Disability "income support"
- Disability insurance
- Disability law
- Disability "legal resources"
- Disabled "social security"
- Discrimination ADA
- Guardianship
- "Legal guardian"

Important Sites

American Civil Liberties Union (ACLU): Disability Rights: Americans with Disabilities Act of 1990: <http://www.aclu.org/DisabilityRights/DisabilityRightslist.cfm?c=69>

American Civil Liberties Union (ACLU): Disability Rights: Discrimination: <http://www.aclu.org/DisabilityRights/DisabilityRightslist.cfm?c=70>

The Arc: Future Planning/Guardianship/Trusts: <http://www.thearc.org/futureplanning.html>

ARCH: A Legal Resource Center for Persons with Disabilities (Canada): <http://www.arch-online.org/>

Department of Justice: Americans With Disabilities Act (ADA): <http://www.ada.gov/>

Australian Human Rights and Equal Opportunity Commission: Disability Rights: <http://www.humanrights.gov.au/disability_rights/>

Department of Health (UK): Caring about Carers: <http://www.carers.gov.uk/>

Disability Alliance: <http://www.disabilityalliance.org/>

Department of Labor (DOL): Employment Standards Administration: Office of Federal Contract Compliance Program: Vietnam Era Veterans' Readjustment Assistance Act (VEVRAA) of 1974: <http://www.dol.gov/esa/regs/compliance/ofccp/fsvevraa.htm>

Disability Rights Commission (UK): <http://www.drc-gb.org/>

Disabilityinfo.gov: Civil Rights: <http://www.disabilityinfo.gov/Civil/>

Disabilityinfo.gov: Income Support: <http://www.disabilityinfo.gov/Income/>

Equal Employment Opportunities Commission (EEOC): Enforcement Guidance: Reasonable Accommodation and Undue Hardship under the Americans with Disabilities Act: <http://www.eeoc.gov/docs/accommodation.html>

Equal Employment Opportunities Commission (EEOC): Federal Laws Prohibiting Job Discrimination: Questions and Answers: <http://www.eeoc.gov/facts/qanda.html>

Independent Living Research Utilization (ILRU): Disability Law Resource Project (DLRP): <http://www.ilru.org/dbtac/>

Internet Resources for Special Children (IRSC): Americans with Disabilities Act (ADA): <http://www.irsc.org/>

Internet Resources for Special Children (IRSC): Laws: <http://www.irsc.org/>

Internet Resources for Special Children (IRSC): Legal Assistance: <http://www.irsc.org/>

National Council on Disability: <http://www.ncd.gov/>

National Guardianship Association: <http://www.guardianship.org/>

Nolo: Law for All: Law Centers: Disability Discrimination FAQ: <http://www.nolo.com/lawcenter/faqs/detail.cfm/objectID/CA070A04-AA25-410C-9532C76CCFECAF57>

Nolo: Law for All: Law Centers: Encyclopedia: Employment Law: <http://www.nolo.com/encyclopedia/emp_ency.html>

Planned Lifetime Advocacy Network (PLAN): Family Resource Guide: <http://www.plan.ca/plan_frg/frg.htm>

RADAR: Health and Social Services: <http://www.radar.org.uk/RANE/Templates/Article1.asp?lHeaderID=211>

RADAR: Legal: <http://www.radar.org.uk/RANE/Templates/Article1.asp?lHeaderID=104>

RADAR: Rights Now: <http://www.radar.org.uk/RANE/Templates/Article1.asp?lHeaderID=92>

RADAR: Social Security: <http://www.radar.org.uk/RANE/Templates/Article1.asp?lHeaderID=115>

Rocky Mountain Disability and Business Technical Assistance Center: *ADA Quiz Book*, 3rd ed.: <http://www.ada-infonet.org/training/quizbook/>

Special Educational Needs and Disability Act 2001 (UK): <http://www.hmso.gov.uk/acts/acts2001/20010010.htm>

Social Security Administration: Benefits for Children with Disabilities: <http://www.ssa.gov/pubs/10026.html>

Social Security Association (SSA): Disability Programs: <http://www.ssa.gov/disability/>

Social Security Association (SSA): Medical/Professional Relations: *Disability Evaluation under Social Security: Blue Book*—January 2003: <http://www.ssa.gov/disability/professionals/bluebook/Contents.htm>

Social Security Association (SSA): Medical/Professional Relations: *Disability Evaluation under Social Security: Blue Book*: Listing of Impairments: Adult Listings (Part A): <http://www.ssa.gov/disability/professionals/bluebook/AdultListings.htm>

Social Security Association (SSA): Medical/Professional Relations: *Disability Evaluation under Social Security: Blue Book*: Listing of Impairments: Childhood Listings (Part B): <http://www.ssa.gov/disability/professionals/bluebook/ChildhoodListings.htm>

U.K.: Special Educational Needs and Disability Act 2001: <http://www.hmso.gov.uk/acts/acts2001/20010010.htm>

U.S. Department of Justice, Civil Rights Division, Disability Rights Section: ADA Information Services: <http://www.usdoj.gov/crt/ada/agency.htm>

Welfare Information Network: <http://www.financeprojectinfo.org/win/>

138. LIFESTYLE CHANGE AND TRANSITIONS

[*See also* "Living with a Chronic Illness," p. 67.]

Recommended Search Terms

- Disability lifestyle "positive adjustment"
- Disability "positive adjustment"
- Disability readjustment
- Disability therapy adjustment
- Disabled "change my life" -insurance
- Disabled counseling adjustment
- Disabled "life change" -insurance
- Disabled lifestyle transition
- Disabled "positive adjustment"
- Disabled readjustment
- Disabled "social adjustment"

Important Sites

Celebration of Wheels: <http://lenmac.tripod.com/>

Cornell University: School of Industrial and Labor Relations: Program on Employment and Disability: Transition from School to Adult Life: <http://www.ilr.cornell.edu/ped/tsal/tsal.html>

U.S. Department of Education: ED.gov: Office for Civil Rights: Students with Disabilities Preparing for Postsecondary Education: <http://www.ed.gov/ocr/transition.html>

Liverpool Trauma Website (Australia): Adjustment to Disability: <http://www.swsahs.nsw.gov.au/livtrauma/public/psycho/adjustment.asp>

Look on the Bright Side Dot Com: <http://www.lookonthebrightside.com/>

National Educational Association of Disabled Students (NEADS)/Association nationale des étudiant(e)s handicapé (e)s au niveau postsecondaire: Moving On: <http://www.neads.ca/movingon/>

National Information Center for Children and Youth with Disabilities (NICHCY): Transition Guides: <http://www.nichcy.org/transitn.asp>

Post-Polio Support: Stages of psychological adjustment to disability: <http://www.postpoliosupport.com/0120%20-%20Stages%20of%20Psychological%20Development%20to%20Disability.pdf>

Scottish Executive: Care and Social Work: Interchange 75: Children's Experiences of Disability: A Positive Outlook: <http://www.scotland.gov.uk/library5/health/ic75-00.asp>

139. MOBILITY

[*See also* "Transportation and Travel," p. 95.]

Recommended Search Terms

- "Adaptive vehicles"
- "Adaptive driving"
- Disability mobility
- Mobility ability ".org"
- "Wheelchair vans"
- "Van conversions"

Important Sites

Ability (UK): Guide Dogs: <http://www.ability.org.uk/Guide_Dogs.html>

AbilityHub: Vehicles and Travel Websites: <http://www.abilityhub.com/links/transportation.htm>

Adaptive Driving Alliance: <http://www.adamobility.com/>

Disability Resource Center (The Boulevard): <http://www.blvd.com/>

Disabled Dealer Magazine: <http://www.disableddealer.com/>

Disabled Drivers Association (DDA) (UK): <http://www.dda.org.uk/>

Laterlife.com: Mobility, Disability, Arthritis, Back Pain, Making Life Easier in Later Life (UK): <http://www.mobility-disability.co.uk/>

New Mobility Magazine: <http://www.newmobility.com/>

Digital Federal Credit Union (DFCU): *StreetWise: Resource Guide for Persons with Disabilities*: Negotiating Tips for Buying or Leasing an Adaptive Vehicle or Accessories: <http://www.dcu.org/streetwise/ability/auto-tips.html>

140. PARENTING

NOTE: "Parenting" is a guide to finding information for disabled parents. For information on children with disabilities, see "Children with Disabilities," p. 85.

Recommended Search Terms

- Disabilities parenting
- Disability "single parents"
- Disabled "lone parents"

Important Sites

Coordinating Council on Juvenile Justice and Delinquency Prevention (OJJDP): Parenting Resources for the 21st Century: Health and Safety: Special Circumstances: Disabilities: <http://www.parentingresources.ncjrs.org/health/disabilities.html>

Disability Cool: Parenting: Parents with Disabilities: <http://www.geocities.com/HotSprings/7319/parent.htm>

Disability Resources Monthly (DRM): DRM WebWatcher (Subjects): Parents with Disabilities: <http://www.disabilityresources.org/PARENTS-WITH.html>

Disabled Parents Network (UK): <http://www.disabledparentsnetwork.org.uk/>

Infinitec: Parenting with a Disability: <http://www.infinitec.org/live/parenting/parenting.htm>

National Family and Parenting Institute (NFPI): Disabled Parents: <http://www.nfpi.org/disabledparents/>

National Women's Health Information Center: 4woman.gov: Women with Disabilities: Parenting and Disabilities: <http://www.4woman.gov/wwd/wwd.cfm?page=70>

Parents with Disabilities Online (Parent Empowerment Network): <http://www.disabledparents.net/>

Project STAR: Parents with Disabilities Program: <http://trfn.clpgh.org/star/>

Special Needs Family Fun and Family Friendly Fun: Disabled parents: <http://www.family-friendly-fun.com/links/disabledparents.html>

Through the Looking Glass: <http://www.lookingglass.org/>

141. PERSONAL PROTECTION, SAFETY, AND AWARENESS

[*See also* "Personal Safety and Domestic Violence," p. 20.]

Recommended Search Terms

- Disabilities "sexual violence"
- Disabilities rape
- Disabilities violence
- Disability abuse
- Disability abuse prevention
- Disabled "self defense"
- Disabled "crime prevention"
- Disabled stalking
- Disabled victim

Important Sites

AdvocateWeb: <http://www.advocateweb.org/>

All Walks of Life (AWOL): <http://www.awol-texas.org/>

All Walks of Life (AWOL): National Organization for Victim Assistance (NOVA) Report: Victim Assistance: Working with Victims of Crime with Disabilities: <http://www.awol-texas.org/articles/article7.html>

Baylor College of Medicine: Center for Research on Women with Disabilities (CROWD): Abuse and Women with Disabilities: <http://www.bcm.tmc.edu/crowd/abuse_women/abuse_women.html>

California Abortion and Reproduction Rights Action League (CARAL): Research Center: Women with Disabilities: <http://www.choice.org/researchcenter/disabilities.html>

City of Fullerton, California: Crime Prevention Tips for the Disabled: <http://www.ci.fullerton.ca.us/police/tips/crimeprv.html>

Deaf Abused Woman Warrior's Web Network (DAWWWN): <http://members.tripod.com/~Deaf-Deb/>

Department of Justice (DOJ): Office on Violence against Women: <http://www.ojp.usdoj.gov/vawo/>

Family Violence against Women with Disabilities (Canada): <http://www.hc-sc.gc.ca/hppb/family violence/html/femdisab_e.html>

International Disabled Self-Defense Association (IDSA): <http://www.defenseability.com/>

National Women's Health Information Center: 4woman .gov: Women with Disabilities: Abuse of People with Disabilities: <http://www.4woman.gov/wwd/wwd.cfm ?page=24>

Violence against Women Online Resources (VAWOR): Abuse and Women with Disabilities: <http://www.vaw .umn.edu/Vawnet/disab.htm>

The Zero: Official Website of Andrew Vachss: Disabled Abuse Resources: <http://www.vachss.com/help_text/ disabled_abuse.html>

142. SEXUALITY

Recommended Search Terms

- Disability intimacy
- Disability sex -xxx -porn -pornography
- Disability "sexual expression"
- Disability sexuality
- Disabled sex -xxx -porn -pornography
- Disabled "sexual expression"
- Disabled "sexual intimacy"
- Disabled sexuality

Important Sites

Baylor College of Medicine: Center for Research on Women with Disabilities (CROWD): <http://www .bcm.tmc.edu/crowd/>

Disability and Sexuality: <http://www.gimpsex.org/>

Disability Cool: Sexuality 'R Us: <http://www.geocities .com/HotSprings/7319/sex.htm>

Disability Online (Australia): Condom for Women—Safe Sex and Contraception: <http://www.disability.vic .gov.au/dsonline/dsarticles.nsf/pages/Condom_for_wo men_safe_sex_and_contraception?OpenDocument>

Disability Resources Monthly (DRM): DRM WebWatcher (Subjects): Sexuality and Disability: <http://www .disabilityresources.org/SEX.html>

Nerve: Special Issue: Sex and Disability: <http://www .nerve.com/SpecialIssues/sexAndDisability/>

Sexual Health and Fertility after Brain and Spinal Cord Impairment: <http://www.scisexualhealth.com/>

Sexual Health Network, Inc.: Sexual Health: <http://www .sexualhealth.com/>

Sexuality Resources and Toys for Disabled Adults (Australia): <http://www.achievableconcepts.com.au/sex _front.htm>

Sexuality Resources and Toys for Disabled Adults (USA): <http://www.achievableconcepts.com/usa_sex_front .htm>

Sexuality Information and Education Council of the United States (SIECUS): Annotated Bibliographies: Sexuality and Disability: <http://www.siecus.org/pubs/ biblio/bibs0009.html>

Youth Information.com: Family and Relationships: Love and Sex: Sexual Expression: <http://www.youth information.com/infopage.asp?snID=528>

143. STATISTICS

Recommended Search Terms

- Disabilities "most common" ".gov"
- Disability statistics ".gov"
- Disability statistics ".org"
- Disabled statistics ".gov"
- Disabled statistics ".org"

Important Sites

AbilityLinks.org: Disability Employment Statistics: <http://www.abilitylinks.org/default.asp?parent id=140>

bridges4kids.org! Education and Disability-related Statistics: <http://www.bridges4kids.org/Stats.html>

Bureau of the Census: Disabilities Affect One-Fifth of All Americans: <http://www.census.gov/prod/3/97pubs/ cenbr975.pdf>

Bureau of the Census: Disability: <http://www.census.gov/ hhes/www/disability.html>

Bureau of the Census: Population Profiles: Disability: <http://www.census.gov/population/www/pop-profile/ disabil.html>

Canadian Council on Social Development: Disability Research Information Page (DRIP): <http://www.ccsd .ca/drip/>

Cornucopia of Disability Information (CODI): Statistics: <http://codi.buffalo.edu/statistics.html>

Disability Resources Monthly (DRM): DRM WebWatcher (Subjects): Statistics: <http://www.disabilityresources .org/STATISTICS.html>

DisabilityInfo.gov: Community Life: Disability Statistics: <http://www.disabilityinfo.gov/Community/47/>

DisabilityInfo.gov: Health: Disability Statistics: <http:// www.disabilityinfo.gov/Health/1111/>

Google Directory: Society: Disabled: Statistics: <http:// directory.google.com/Top/Society/Disabled/Statistics/>

Internet Resources for Special Children (IRSC): News, Media and Statistics: Statistics: <http://www.irsc .org/>

National Center for Health Statistics (NCHS): Classification of Diseases, Functioning, and Disability: <http://www.cdc.gov/nchs/icd9.htm>

National Center for Health Statistics (NCHS): National Health Interview Survey on Disability (NHIS-D): <http://www.cdc.gov/nchs/about/major/nhis_dis/nhis_dis.htm>

National Center for Health Statistics (NCHS): FastStats A to Z: Disabilities/Impairments: <http://www.cdc.gov/nchs/fastats/disable.htm>

National Center for the Dissemination of Disability Research (NCDDR): <http://www.ncddr.org/>

National Institute on Disability and Rehabilitation Research: Access to Disability Data: An InfoUse Project: <http://www.infouse.com/disabilitydata/>

Sociometrics: Data Archives: Research Archive on Disability in the United States (RADIUS): <http://www.socio.com/data_arc/radius_0.htm>

United Nations Statistics Division: <http://unstats.un.org/unsd/>

University of California, San Francisco: Disability Statistics Center: <http://dsc.ucsf.edu/>

International Center for Disability Information: Disability Tables: <http://www.icdi.wvu.edu/disability/tables.html>

Workwithus.org (Scotland): Disability Statistics: <http://www.workwithus.org/charities-scotland/disability/disability-statistics.htm>

144. ADAPTIVE OR ASSISTIVE TECHNOLOGIES

[*See also* "Internet Access for Persons with Disabilities," vol. 1, p. 12.]

Recommended Search Terms

- Adaptive engineering
- "Adaptive technologies"
- "Adaptive technology"
- "Assistive technologies"
- "Assistive technology"
- Disabilities technologies
- Disabilities technology
- Disabled technologies
- Disabled technology
- Handicapped technology
- Rehabilitation engineering
- Rehabilitation technology

Important Sites

Ability Hub: Assistive Technology Solutions: <http://www.abilityhub.com/>

Ability Resources, Inc.: <http://ability-resources.org/>

Alliance for Technology Access: The Alliance for Technology Access: <http://www.ataccess.org/>

American Library Association (ALA): Products and Publications: Adaptive Technology for the Internet: Making Electronic Resources Accessible to All (The Online Version): <http://www.ala.org/editions/openstacks/insidethecovers/mates/mates_toc.html>

Accessibility Forum: <http://www.accessibilityforum.org/>

University of Washington: AccessIT: National Center on Accessible Information Technology in Education: <http://www.washington.edu/accessit/>

Americans with Disabilities Act (ADA) and IT: Technical Assistance Centers: ADA Technical Assistance Program: <http://www.adata.org/>

AssistiveTech.net: <http://www.assistivetech.net/>

California State University, Northridge: Center On Disabilities: <http://www.csun.edu/cod/>

Centre for Educational Technology Interoperability Standards (CETIS): <http://www.cetis.ac.uk/>

Digital Federal Credit Union (DFCU): *StreetWise: Resource Guide for Persons with Disabilities*: Adaptive Computing: <http://www.dcu.org/streetwise/ability/computing-index.html>

Disability Equipment Register: <http://dialspace.dial.pipex.com/town/square/ae208/>

Disabilityinfo.gov: Technology: <http://www.disabilityinfo.gov/Technology/>

Disability Resources Monthly (DRM): DRM WebWatcher (Subjects): Assistive Technology: <http://www.disabilityresources.org/AT.html>

Equal Access to Software and Information (EASI): <http://www.rit.edu/~easi/>

Federal Communications Commission (FCC): Consumer and Governmental Affairs Bureau: Disabilities Issues: <http://www.fcc.gov/cgb/dro/>

Federal Communications Commission (FCC): Consumer and Governmental Affairs Bureau: Disabilities Issues: Section 255: <http://www.fcc.gov/cgb/dro/section255.html>

Georgia Institute of Technology: Center for Assistive Technology and Environmental Access: Information Technology and Technical Assistance Training Center (ITTATC): <http://www.ittatc.org/>

Google Directory: Society: Disabled: Assistive Technology: <http://directory.google.com/Top/Society/Disabled/Assistive_Technology/>

Oklahoma ABLE Tech: <http://okabletech.okstate.edu/>

Rehabilitation Engineering and Assistive Technology Society of North American (RESNA): <http://www.resna.org/>

Rehabilitation, Research and Training Center (RRTC): Health and Wellness Consortium: <http://www.healthwellness.org/>

95

Living with a Disability

U.S. Department of Agriculture (USDA) TARGET Center: <http://www.usda.gov/oo/target.htm>
Smart Thinking: <http://www.usda.gov/oo/target/>
TechDis (UK): <http://www.techdis.ac.uk/>
University of Wisconsin, Madison: College of Engineering: Trace Center: <http://www.tracecenter.org/>
UsableNet: Website Testing Systems: <http://www.usable net.com/>
World Association for Persons with Disabilities (WAPD): Assistive Device Lab: <http://www.wapd.org/assistive/>

145. Transportation and Travel

[*See also* "Moblility," p. 91.]

Recommended Search Terms

- Accommodation "public transit"
- Accessible "public transit"
- Disability "public transit"
- Disabled "public transit"
- Accommodation "transit authority"
- Accessible "transit authority"
- Disability "transit authority"
- Disabled "transit authority"
- Accommodation holiday
- Accessible holiday
- Disability holiday
- Disabled holiday
- Accommodation travel
- Accessible travel
- Disability travel
- Disabled travel
- Accommodation transportion
- Accessible transportion
- Disability transportion
- Disabled transportion
- Accommodation vacation
- Accessible vacation
- Disability vacation
- Disabled vacation

Important Sites

AbilityHub: Vehicles/Travel Websites: <http://www.ability hub.com/links/transportation.htm>
Action for Leisure (UK): <http://www.actionforleisure.org.uk/>
British Broadcasting Corporation (BBC): Lifestyle: Disabled Traveler (UK): <http://www.bbc.co.uk/holiday/disabled_traveller/>
Digital Federal Credit Union (DFCU): *StreetWise: Resource Guide for Persons with Disabilities*: <http://www.dcu.org/streetwise/ability/>

Disabilityinfo.gov: Transportation: <http://www.disability info.gov/Transportation/>
Easter Seals: Project ACTION (Accessible Community Transportation in Our Nation): <http://projectaction.easter-seals.org/site/PageServer?pagename=ESPA _homepage>
Equip for Equality: Public Transportation Issues: <http://www.equipforequality.org/headerg.html>
Google Directory: Society: Disabled: Travel: <http://directory.google.com/Top/Society/Disabled/Travel/>
HalfthePlanet: <http://halftheplanet.org/>
Moss Rehab Resource Net: Accessible Travel: <http://www.mossresourcenet.org/travel.htm>
National Information Center for Children and Youth with Disabilities (NICHCY): Travel Training for Youth with Disabilities: <http://www.nichcy.org/pubs/transum/ts9 txt.htm>
RADAR: Holiday Accommodation Website: <http://www.radarsearch.org/>
RADAR: Transport: <http://www.radar.org.uk/RANE/Templates/Article1.asp?lHeaderID=125>

146. Women with Disabilities

Recommended Search Terms

- Girl disability -xxx -porn -pornography
- Woman [name of a specific disability]
- Woman disabilities
- Woman disabilities "self esteem"
- Woman disabilities "sexual safety"
- Woman disabled -xxx -porn -pornography
- Woman handicapped -xxx -porn -pornography
- Women [name of a specific disability]
- Women disability
- Women disabled -xxx -porn -pornography
- Woman handicapped -xxx -porn -pornography
- Woman handicapped "sexual safety"

Important Sites

ABLED! Woman: <http://abledwomen.org/>
Baylor College of Medicine: Center for Research on Women with Disabilities (CROWD): <http://www.bcm.tmc.edu/crowd/>
Breast Health Access for Women with Disabilities (BHAWD): <http://www.bhawd.com/>
Center for Research on Women with Disabilities (CROWD): National Study on Women with Physical Disabilities: <http://www.bcm.tmc.edu/crowd/national_study/national_study.html>
Disabled Women's Network (DAWN) Canada: <http://www.dawncanada.net/>
GimpGirl Community: <http://www.gimpgirl.com/>

LadyAmp.com for the Woman Amputee: <http://ladyamp .netfirms.com/>

National Women's Health Information Center: 4woman .gov: Women with Disabilities: <http://www.4woman .gov/wwd/>

National Women's Health Information Center: 4woman .gov: Women with Disabilities: Parenting and Disabilities: <http://www.4woman.gov/wwd/wwd.cfm?page= 70>

Women with Disabilities Australia (WWDA): <http://www .wwda.org.au/>

DISABILITY HOTLINES

NOTE: Many businesses and organizations of general interest will have a special phone line or TDD TTY line to use in lieu of voice lines. Their Web sites or advertising materials often list these numbers as a "disability hotline". A search for hotlines will therefore retrieve large numbers of phone numbers for companies who would love to sell something. If you have a specific organization or topic in mind, it is best to combine that with the recommended search strings.

Recommended Search Terms

- Disabilities hotlines
- Disability hotline
- TDD [use with another more specific subject term, or business or organization name]
- TTY [use with another more specific subject term, or business or organization name]
- "V/TDD"
- "V/TTY"
- "Voice/TDD"
- "Voice/TTY"

Online Directories

Blue Pages (U.S. Federal Government): <http://bp.fed .gov/>

Federal TTY Directory: <http://www.pueblo.gsa.gov/cic _text/misc/ustdd/tty.htm>

HUD 800 Numbers: <http://www.hud.gov/directory/800/ 800num1.cfm>

HOTLINES

ABLEDATA: National Database of Assistive Technology: 1-800-272-0216

Canadian Association for Community Living (CACL): 1-800-856-2207; (416) 661-5701 (Fax); (416) 661-2023 (TTY)

Dial UK: 01302 310123

Equal Employment Opportunity Commission (EEOC): 1-800-669-4000; 1-800-669-6820 (TDD)

HEATH: The National Clearinghouse on Postsecondary Education for Individuals with Disabilities: 1-800-544-3284

Housing and Urban Development (HUD): 1-800-245-2691

Housing and Urban Development (HUD): Information en Español: 1-800-685-8470

Job Accommodation Network: 1-800-526-7234 (V/TTY)

National Organization on Disability: (202) 293-5960, or e-mail: <ability@nod.org>

National Information Center for Children and Youth with Disabilities (English/Spanish): 1-800-695-0285 (TTY); (202) 884-8441 (Fax), or e-mail: <nichcy@aed.org>

National Institute on Deafness: 1-800-241-1044; 1-800-241-1055 (TDD)

Office of Disabled American Veterans Affairs: 1-800-827-1000

SpecialLink (National Centre for Child Care Inclusion) (Canada): 1-800-840-LINK; (902) 562-1662; (902) 539-9117 (Fax)

Supplemental Security Income for the Disabled: 1-800-772-1213

U.S. Access Board: 1-800-872-2253

FAQs

Best General Disability FAQs

Disability Resources Monthly (DRM): The FAQ Page: <http://www.disabilityresources.org/DRMfaq.html>

Disability Resources Monthly (DRM): The FAQ Page: Alphabet Soup: Disability-Related Acronyms: <http:// www.disabilityresources.org/ABC.html>

Examples of Special Disability Topic FAQs

AbleProject.org: Frequently Asked Questions: <http:// www.ableproject.org/ableproject/company/faq.asp>

Boston Public Library: Higher Education Information Center (HEIC): Financial Aid FAQs for Disabled: <http://www.heic.org/disabled.htm>

Council for Disability Rights (CDR): The Americans with Disabilities Act (ADA): Civil Rights for People with Disabilities: <http://www.disabilityrights.org/adatoc .htm>

Council for Disability Rights (CDR): The CDR Guide to Disability Rights: <http://www.disabilityrights.org/faq .htm>

Department for Work and Pensions (DWP) (UK): Disability: Frequently Asked Questions: <http://www.disability.gov.uk/faq.htm>

Department of Labor (DOL): Employment and Training Administration: disAbility Online: Frequently-Asked Questions: <http://wdsc.doleta.gov/disability/faq.cfm>

Disability Resources Monthly (DRM): Regional Resources Directory (States): <http://www.disabilityresources.org/DRMreg.html>

Disability Resources Monthly (DRM): Librarian's Connections: <http://www.disabilityresources.org/DRMlibs.html>

Disability Rights Commission (UK): Frequently Asked Questions: <http://www.drc-gb.org/whatwedo/faqs.asp>

Educational Testing Service (ETS): Disabilities and Testing: Frequently Asked Questions: <http://www.ets.org/disability/faq.html>

U.S. Equal Employment Opportunity Commission (EEOC): Federal Laws Prohibiting Job Discrimination Questions and Answers: <http://www.eeoc.gov/facts/qanda.html>

National Information Center for Children and Youth with Disabilities (NICHCY): Frequently Asked Questions: <http://www.nichcy.org/faqs.htm>

National Organization of Social Security Claimants' Representatives (NOSSCR): Social Security Disability: Frequently Asked Questions: <http://www.nosscr.org/faqind.html>

Raise-Up: Employers' Frequently Asked Questions: <http://www.raiseup.org/html/FAQ.php>

PUBLICATIONS ON THE INTERNET ABOUT DISABILITIES OR FOR PERSONS WITH DISABILITIES

NOTE: This topic area has an unusually large number of publications available both in print and online, as well as several excellent publications that are electronic only. This is a small sampling of the titles available that are of general interest; for professionals; for specific age groups, specific disabilities, or other special interests; and indicative of the unusual range of topics available. Also included are special theme issues in publications with a broader scope. Chances are fairly good that if you have a special interest not shown here and search for that topic with a selection of words like "newsletter," "journal," or "magazine," you will find something relevant.

Abilities (Canadian Abilities Foundation): <http://www.abilities.ca/>

Access Board: Access Currents: <http://www.access-board.gov/news/Access%20Currents/General.htm>

American Academy of Orthotists and Prosthetists: *Journal of Prosthetics and Orthotics*: JPO Online Library: <http://www.oandp.org/jpo/>

American Civil Liberties Union (ACLU): Briefing Paper #21 on Disabilities Rights: <http://www.aclu.org/DisabilityRights/DisabilityRights.cfm?ID=9474&c=18>

The Boulevard: Accent on Living Magazine: <http://www.blvd.com/accent/>

Deaf Magazine: <http://www.deaf-magazine.org/>

Deaf Queer Resource Center: FLASH: <http://www.deafqueer.org/ctnmagazine/FLASH/>

Department of Veterans Affairs (VA): VA Rehabilitation Research and Development Service: *Journal of Rehabilitation Research and Development* (*JRRD*): <http://www.vard.org/jour/jourindx.htm>

Disability Central: *ActiveTeen*: <http://www.disabilitycentral.com/>

Disability Now: <http://www.disabilitynow.org.uk/news.htm>

Disability Resources Monthly (DRM): <http://www.disabilityresources.org/>

E-bility: <http://ebility.com/>

Enabled Online: <http://www.enabledonline.com/>

Equip for Equality: Equalizer Online: <http://www.equipforequality.org/equalizer/>

European League of Stuttering Associations (ELSA): *The Voice of ELSA* (Newsletter): <http://www.mmedia.is/~benben/ELSA/voe/voice.html>

Exceptional Parent: *EP Magazine*: <http://www.eparent.com/>

Manifesto (Institute on Disability Culture): The Latest Manifesto: <http://www.dimenet.com/disculture/manifesto/>

Mouth Magazine: Voice of the Disability Nation: <http://www.mouthmag.com/>

National Center for the Dissemination of Disability Research (NCDDR): Brochures and Posters: <http://www.ncddr.org/du/products/bp.html>

National Center for the Dissemination of Disability Research (NCDDR): Research Exchange Newsletter: <http://www.ncddr.org/du/researchexchange/>

National Stuttering Association: Letting Go (Newsletter): <http://www.nsastutter.org/lettinggo.html>

New Mobility: <http://www.newmobility.com/>

Paralinks Electronic Magazine: <http://www.paralinks.net/>

PN/Paraplegia News: <http://www.sportsnspokes.com/pn/library.htm>

Ragged Edge Magazine Online (The Disability Rag): <http://www.ragged-edge-mag.com/>

Reach Out Magazine: <http://www.reachoutmag.com/>

Research and Practice for Persons with Severe Disabilities: <http://www.tash.org/publications/jash/>

Ricability (UK): <http://www.ricability.org.uk/>
Special Child: For Parents of Children with Disabilities: <http://www.specialchild.com/>
Sports 'N' Spokes Magazine: <http://www.pvamagazines .com/sns/>
Vanier Institute of the Family: *Transition Magazine*: Back Issues: Families Living with Disability: <http://www.vi family.ca/library/transition/321/321.html>

MEDICAL SPECIALTIES

NOTE: Virtually every medical specialty in existence serves persons with disabilities but certain specialties have a greater focus on the special needs of persons with disabilities. This list is highly selective, not comprehensive, and may not include the medical specialty most relevant to your interests.

Kinesiology; Occupational medicine; Orthotics; Physiatrics; Physical medicine; Prosthetics; Rehabilitation; Rehabilitation engineering; Rehabilitation medicine; Vocational rehabilitation

PROFESSIONAL ORGANIZATIONS

American Academy of Physical and Rehabilitation Medicine (AAPMR): <http://www.aapmr.org/>
American Congress of Rehabilitation Medicine (ACRM): <http://www.acrm.org/>
Association of Medical Professional with Hearing Losses (AMPHL): <http://www.amphl.org/>
Association of Rehabilitation Nurses: <http://www.rehab nurse.org/>
International Association for the Scientific Study of Intellectual Disabilities (IASSID): <http://www.iassid.org/>
National Rehabilitation Association: <http://www.national rehab.org/>
Rehabilitation Engineering and Assistive Technology Society of North American (RESNA): <http://www.resna .org/>
Rehabilitation International: <http://www.rehab -international.org/>

PATIENT SUPPORT ORGANIZATIONS/ DISCUSSION GROUPS

NOTE: There are an almost infinite number of these. You may wish to search for support groups, discussion groups, or mailing lists for a specific topic or browse the collections of support groups listed in "Tools and Support: Where to Ask Questions." p. 147, vol. 1.

American Association of People with Disabilities (AAPD): <http://www.aapd.com/>
American Disability Association: <http://www.adanet .org/>

American Self-Help Group Clearinghouse: <http://www .selfhelpgroups.org/>
Directory of UK Self Help Groups and Support Organisations: <http://www.doctor.gp/help/>
Disability Forum: <http://handicap.bfn.org/>
Disability Resources Monthly (DRM): The DRM Web-Watcher (Subjects): Listservs: <http://www.disability resources.org/LISTSERVS.html>
Easter Seals: <http://www.easter-seals.org/>
Everyday Warriors: <http://www.everydaywarriors.com/>
Google Directory: Health: Support Groups: Disability: <http://directory.google.com/Top/Health/Support _Groups/Disability/>
Google Directory: Society: Disabled: <http://directory .google.com/Top/Society/Disabled/>
New Horizons Unlimited, Inc.: <http://www.new-horizons .org/>
Open Directory Project (DMOZ): Society: Disabled: Mailing Lists: <http://dmoz.org/Society/Disabled/Mailing _Lists/>
People with disAbilities in Today's World: <http://www .geocities.com/pwdliny/>
Support Central: <http://members.tripod.com/~Koko Baby/supportcentral.html>
Women with Disabilities Australia (WWDA): <http://www .wwda.org.au/>
World Association of Persons with Disabilities (WAPD) [Multilingual]: <http://www.wapd.org/>

BEST ONE-STOP SHOPS

American Disability Association (ADA): <http://www .adanet.org/>
Americans with Disabilities Act (ADA) Home Page: <http://www.ada.gov/>
American Disability Association (ADA): Information Center for the Mid-Atlantic Region: <http://www.adainfo .org/>
British Broadcasting Corporation (BBC): Ouch!: <http:// www.bbc.co.uk/ouch/>
British Broadcasting Corporation (BBC): Watchdog: Guides to: Disability: <http://www.bbc.co.uk/ watchdog/guides_to/disability/>
Cornucopia of Disability Information (CODI): <http:// codi.buffalo.edu/>
Dial UK: Disability Information and Advice Line Network: <http://www.dialuk.org.uk/>
Disability Information Services: <http://www.a-z.org/dis/>
Disabilityinfo.gov: <http://www.disabilityinfo.gov/>
Disability Resources Monthly (DRM): <http://www .disabilityresources.org/>
Google Directory: Society: Disabled: <http://directory .google.com/Top/Society/Disabled/>
Half the Planet: <http://halftheplanet.org/>

healthfinder: Health Library: Prevention and Wellness: Disabilities: <http://www.healthfinder.gov/scripts/SearchContext.asp?topic=246&super=112&Branch=5>

Job Accommodation Network (JAN): <http://janweb.icdi.wvu.edu/>

Library of Congress: National Library Service for the Blind and Physically Handicapped (NLS): <http://lcweb.loc.gov/nls/>

MedlinePlus: Amputees: <http://www.nlm.nih.gov/medlineplus/amputees.html>

MedlinePlus: Disabilities: <http://www.nlm.nih.gov/medlineplus/disabilities.html>

National Organization on Disability: <http://www.nod.org/>

The National Rehabilitation Information Center (NARIC): <http://www.naric.com/>

Royal Association for Disability and Rehabilitation (RADAR) (UK): <http://www.radar.org.uk/>

Youreable.com (UK): <http://www.yourable.com/>

References

1. For an example of such a debate, see Snow, Randy. "Timeout: The G-Word." Sports 'N' Spokes. (2002, June). Retrieved February 22, 2003, from <http://www.sportsnspokes.com/sns/Articles/06.02/Timeout.htm>.

Part X: Pain and Pain Management

P. F. Anderson

[*See also* "Tools and Support," p. 133, vol. 1; "Living with a Chronic Illness," p. 67; "Cancers," p. 12, vol. 2.]

Special Searching Issues for This Topic

The treatment of the concept of pain is unusual in health information searching in that there is little variety in the terms used to describe the concept. Most people seem to agree that pain is pain is pain, and that there is only one way in English to spell the word. This makes searching both easier and harder. It is easier because you do not need a lot of different words to describe the idea, and you do not need to try a host of terms to find more information. The downside is that it is harder is to avoid retrieving irrelevant materials. For example, a search in Google for just the word "pain"[1] retrieves, among the top

10 results, a horror magazine and a computer technology resource.

Much of the most helpful information about resources for locating help or standards for how pain should be managed come from government and nonprofit organizations. To focus a search more towards these types of resources (government or nonprofit sources), you may wish to add to your search string either (but not both) of the following two search strings:

- ".gov"
- ".org"

Unfortunately, these strategies would limit finding much of the excellent information about support groups, personal experience, and coping that are located on commercial servers or inexpensive Web provider services such as AOL, Geocities, or Yahoo. These resources can be more difficult to find with a search engine, and it can be very difficult to tell from search engine listings which of these are helpful and which are simply a tale someone is telling in which pain plays a part, for example, someone's diary of a bad toothache.

For such resources, or as a general starting strategy, you would want to begin with the links mentioned in this chapter, or go to collections of links or resources to see what has been reviewed and chosen as quality resources. A good strategy would be to begin by exploring the links listed under "Best One-Stop Shops" for pain information. These sources contain excellent information about the resources available to prevent patients from suffering needlessly.

Abbreviations Used in This Section

AAFP = American Academy of Family Physicians
AAPM = American Academy of Pain Professionals
AHRQ = Agency for Healthcare Research and Quality
APF = American Pain Foundation
DHHS = Department of Health and Human Services
NIH = National Institutes of Health

Procedures and Special Topics

147. General

Recommended Search Terms

- Pain
- Pain management

Important Sites

Agency for Healthcare Research and Quality (AHRQ): *Making Health Care Safer: A Critical Analysis of Patient Safety Practices*: Chapter 37: Pain Management (Erica Brownfield, MD): <http://www.ahcpr.gov/clinic/ptsafety/chap37a.htm>

Arkansas Coalition for Patient Rights and Chronic Pain Management: <http://www.arpaincoalition.com/>

Canadian Pain: <http://www.canadianpain.com/>

Mayo Foundation for Medical Education and Research: Pain Management Center: You Have Chronic Pain: Now What?: <http://www.mayoclinic.com/invoke.cfm?id=PN00048>

National Institute of Neurological Disorders and Stroke (NINDS): Disorders: Chronic Pain Information Page: <http://www.ninds.nih.gov/health_and_medical/disorders/chronic_pain.htm>

Pain Concern (UK): <http://www.painconcern.org.uk/>

Pain World (Australia): <http://www.painworld.zip.com.au/>

Purdue Pharma L.P.: Partners against Pain: <http://www.partnersagainstpain.com/>

148. ACUTE PAIN

Recommended Search Terms

- Acute pain management
- "Acute pain" treatment
- "Debilitating pain" management
- "Excruciating pain" control -xxx -porn
- "Severe pain" therapies

Important Sites

Agency for Healthcare Research and Quality (AHRQ): Acute Pain Management: Operative or Medical Procedures and Trauma, Clinical Practice Guideline: <http://www.ahcpr.gov/clinic/medtep/acute.htm>

American Academy of Pediatrics (AAP) Policy Statement: The Assessment and Management of Acute Pain in Infants, Children, and Adolescents: <http://www.aap.org/policy/9933.html>

American Association of Endodontists (AAE): Management of Acute Pain: <http://www.aae.org/ss95ecfe.html>

Virtual Children's Hospital: Acute Pain Management for Pediatric Patients: <http://www.vh.org/pediatric/provider/pediatrics/PediatricPainMgmt/index.html>

149. CANCER PAIN

[*See also* "Cancers," p.12, vol. 2.]

Recommended Search Terms

- "Cancer pain"
- "Cancer pain" management
- Stop cancer pain
- Treat cancer pain

Important Sites

Beth Israel Medical Center: Department of Pain Medicine and Palliative Care: Stop Pain.org: Pain Palliative Care: <http://www.stoppain.org/palliative_care/>

Cancer-Pain.org: <http://www.cancer-pain.org/>

Cancer-Pain.org: Understanding Cancer Pain: What to Tell Your Doctor: <http://www.cancer-pain.org/understanding/tell.html>

Johns Hopkins Medical Institutions: Kimmel Comprehensive Cancer Center: Cancer Pain: Common Patient Questions: <http://www.hopkinskimmelcancercenter.org/clientpages/onc_fastfacts_pain.cfm>

Medical College of Wisconsin: HealthLink: Get Relief from Cancer Pain: <http://healthlink.mcw.edu/article/926794802.html>

National Cancer Institute: Cancer.gov: Pain Control: A Guide for People with Cancer and Their Families: <http://www.nci.nih.gov/cancerinfo/paincontrol/>

OncologyChannel.com: Pain: Types: <http://www.oncologychannel.com/pain/types.shtml>

Texas Children's Hospital: Texas Children's Cancer Center: Cancer Pain Management in Children: <http://www.childcancerpain.org/>

World Health Organization: Global Communications Program: Cancer Pain Release: <http://www.whocancerpain.wisc.edu/>

Wisconsin Pain Initiative (WPI): <http://www.aacpi.wisc.edu/wcpi/>

150. CHRONIC PAIN

Recommended Search Terms

- Chronic pain
- Ongoing pain

Important Sites

American Chronic Pain Association (ACPA): <http://www.theacpa.org/>

Beth Israel Medical Center: Department of Pain Medicine and Palliative Care: Stop Pain.org: <http://www.stoppain.org/>

Chronic Illness Alliance Inc. (Australia): <http://www.chronicillness.org.au/>

Chronic Pain Association of Canada (CPAC): <http://ecn.ab.ca/cpac/>

Chronic Pain Clearinghouse: [requires password] <http://painmanagementtheory.homestead.com/>

Chronic Pain Foundation: <http://www.chronicpainfoundation.org/home/>

Chronic Pain and Illness Life-line: <http://members.tripod.com/~Catnip100/intro.html>

Chronic Pain Support Group: <http://www.chronicpainsupport.org/>

Out of Pain Support Group: Chronic Pain Support Group: <http://www.outofpain.com/>

Pain Connection: Chronic Pain Outreach Center, Inc.: <http://www.pain-connection.com/>

University of Iowa: College of Nursing: Pain: International Center for the Control of Pain in Children and Adults: <http://adultpain.nursing.uiowa.edu/>

Veritas: Chronic Pain: Find Clinical Trials: <http://www.veritasmedicine.com/chronic_pain/>

151. END-OF-LIFE PAIN

Recommended Search Terms

- Pain "end of life"
- Pain hospice
- Pain "palliative care"
- Pain "palliative treatment"

Important Sites

AARP (American Association of Retired Persons): End of Life Issues: <http://www.aarp.org/endoflife/>

American Pain Society (APS): Advocacy and Policy: Treatment of Pain at the End of Life: <http://www.ampainsoc.org/advocacy/treatment.htm>

Americans for Better Care of the Dying: <http://www.abcd-caring.org/>

The City of Hope Pain/Palliative Care Resource Center: <http://www.cityofhope.org/prc/>

End of Life/Palliative Education Resource Center (EPERC): <http://www.eperc.mcw.edu/start.cfm>

152. PHANTOM PAIN

Recommended Search Terms

- "Phantom pain"
- "Phantom limb pain"
- Post-amputation pain

Important Sites

Amputee Web Site: Phantom Pain and How to Deal With It: <http://www.amputee-online.com/amputee/phantom.html>

Beth Israel Medical Center: Department of Pain Medicine and Palliative Care: Stop Pain.org:

Disability Information Services: Phantom Pain: What Causes Phantom Pain: <http://www.a-z.org/dis/phantom.htm>

Pain Medicine and Palliative Care: Phantom and Stump Pain: <http://www.stoppain.org/pain_medicine/phantom.html>

153. POSTOPERATIVE PAIN

Recommended Search Terms

- Pain "after surgery" treatment
- "Post-op" pain
- "Post-op" "pain relief"
- "Post-operative pain"
- "Post-surgery pain"
- "Post-surgical pain"

Important Sites

Ask Your Surgeon: <http://www.askyoursurgeon.com/>

Ask Your Surgeon: Post-Op Pain Relief: <http://askyoursurgeon.com/inthenews.lasso/>

eMedicine: Pain after Surgery (Michael J. Ameres, MD): <http://www.emedicine.com/aaem/topic503.htm>

MedlinePlus: Medical Encyclopedia: Post Surgical Pain Treatment: <http://www.nlm.nih.gov/medlineplus/ency/article/002128.htm>

Neck Reference: FAQs: Will I Have Pain after Surgery?: <http://www.neckreference.com/faq-painafter.html>

154. ASSESSMENT, MEASUREMENT, AND DIAGNOSIS

Recommended Search Terms

- Assessing pain
- "Assessment tools" pain
- "How bad is" pain
- Measuring pain
- "Pain assessment"
- "Pain assessment" tool
- Pain describe
- Pain description
- Pain diagnosis
- Pain diagnostic
- "Pain measurement"
- "Pain measurement" tools
- Pain severity

Important Sites

American Geriatrics Society: Daily Pain Diary: <http://www.americangeriatrics.org/education/daily_pain_diary.pdf>

Cleveland Clinic: Pain Management Department: <http://www.clevelandclinic.org/painmanagement/eval_treat/>

Handbook for Mortals: Controlling Pain (Joanne Lynn, M.D.): Types of Pain: Severity of Pain: <http://www.mywhatever.com/cifwriter/library/mortals/mort2497.html>

Hospice Net: Pain: What Is It?: <http://www.hospicenet.org/html/what_is_pain.html>

Pain Assessment Resources: <http://www.painassessmentresources.com/>

University of Minnesota Cancer Center: Describing Cancer Pain: <http://www.cancer.umn.edu/page/patients/paindes.html>

University of Utah: Pain Management Center: Pain Measurement: <http://medlib.med.utah.edu/pain_center/education/outlines/measure.html>

155. CHILDREN'S PAIN

Recommended Search Terms

- "Acute pain" child
- "Acute pain" children
- Pain child treatment
- Pain children management
- Pediatric pain
- "Pediatric pain"

Important Sites

American Academy of Family Physicians (AAFP): Self-Care on familydoctor.org: Flowcharts: Chest Pain in Infants and Children: <http://familydoctor.org/flowcharts/525.html>

American Academy of Pediatrics (AAP) Policy Statement: The Assessment and Management of Acute Pain in Infants, Children, and Adolescents: <http://www.aap.org/policy/9933.html>

International Center for the Control of Pain in Children and Adults: Medications: Kids: Pain Medicine: Specific Information: <http://adultpain.nursing.uiowa.edu/resources/kids_meds.htm>

Pediatric Pain: Science Helping Children (Canada): <http://www.dal.ca/~pedpain/>

Virtual Children's Hospital: Acute Pain Management for Pediatric Patients: <http://www.vh.org/pediatric/provider/pediatrics/PediatricPainMgmt/index.html>

156. FINDING A PAIN CLINIC

Recommended Search Terms

- Find pain management [add your geographic area or location]
- Find pain professional
- "Pain clinic" [add your geographic area or location]
- "Pain clinics"

Important Sites

American Academy of Pain Management (AAPM): Find an Academy Member Professional: <http://www.aapainmanage.org/search/MemberSearch.php>

American Pain Foundation (APF): *Finding Help for Your Pain: A Pain Resource Guide*: <http://www.painfoundation.org/downloads/FindingCare.pdf>

Dannemiller Foundation: Pain Clinics: <http://www.pain.com/sections/consumer/painclinics/>

Facial Neuralgia Resources: United States Pain Clinics and Specialists: Treatment Centers/Pain Clinics: <http://facial-neuralgia.org/support/pain-us.html>

Google Directory: Health: Medicine: Medical Specialties: Pain Management: Clinics and Practices: <http://directory.google.com/Top/Health/Medicine/Medical_Specialties/Pain_Management/Clinics_and_Practices/?il=1>

healthfinder: Find a Pain Management Professional: <http://www.healthfinder.gov/Scripts/ShowDocDetail.asp?doc=4904&lang=1>

North American Chronic Pain Association of Canada (NACPAC): Directory of Canadian Pain Clinics and Pain Specialists: <http://www.chronicpaincanada.org/nacpac04.htm>

North American Chronic Pain Association of Canada (NACPAC): Links to Directories of American Pain Clinics: <http://www.chronicpaincanada.org/nacpac04a.htm>

157. FUNDING AND SUPPORT FOR PAIN AND PAIN TREATMENT

[*See also* "Tools and Support," p. 133, vol. 1.]

Recommended Search Terms

- Funding pain medication
- Pain medication funding
- Paying for pain medication
- "Medication program" pain
- "Medication program" [name of medicine]
- "Patient assistance program" pain
- "Patient assistance program" [name of medicine]

Important Sites

National Foundation for the Treatment of Pain: <http://www.paincare.org/>

NeedyMeds.com: <http://www.needymeds.com/>

Open Directory Project (DMOZ): Health: Support Groups: Conditions and Diseases: Chronic Pain: <http://dmoz.org/Health/Support_Groups/Conditions_and_Diseases/Chronic_Pain/>

Robert Wood Johnson Foundation: RxAssist: <http://www.rxassist.org/>

Society for Ongoing Relief of Chronic Excruciating Pain: <http://www.sorcep.com/>

158. Pain by Body Location

[*See also* "Headache and Migraine," p. 82, vol. 2, or under specific disease topics.]

NOTE: The following are examples of types of searches or of language you might use to find information on pain in a specific area of the body or with a specific diagnosis. These are only a few of the terms possible. Ask your doctor to write down your diagnosis.

Recommended Search Terms

- "Back pain"
- "Carpal tunnel syndrome"
- "Complex regional pain syndrome"
- Fibromyalgia
- Headache
- "Muscle pain"
- Myalgia
- "Neck pain"
- "Nerve pain"
- Neuralgia
- "Orofacial pain"
- Osteoarthritis
- Pain [anatomical term]
- Pain management [type of pain] [anatomical term]
- Pain management [diagnosis]
- "Referred pain"
- "Reflex sympathetic dystrophy"
- Shingles +pain
- Shingles "herpes zoster"
- Shingles "varicella-zoster"
- Shingles zoster

Important Sites

American Academy of Family Physicians (AAFP): Information from Your Family Doctor: Complex Regional Pain Syndrome: <http://familydoctor.org/handouts/238.html>

American Academy of Orofacial Pain (AAOP): <http://www.aaop.org/>

American RSDHope Group (Reflex Sympathetic Dystrophy Syndrome): <http://www.rsdhope.org/>

Arthritis Foundation: Diseases: Osteoarthritis (OA): <http://www.arthritis.org/conditions/DiseaseCenter/oa.asp>

Coccydynia: Referred Pain: <http://www.coccyx.org/whatisit/referred.htm>

Carpal Tunnel Syndrome: What Information Do You Need?: <http://www.ctsplace.com/>

Fibromyalgia.com: <http://www.fibromyalgia.com/>

Fibromyalgia Network: <http://www.fmnetnews.com/>

Inlet Medical: Pelvic Health: Where to Start?: <http://www.dyspareunia.org/>

MedlinePlus: Osteoarthritis: <http://www.nlm.nih.gov/medlineplus/osteoarthritis.html>

MedlinePlus: Shingles (Herpes zoster): <http://www.nlm.nih.gov/medlineplus/shinglesherpeszoster.html>

National Institute of Neurological Disorders and Stroke (NINDS): Carpal Tunnel Syndrome Information Page: <http://www.ninds.nih.gov/health_and_medical/disorders/carpal_doc.htm>

National Institute of Neurological Disorders and Stroke (NINDS): Complex Regional Pain Syndrome (also called Reflex Sympathetic Dystrophy Syndrome) Information Page: <http://www.ninds.nih.gov/health_and_medical/disorders/reflex_sympathetic_dystrophy.htm>

National Institute of Neurological Disorders and Stroke (NINDS): Shingles Information Page: <http://www.ninds.nih.gov/health_and_medical/disorders/shingles_doc.htm>

Reflex Sympathetic Dystrophy Association of California (RSDA): <http://www.rsdsa-ca.org/>

Reflex Sympathetic Dystrophy Syndrome Association of America (RSDSA): <http://www.rsds.org/>

Spine-Health.com: Pain Management: <http://www.spine-health.com/search/pain01.html>

Trigeminal Neuralgia Association Homepage: <http://www.tna-support.org/>

Vulvar Pain Foundation: <http://www.vulvarpainfoundation.org/>

159. Research

Recommended Search Terms

- Pain grants funding
- Pain research

Important Sites

Canadian Institute for the Relief of Pain and Disability (CIRPD): <http://www.icpro.org/>

Pain Relief Foundation (UK): <http://www.painrelief foundation.org.uk/>

Pain Research and Management (Canada): <http://www.pulsus.com/Pain/home.htm>

160. TREATMENT

General

Recommended Search Terms

- Pain management
- "Pain relief"
- Pain treatment
- "Treatment of pain"

Important Sites

Agency for Healthcare Research and Quality (AHRQ): Evidence Report/Technology Assessment: Number 35: Management of Cancer Pain: <http://www.ahcpr.gov/clinic/epcsums/canpainsum.htm>

Cleveland Clinic: Pain Management Department: <http://www.clevelandclinic.org/painmanagement/eval_treat/>

Injury Resources: <http://www.injuryresources.com/>

Medical College of Wisconsin: HealthLink: New Standards for Assessment and Treatment of Pain: <http://healthlink.mcw.edu/article/977857835.html>

National Foundation for the Treatment of Pain: <http://www.paincare.org/>

Open Directory Project (DMOZ): Health: Medicine: Medical Specialties: Pain Management: <http://dmoz.org/Health/Medicine/Medical_Specialties/Pain_Management/>

PainNet: <http://www.painnet.com/>

University of Southern California: USC Pain Center: <http://www.helpforpain.com/>

Medications

Recommended Search Terms

- "Pain meds"
- "Pain medication"
- Pain therapeutics

Important Sites

Cancer-Pain.org: Cancer Pain Treatments: Pain Medication Delivery: <http://www.cancer-pain.org/treatments/medication.html>

International Center for the Control of Pain in Children and Adults: Medications: Adults: Medicines Used for Pain: <http://adultpain.nursing.uiowa.edu/resources/adultmed.htm>

International Center for the Control of Pain in Children and Adults: Medications: Kids: Pain Medicine: Specific Information: <http://adultpain.nursing.uiowa.edu/resources/kids_meds.htm>

MedlinePlus Medical Encyclopedia: Pain Medications: <http://www.nlm.nih.gov/medlineplus/ency/article/002123.htm>

National Institute on Drug Abuse (NIDA): InfoFacts: Prescription Drugs and Pain Medications: <http://www.nida.nih.gov/Infofax/PainMed.html>

Non-drug Treatments

[*See also* "Alternative/Complementary Health Sources," p. 44.]

NOTE: Recommended search terms are only to illustrate useful search strings; they are not recommendations for pain treatment.

Recommended Search Terms

- Pain relief surgery
- Pain treatment surgery
- Pain relief acupuncture
- Pain relief "alternative treatments"
- Pain relief biofeedback
- Pain relief massage
- Pain relief meditation
- Pain relief "non-drug"
- Pain relief "non-pharmaceutical"
- Pain relief "non-pharmacological"
- Pain relief visualisation
- Pain relief visualization

Important Sites

Back Pain Relief the Ultimate Guide (Robert Miller): Meditation: <http://www.backpainalternatives.com/meditation.htm>

Cancer-Pain.org: Cancer Pain Treatments: Alternative/Complementary Methods: <http://www.cancer-pain.org/treatments/alternative.html>

CancerSymptoms.org: Symptoms: Pain: <http://www.cancersymptoms.org/symptoms/pain/manage/non-pharmacological.php>

Center for Well-Being: Chronic Pain Relief: <http://www.centerforwellbeing.com/Chronic_Pain_Relief/chronic_pain_relief.html>

Childbirth.org: Pain Relief in Labor: <http://www.childbirth.org/articles/labor/painrelief.html>

Memorial Sloan Kettering Cancer Center (MSKCC): Integrative Medicine: Individual Therapies: <http://www.mskcc.org/mskcc/html/1987.cfm>

National Center for Complementary and Alternative Medicine (NCCAM): Acupuncture Information and Resources: <http://nccam.nih.gov/health/acupuncture/>

National Institute for Arthritis and Musculoskeletal and Skin Diseases (NIAMSD): Health Information: Questions and Answers about Arthritis Pain: <http://www.niams.nih.gov/hi/topics/arthritis/arthpain.htm>

Pain Support (UK): Survival Skills: <http://www.painsupport.co.uk/survivalskills/survbody.htm>

HOTLINES

American Chronic Pain Association (ACPA):
1-800-533-3231, or e-mail: <ACPA@pacbell.net>
American Council for Headache Education (ACHE):
1-800-255-ACHE/1-800-255-2243, or e-mail: <achehq@talley.com>
American Pain Foundation (APF):
1-888-615-PAIN/1-888-615-7246, or e-mail: <info@painfoundation.org>
National Headache Foundation (NHF):
1-888-NHF-5552/1-888-643-5552, or e-mail: <info@headaches.org>
Pain Advocacy:
1-800-846-7444
Pain Advocate Foundation:
1-800-532-5274

FAQs

American Academy of Pain Management (AAPM): Pain Patient Information: <http://www.aapainmanage.org/info/Patients.php>

American Chronic Pain Association: Frequently Asked Questions: <http://www.theacpa.org/faqs.htm>

Pain Management and Rehabilitation Medical Services of New York: Frequently Asked Questions (FAQs) about Chronic Pain and Pain Management: <http://www.painmanagementny.com/educ_faqs.html>

Decatur Memorial Hospital: Pain Management Frequently Asked Questions: <http://www.dmhcares.org/services/pain/>

Medical Services of New York: Pain Management and Rehabilitation: Frequently Asked Questions (FAQs) about Chronic Pain and Pain Management: Pain-Pal: Pain Management: Chronic Pain FAQ: <http://www.pain-pal.com/faq.html>

Spine Universe: Pain Management FAQs: <http://www.spineuniverse.com/community/board1/archive_pain manage.html>

Yale University: Yale Center for Pain Management: Myofascial Pain: FAQ: <http://gasnet.med.yale.edu/local/pain/html/faq.html>

PAIN PUBLICATIONS ON THE INTERNET

Agency for Healthcare Research and Quality (AHRQ): *Making Health Care Safer: A Critical Analysis of Patient Safety Practices*: Chapter 37. Pain Management (Erica Brownfield, MD): <http://www.ahcpr.gov/clinic/ptsafety/chap37a.htm>

American Pain Foundation (APF): *Finding Help for Your Pain: A Pain Resource Guide*: <http://www.painfoundation.org/downloads/FindingCare.pdf>

Chronic Pain Support Group (CPSG): Chronic Pain News Letters: <http://chronicpainsupport.org/newsletters.html>

From Patient to Patient: A Survival Guide: <http://www.geocities.com/bhchcactus/patient.htm>

International Pelvic Pain Society, and Inlet Medical: Periscope: <http://www.dyspareunia.org/html/newsletter.htm>

Vulvar Pain Newsletter: <http://www.vulvarpainfoundation.org/vpfnewsletter.htm>

SHOULD YOU SEE A DOCTOR?

American Academy of Family Physicians (AAFP): Self-Care on familydoctor.org: Flowcharts: Abdominal Pain, Acute: <http://familydoctor.org/flowcharts/527.html>

American Academy of Family Physicians (AAFP): Self-Care on familydoctor.org: Flowcharts: Abdominal Pain, Chronic: <http://familydoctor.org/flowcharts/528.html>

American Academy of Family Physicians (AAFP): Self-Care on familydoctor.org: Flowcharts: Chest Pain, Acute: <http://familydoctor.org/flowcharts/523.html>

American Academy of Family Physicians (AAFP): Self-Care on familydoctor.org: Flowcharts: Chest Pain, Chronic: <http://familydoctor.org/flowcharts/524.html>

American Academy of Family Physicians (AAFP): Self-Care on familydoctor.org: Flowcharts: Chest Pain in Infants and Children: <http://familydoctor.org/flowcharts/525.html>

American Academy of Family Physicians (AAFP): Self-Care on familydoctor.org: Flowcharts: Ear Problems: <http://familydoctor.org/flowcharts/507.html>

American Academy of Family Physicians (AAFP): Self-Care on familydoctor.org: Flowcharts: Lower Back Pain: <http://familydoctor.org/flowcharts/531.html>

American Academy of Family Physicians (AAFP): Self-Care on familydoctor.org: Flowcharts: Menstrual Cycle Problems: <http://familydoctor.org/flowcharts/538.html>

American Academy of Family Physicians (AAFP): Self-Care on familydoctor.org: Flowcharts: Neck Pain: <http://familydoctor.org/flowcharts/513.html>

Lactose.co.uk: Irritable Bowel Syndrome: When Should I See a Doctor?: <http://www.lactose.co.uk/ibs/seedoctor.html>

University of California, Irvine: Headaches: When to See a Doctor: <http://www.ucihealth.com/News/UCI%20Health/headach2.htm>

Medical Specialty

Pain management

Professional Organizations

American Academy of Pain Management: <http://www.aapainmanage.org/>

American Academy of Pain Medicine: <http://www.painmed.org/>

American Chronic Pain Association (ACPA): <http://www.theacpa.org/>

American Pain Society (APS): <http://www.ampainsoc.org/>

American Pain Foundation (APF): <http://www.painfoundation.org/>

American Society of Pain Management Nurses (ASPMN): <http://www.aspmn.org/>

Institute for the Study and Treatment of Pain (iSTOP) (Canada): <http://www.istop.org/>

International Association for the Study of Pain (IASP): <http://www.iasp-pain.org/>

North American Chronic Pain Association of Canada (NACPAC): <http://www.chronicpaincanada.org/>

Pain Society (UK): <http://www.painsociety.org/>

Society for Pain Practice Management (SPPM): <http://www.sppm.org/>

Patient Support Organizations/Discussion Groups

Back Pain Support Group: <http://www.backpainsupportgroup.com/>

Beth Israel Medical Center: Department of Pain Medicine and Palliative Care: Stop Pain.org: <http://www.stoppain.org/>

Chronic Pain and Illness Lifeline: <http://members.tripod.com/~Catnip100/intro.html>

Fibromyalgia Personal Support Centre: Support: <http://www.fmpsc.org/support/support.htm>

Google Directory: Health: Support Groups: Conditions and Diseases: Chronic Pain: <http://directory.google.com/Top/Health/Support_Groups/Conditions_and_Diseases/Chronic_Pain/>

Best One-Stop Shops

American Chronic Pain Association (ACPA): <http://www.theacpa.org/>

American Council for Headache Education (ACHE): <http://www.achenet.org/>

American Pain Foundation (APF): <http://www.painfoundation.org/>

healthfinder: Health Library: Prevention and Wellness: Pain: <http://www.healthfinder.gov/scripts/SearchContext.asp?topic=624&super=112&Branch=5>

healthfinder: Health Library: Prevention and Wellness: Pain Management: <http://www.healthfinder.gov/scripts/SearchContext.asp?topic=1058&super=112&Branch=5>

healthfinder: Health Library: Diseases and Conditions: Pain: <http://www.healthfinder.gov/scripts/SearchContext.asp?topic=624&super=113&Branch=5>

healthfinder: Health Library: Diseases and Conditions: Pain Management: <http://www.healthfinder.gov/scripts/SearchContext.asp?topic=1058&super=113&Branch=5>

MedlinePlus: Pain: <http://www.nlm.nih.gov/medlineplus/pain.html>

National Foundation for the Treatment of Pain: <http://www.paincare.org/>

National Headache Foundation: <http://www.headaches.org/>

References

1. Google Search on "Pain," Retreived February 2003.

Part XI: Hospice and End-of-Life Care

Sarah Brick Archer

Special Searching Issues for This Topic

Perhaps the most fundamental human decision is choosing how to die. Hospice care provides a core of various health professionals and volunteers that enable a terminally ill patient with six months or less to live the ability to return home and live the remainder of his/her life to the fullest. The goal of hospice is to minimize pain and discomfort and to emphasize the family and the hope of living, not the despair of dying. Hospice care is holistic in scope, because it provides for the spiritual and psychological needs of the patient as well as the medical. It is also an economical approach to medical care, because at-home care is generally less expensive than institutionalized care.

The concept of hospice care was conceived in the 1960s, with the first hospice services provided in the United States during the 1970s. A Hospice Patient's Bill of Rights <http://www.hospice-america.org/billofrights.html> ensures that patients are involved in decision making and that their dignity, privacy, and quality of care are safeguarded.

What to Ask

It is important to identify the specific aspects about hospice that are of interest. For example, is there a need for information on eligibility, locating a facility, or bereavement counseling?

Where to Start

Unlike some specific diseases, good resources on hospice can be located by doing a Google search. Additional resources can be located using MedlinePlus and healthfinder. While searching for information on hospice, a Google search may reveal home pages for specific hospice care facilities that may not be relevant to all patrons. Look for national organizations, as they will provide good, generic resources applicable to all patients. Since many hospice patients have cancer, there are resources about hospice available on pages pertaining to cancer.

Additional Search Strategies

Use multiple search engines to locate resources available through national organizations and associations.

Topic Profile

Who

A patient who chooses to enter a hospice program who has been certified by a physician as having a terminal illness with six months or less to live. Originally, many of the hospice patients had cancer, but now many diseases are represented.

What

Hospice is a concept of care that tries to meet the medical, psychological, and spiritual needs of terminally ill patients to enable them to die on their own terms.

Where

The majority of patients receive hospice services in their homes, but some patients receive care through designated hospitals, skilled nursing facilities, or special hospice inpatient facilities. Hospice programs are available in approximately 100 countries throughout the world.

When

The need for hospice care affects patients of all ages. Patients can be recertified if they live beyond the initial six months and can be returned to curative treatments if the illness goes into remission.

Abbreviations Used in This Section

AAFP = American Academy of Family Physicians
ACS = American Cancer Society
AHF = American Hospice Foundation
ASCP = American Society of Consultant Pharmacists
HFA = Hospice Foundation of America
NAHC = National Association for Home Care
NHPCO = National Hospice and Palliative Care Organization

Procedures and Special Topics

161. General

Recommended Search Terms

- "Advanced directives"
- Bereavement
- "Death and dying"
- "Death with dignity"
- "End of life"
- "End of life care"
- "Home care agencies"
- Homecare
- Hospice
- "Hospice care"
- "Living wills"
- "Palliative care"
- "Respite care"
- "Terminal illness"

Important Sites

Family Caregiver Alliance: Fact Sheets and Publications: Caregiving Issues and Strategies: Community Care Options: <http://www.caregiver.org/caregiver/jsp/content_node.jsp?nodeid=394>
Family Caregiver Alliance: Fact Sheets and Publications: Caregiving Issues and Strategies: Hiring In-Home Help: <http://www.caregiver.org/caregiver/jsp/content_node.jsp?nodeid=407>
Family Caregiver Alliance: Fact Sheets and Publications: Caregiving Issues and Strategies: Out-of-Home Care

Options: <http://www.caregiver.org/caregiver/jsp/content_node.jsp?nodeid=411>

Hospice Association of America: <http://www.hospice-america.org/home.html>

Hospice Foundation of America (HFA): <http://www.hospicefoundation.org/>

International Association for Hospice and Palliative Care (IAHPC): <http://www.hospicecare.com/>

National Hospice and Palliative Care Organization (NHPCO): <http://www.nhpco.org/>

162. LOCATING HOSPICE CARE

Recommended Search Terms

- "Home care agencies"
- Hospice directories
- Hospice directory
- "Palliative care directory"
- "Palliative care directories"

Important Sites

Hospice Information: Find a Hospice: International Directory <http://www.hospiceinformation.info/findahospice/international.asp>

National Association for Home Care (NAHC): Member Home Care and Hospice State Associations: <http://www.nahc.org/Consumer/stassn.html>

National Hospice and Palliative Care Organization (NHPCO): Find a Hospice Program: <http://www.nhpco.org/Directory/>

163. MANAGING PAIN IN HOSPICE CARE

Recommended Search Terms

- "End of life" "pain management"
- Hospice "pain management"
- Hospice "pain control"
- Hospice "pain relief"
- Hospice "pain medications"

Important Sites

American Academy of Family Physicians (AAFP): *American Family Physician*: Challenges in Pain Management at the End of Life <http://www.aafp.org/afp/20011001/1227.html>

American Society of Consultant Pharmacists (ASCP): Pain Management Consulting Page <http://www.ascp.com/public/pr/pain/>

Growth House: Pain Management: <http://www.growthhouse.org/pain.html>

Ted Mann Family Resource Center: "Pain Management and Hospice Care: Solutions and Help" <http://cancerresources.mednet.ucla.edu/5_info/5c_archive_lec/1995/painhospice.htm>

164. HANDLING GRIEF AND BEREAVEMENT IN HOSPICE CARE

Recommended Search Terms

- Hospice bereavement
- Hospice grief
- Hospice "grief counseling"

Important Sites

American Hospice Foundation (AHF): Grief and Faith: Spiritual Paths through Faith: <http://www.americanhospice.org/faith.htm>

Growth House: Grief and Bereavement: <http://www.growthhouse.org/death.html>

Hospice Foundation of America (HFA): Grief Resource Page: <http://www.hospicefoundation.org/grief/index.htm>

HOTLINE

Elder Care Locator: 1-800-677-1116

FAQs

American Cancer Society (ACS): Managing Day to Day: What Questions Should I Ask about Hospice Care?: <http://www.cancer.org/docroot/eto/content/eto_2_5x_what_questions_should_i_ask_about_hospice_care.asp?sitearea=mlt>

Hospice Association of America: Hospice Fact Sheet: <http://www.hospice-america.org/facts.html>

HOSPICE AND END-OF-LIFE CARE PUBLICATIONS ON THE INTERNET

Hospice Foundation of America (HFA): HFA e-Newsletter: <http://www.hospicefoundation.org/signup.htm>

Last Acts e-Newsletter: <http://www.lastacts.org/>

Peds@Home: An Electronic Newsletter about Providers of Hospice Care for Children: <http://www.nahc.org/NAHC/Peds/peds.html>

MEDICAL SPECIALTIES

NOTE: When searching for information on hospice personnel, try counseling (U.S. spelling) as well as counseling (UK spelling).

Bereavement counseling; Bereavement support; Bereavement therapy; Bereavement therapist; Clinical social worker (Hospice); End-of-Life Physician; Family support worker; Home care aides; Home health aide; Home health nurse; Homemaker services; Home health social worker; Hospice certified nursing assistant; Hospice licensed nursing assistant; Hospice chaplain; Hospice clergy; Hospice counseling; Hospice counseling; Hospice counselor; Hospice dietary counseling; Hospice dietary therapist; Hospice medical director; Hospice nurse manager; Hospice nursing; Hospice nurse; Hospice occupational therapist; Hospice occupational therapy; Hospice pharmacist; Hospice physical therapist; Hospice physical therapy; Hospice physician; Hospice registered nurse; Hospice social work; Hospice social worker; Hospice speech-language therapist; Hospice speech-language therapy; Hospice speech therapist; Hospice speech therapy; Hospice spiritual counseling; Grief counseling; Grief therapist; Grief support services; Grief therapy; Loss therapy; Loss therapist; Medical social worker (Hospice); Palliative care physician; Pre-hospice counseling; Home care aides; Personal hygiene assistant; Primary care physician; Transitional counseling

PROFESSIONAL ORGANIZATION(S):

American Academy of Hospice and Palliative Medicine (AAHPM): <http://www.aahpm.org/>
Hospice Association of America (HAA): <http://www.hospice-america.org/home.html>
Hospice Foundation of America (HFA): <http://www.hospicefoundation.org/>
International Association for Hospice and Palliative Care: <http://www.hospicecare.com/>
National Hospice and Palliative Care Organization (NHPCO): <http://www.nhpco.org/>
National Hospice Foundation (NHF): <http://www.hospiceinfo.org/>

PATIENT SUPPORT ORGANIZATION/ DISCUSSION GROUP

Last Acts Discussion List: <http://www.lastacts.org/>

BEST ONE-STOP SHOPS

Growthhouse.org: <http://www.growthhouse.org/>
Hospice Association of America: <http://www.hospice-america.org/home.html>
Hospice Foundation of America: <http://www.hospicefoundation.org/>
MedlinePlus: Hospice Care: <http://www.nlm.nih.gov/medlineplus/hospicecare.html>

Life Stages and Reproduction

Part I: Newborn and Postpartum Health Issues

Nancy J. Allee

SPECIAL SEARCHING ISSUES FOR THIS TOPIC

This section is the first in the series on finding health information on the Internet by age or gender, or, as we prefer to describe it, by life stage. This chapter will be of primary interest to expectant and new parents and other caregivers. The arrival of a baby is an exciting, life-changing experience, and there are numerous resources available on the Internet to help prepare for this event. Parents may want to explore many of these sites prior to the baby's arrival to become familiar with the types of resources and information offered in addition to consulting the sites once the baby is born. The Web sites recommended below represent credible, reliable sources; however, it is always important to evaluate information from the Internet, and, in the case of infants and newborns, it is essential to confer with your pediatrician about any health questions and concerns.

What to Ask

An initial issue to consider when approaching the Internet for health information on infants is where you are in the process. Are you a new parent preparing for the arrival of a newborn? In this case, you may want to explore sites about what to expect when the baby arrives. Do you have questions about taking care of the baby, such as how to burp, bathe, and diaper the baby, or questions about childproofing your home? Are you looking for the latest research to help decide whether to breastfeed or bottle feed or whether to immunize your child? Or has the baby already arrived, and you are wondering how to childproof your home and how to determine if your child's development is progressing normally.? There are Web sites that provide information on each of these issues and more. Additionally, information is included on common illnesses of infanthood.

Where to Start

Begin by exploring the sites in the "Best One Stop Shops" and "General" sections to become familiar with the kinds of information they include. If you are looking for Web sites on a particular topic, you will also want to review the Web sites featured under "Procedures and Special Topics" below. Usually, it is best to begin searching

under Web sites specifically dedicated to providing health information, such as healthAtoZ, MayoClinic, Medline-Plus, NOAH, and others before searching in general search engines.

Additional Search Strategies

It is important to distinguish between the terms used to describe young children when searching for health information. Typically, information about infants can be found using terms such as "infants," "newborns," or "babies." "Toddler" may also be used. When visiting a health information site, first look for a topics section by life stage. If there is no section for infants, try looking under children's health, women's health, and pregnancy and postpartum care. If you are looking for information on common illnesses of babyhood, this information can also vary by Web site, so you may need to visit several health sites to find the exact illness for which you are searching. Remember that more than one term may be used to describe a condition, so you will want to become familiar with common terms as well as clinical. For instance, "cradle cap" is also known as "infantile seborrhoeic dermatitis." Also remember that professional organizations, such as the American Academy of Pediatrics, and government organizations, such as the National Institute of Child Health and Human Development, may have resources of interest to new parents. Finally, there are several other sections in this guide that are particularly relevant to issues related to newborns, infants, and parenting., including "Women's Health," (p. 136); "Pregnancy," (p. 144); and "Men's Health" (p. 130).

TOPIC PROFILE

Who

Infants, generally defined as children between 1 and 23 months of age. Newborns are defined as infants during the first month following birth.

What

A broad category of health topics for parents and caregivers.

Where

Overall health and wellness of infants and newborns.

When

During the stage of infancy, following birth and preceding early childhood.

ABBREVIATIONS USED IN THIS SECTION

AAP = American Academy of Pediatrics

ACOG = American College of Obstetricians and Gynecologists

CDC = Centers for Disease Control and Prevention

CPSC = Consumer Product Safety Commission

FAQ = Frequently Asked Questions

FDA = Food and Drug Administration

FNS = Food and Nutrition Service

IAC = Immunization Action Coalition

IOM = Institute of Medicine

NCHS = National Center for Health Statistics

NOAH = New York Online Access to Health

PCC = Physician's Computer Company

SIDS = Sudden Infant Death Syndrome

USDA = United States Department of Agriculture

WIC = Women, Infants, and Children

PROCEDURES AND SPECIAL TOPICS

1. GENERAL

Recommended Search Terms

- Babies' health
- Baby health
- Baby's health
- "Infant and newborn"
- "Infant health"
- "Infants and children"
- "Infant's health"
- "Infants health"
- "Infant's health" guide
- "Infant's health" "health links"
- "Infant's health" information
- "Infant's health" issues
- "Infant's health" prevention
- "Infant's health" "risk factors"
- "Infant's health" topics
- "Infant's health" trends
- "Kids health"
- Newborn baby
- Newborn health
- Newborns
- Newborn's health
- Newborn infants

Important Sites

Aetna InteliHealth: Babies' Health: Guiding Your Child through the Infant Years: <http://sushi.intelihealth.com/IH/ihtIH/WSIHW000/29010/29010.html>

aHealthyMe!: Children's Health: Baby Health (to Age 1): <http://www.ahealthyme.com/topic/babyshealth>

Centers for Disease Control and Prevention (CDC): Health Topic: Infants and Children: <http://www.cdc.gov/health/nfantsmenu.htm>

healthAtoZ: Health Channels: Children's Health: Babies: <http://www.healthatoz.com/healthatoz/atoz/hc/chi/baby/babyindex.html>

healthfinder: Just for You: Infants: <http://www.healthfinder.gov/justforyou/justforyou.asp?KeyWordID=167&branch=1>

Healthykids.com: Kids' Health Basics: <http://www.healthykids.com/hk/category.jhtml?categoryid=/templatedata/hk/category/data/HK164.xml>

KidsHealth: Parents: Pregnancy and Newborns: <http://kidshealth.org/parent/pregnancy_newborn/>

MayoClinic.com: Baby's Health Center: <http://www.mayoclinic.com/>

MedlinePlus: Infant and Toddler Health: <http://www.nlm.nih.gov/medlineplus/infantandtoddlerhealth.html>

New York Online Access to Health (NOAH): Ask NOAH About: Newborns to 2 Years: <http://www.noah-health.org/english/pregnancy/newborn.html>

Stanford Health Library: Health Topics: Child and Adolescent Health: <http://healthlibrary.stanford.edu/resources/internet/bodysystems/childrenshealth.html>

2. COMMON DISEASES, ILLNESSES, AND CONDITIONS

Recommended Search Terms

- Baby acne
- Baby "ear infections"
- Colic
- Conjunctivitis
- Cradle cap
- Diaper rash
- Ear tubes
- Infant fever
- Jaundice
- Oral thrush
- Pinkeye

Important Sites

aHealthyMe!: Children's Health: Baby Ills and Conditions: <http://www.ahealthyme.com/topic/topic13351;jsessionid=BXEGVAMENMYWECTYAIRS4EQ>

American Academy of Family Physicians (AAFP): Family Doctor: Common Conditions in Children: <http://www.familydoctor.org/x5323.xml>

American Academy of Family Physicians (AAFP): Family Doctor: Everyday Illnesses and Injuries: <http://www.kidshealth.org/PageManager.jsp?dn=familydoctor&lic=44&ps=303&cat_id=45>

American Academy of Family Physicians (AAFP): Family Doctor: Special Conditions in Children: <http://www.familydoctor.org/x5336.xml>

AskDrSears.com: Childhood Illness Index: <http://www.askdrsears.com/html/8/T080100.asp>

Immunization Action Coalition (IAC): Recommended Childhood and Adolescent Immunization Schedule—United States, 2003: <http://www.immunize.org/cdc/child-schedule.pdf>

KidsHealth: Parents: Infections: <http://kidshealth.org/parent/infections/>

MayoClinic.com: Baby's Health Center: Common Problems: <http://www.mayoclinic.com/>

MedicineNet.com: Focus on Healthy Kids: Pediatric Medical Information: <http://www.medicinenet.com/healthy_kids/focus.htm>

New York Online Access to Health (NOAH): Ask NOAH About: Newborns to 2 Years: Infant Care/Parenting: Common Medical Conditions: <http://www.noah-health.org/english/pregnancy/newborn.html>

3. NEWBORN CARE

Recommended Search Terms

- Apgar scores
- "Baby car safety"
- Baby "what to expect"
- "Babyproofing your home"
- Baby's checkup
- Baby's "first few weeks"
- Baby "bath safety"
- "Bringing baby home"
- "Bringing your baby home"
- "Burping your baby"
- Burping baby "how to"
- Burping baby tips
- Childproof house
- "Childproofing your home"
- Circumcision
- Infant car seats
- Infant care
- Infant safety
- Neonatal care
- Newborn care
- "Newborn care"
- Newborn "medical care"

- Newborn screening tests
- Prenatal care
- Post-natal care
- Postnatal care
- "Toy safety" infants
- Umbilical cord care
- Uncircumcised penis "care of"

Important Sites

Aetna InteliHealth: Babies' Health: Guiding Your Child through the Early Years: Childproofing Your Home: <http://www.intelihealth.com/>

American Academy of Pediatrics (AAP): Circumcision Policy Statement (RE9850): <http://www.aap.org/policy/RE9850.html>

Consumer Product Safety Commission (CPSC): Childproofing Your Home: 12 Safety Devices to Protect Your Children: <http://www.cpsc.gov/cpscpub/pubs/grand/12steps/12steps.html>

Consumer Product Safety Commission (CPSC): Which Toy for Which Child: A Consumer's Guide for Selecting Suitable Toys: <http://www.cpsc.gov/cpscpub/pubs/285.pdf>

healthAtoZ: Healthy Lifestyles: Safety and Prevention: Child Safety: Infant and Car Seat Safety: <http://www.healthatoz.com/healthatoz/Atoz/hl/sp/chil/carsafety.html>

keepkidshealthy.com: Safety: Car Seat Safety Guide: Car Seat Ease of Use Ratings: <http://www.keepkidshealthy.com/welcome/safety/car_seats_safety/car_seat_ratings.html>

KidsHealth: Parents: Pregnancy and Newborns: Baby Basics: Burping Your Baby: <http://kidshealth.org/parent/pregnancy_newborn/basics/burping.html>

KidsHealth: Parents: Growth and Development: Growing Up: Teething Tots: <http://kidshealth.org/parent/growth/growing/teething.html>

KidsHealth: Parents: Pregnancy and Newborns: Medical Care and Your Baby: What is the Apgar Score? <http://kidshealth.org/parent/pregnancy_newborn/medical_care/apgar.html>

MayoClinic.com: Baby's Health Center: New Arrival: Bringing Baby Home: <http://www.mayoclinic.com/>

MayoClinic.com: Baby's Health Center: Newborn Care: <http://www.mayoclinic.com/>

MayoClinic.com: Baby's Health Center: Newborn Screening Tests: <http://www.mayoclinic.com/>

Medem: Medical Library: American Academy of Pediatrics: Care of the Uncircumcised Penis: <http://www.medem.com/>

Medem: Medical Library: Medem Learning Center: Circumcision: <http://www.medem.com/>

MedicineNet.com: Doctor's Views A–Z List: Healthy Kids: Newborn Screening Tests: <http://www.medicinenet.com/script/main/art.asp?articlekey=10104>

MedicineNet.com: Procedures and Tests A–Z List: Hearing: Newborn Infant Hearing Screening: <http://www.medicinenet.com/Newborn_Infant_Hearing_Screening/article.htm>

MedlinePlus: Infant and Newborn Care: <http://www.nlm.nih.gov/medlineplus/infantandnewborncare.html>

4. NEWBORN DEVELOPMENT

Recommended Search Terms

- Child development infants
- "Development disorders" infants
- "Development milestones" infants
- "Development milestones" months
- "Developmental milestones" newborns
- Infant development
- Infant development complications
- "Infant development" problems
- Growth charts
- Movement coordination infant
- Neonatal development
- Newborn development
- Normal growth development infants
- Normal newborns
- Potty training
- Premature babies development
- "Premature birth" development
- Teething
- Toilet training
- "What's normal" newborns

Important Sites

aHealthyMe!: Children's Health: Development and Behavior: <http://www.ahealthyme.com/topic/childdevelopment>

Centers for Disease Control and Prevention (CDC): National Center for Health Statistics (NCHS): 2000 CDC Growth Charts: United States: <http://www.cdc.gov/growthcharts/>

Keepkidshealthy.com: Childrens Growth Charts: <http://www.keepkidshealthy.com/growthcharts/>

KidsHealth: Growth and Development: <http://kidshealth.org/parent/growth/>

MayoClinic.com: Baby's Health Center: Infant Development: What Happens during the First 3 Months: <http://www.mayoclinic.com/>

MedlinePlus: Infant and Toddler Development: <http://www.nlm.nih.gov/medlineplus/infantandtoddlerdevelopment.html>

MedlinePlus: Premature Babies: <http://www.nlm.nih.gov/medlineplus/prematurebabies.html>

Merck Manual, 2nd home ed.: Section 23. Children's Health Issues: Chapter 263. Normal Newborns and Infants: <http://www.merck.com/mrkshared/mmanual_home2/sec23/ch263/ch263a.jsp>

Merck Manual, 2nd home ed: Section 23. Children's Health Issues: Chapter 267. Problems in Infants and Very Young Children: <http://www.merck.com/mrkshared/mmanual_home2/sec23/ch267/ch267a.jsp>

Merck Manual, 2nd home ed: Section 23. Children's Health Issues: Chapter 264. Problems in Newborns: <http://www.merck.com/mrkshared/mmanual_home2/sec23/ch264/ch264a.jsp>

5. NEWBORN HEALTH

Recommended Search Terms

- Babies' health
- Baby "what to expect"
- Baby's checkup
- Baby's "first few weeks"
- Circumcision
- Infant care
- Infant health
- Infant development
- "Infant and newborn"
- Infant safety
- Newborn baby
- Newborn care
- Newborn infants
- Newborns
- Prenatal care
- Premature babies

Important Sites

aHealthyMe!: Children's Health: Baby Health (to Age 1): <http://www.ahealthyme.com/topic/babyshealth>

Aetna InteliHealth: Babies' Health: Guiding Your Child Through the Infant Years: <http://www.intelihealth.com/IH/ihtIH/WSIHW000/29010/29010.html>

MayoClinic.com: Newborn Care: <http://www.mayoclinic.com/findinformation/conditioncenters/subcenters.cfm?objectid=8A8B4F6B-A8CE-4B8D-9E0EB2FF90A44915>

MedlinePlus: Infant and Toddler Health: <http://www.nlm.nih.gov/medlineplus/infantandtoddlerhealth.html>

Merck Manual: Infections in Newborns and Infants: <http://www.merck.com/mrkshared/mmanual_home/sec23/253.jsp>

Merck Manual, 2nd home ed.: Section 23. Children's Health Issues: Chapter 272. Bacterial Infections: <http://www.merck.com/mrkshared/mmanual_home2/sec23/ch272/ch272a.jsp>

Merck Manual, 2nd home ed: Section 23. Children's Health Issues: Chapter 273. Viral Infections: <http://www.merck.com/mrkshared/mmanual_home2/sec23/ch273/ch273a.jsp>

Merck Manual, 2nd home ed: Section 23. Children's Health Issues: Problems in Newborns: <http://www.merck.com/mrkshared/mmanual_home/sec23/252.jsp>

6. NUTRITION

Recommended Search Terms

- Baby "enough milk"
- Baby "enough to eat"
- Baby formula
- Bottlefeeding
- Breastfeeding
- Breastfeeding research
- Breast milk
- Breast milk research
- Breast pumps
- Finger feeding
- Good "latch on"
- Infant formula
- Infant nursing
- Infants nutrition
- "Lactation consultant"
- Solid foods infants
- "Vegetarian diets" infants
- "Vegetarian infants"

Important Sites

Aetna InteliHealth: Babies' Health: Guiding Your Child through the Infant Year: Introducing Solid Foods: <http://www.intelihealth.com/IH/ihtIH/WSIHW000/29010/29741/333044.html?d=dmtChildGuide>

American Academy of Pediatrics (AAP): Advocacy: AAP Breastfeeding Resources: <http://www.aap.org/advocacy/bf/aapbrres.htm>

American Academy of Pediatrics (AAP): News Release: AAP Report: Infants Need Vitamin D Supplementation: <http://www.aap.org/advocacy/archives/aprvitamin.htm>

American Academy of Pediatrics (AAP): Policy Statement: Breastfeeding and the Use of Human Milk (RE9729): <http://www.aap.org/policy/re9729.html>

American Academy of Pediatrics (AAP): A Woman's Guide to Breastfeeding: <http://www.aap.org/family/brstguid.htm>

AskDrSears.com: Breastfeeding: Proper Positioning and Latch-On Skills: <http://www.askdrsears.com/html/2/T021000.asp>

Baylor College of Medicine: Children's Nutrition Research Center: Consumer News: Facts and Answers: Breastfeeding: <http://www.bcm.tmc.edu/cnrc/consumer/archives/factsanswers.html#breastfeeding>

Lactation Education Resources: Latch-on: Signs of a good latch-on: <http://www.leron-line.com/Latch-on.htm>

Medem: Medical Library: American Academy of Pediatrics: Bottlefeeding: <http://www.medem.com/>

Medem: Medical Library: Medem Learning Center: Infant Nutrition: <http://www.medem.com/>

MedicineNet.com: Focus Topics: Healthy Kids: Newborn Care: Infant Formulas: <http://www.medicinenet.com/Infant_Formulas/page1.htm>

MedlinePlus: Breast Feeding: <http://www.nlm.nih.gov/medlineplus/breastfeeding.html>

Nutrition.gov: Lifecycle Issues: Children: <http://www.nutrition.gov/>

ParentingWeb: ParentingWeb's Guide to Breastfeeding Basics: Latching On: <http://www.parentingWeb.com/lounge/bf_basics/latchon.htm>

7. POSTPARTUM CARE

Recommended Search Terms

- Kegel exercises
- Postpartum care
- Postpartum checkup
- Postpartum coping
- Postpartum fitness
- Postpartum pain
- Postpartum recovery
- Postpartum weight loss

Important Sites

aHealthyMe!: Children's Health: Postpartum: <http://www.ahealthyme.com/topic/postpartum>

BabyCenter: Baby: Postpartum Fitness: <http://www.babycenter.com/baby/postpartumfitness/index>

BabyCenter: Baby: Postpartum Recovery: <http://www.babycenter.com/baby/physrecovery/index>

Depression after Delivery: Postpartum Depression: <http://www.depressionafterdelivery.com/>

healthAtoZ: Diseases and Conditions: Postpartum Depression: <http://www.healthatoz.com/healthatoz/Atoz/dc/caz/ment/depr/postpart.html>

KidsHealth: Parents: Pregnancy and Newborns: Pregnancy and Childbirth: Recovering from Delivery: <http://kidshealth.org/parent/pregnancy_newborn/pregnancy/recovering_delivery.html>

MayoClinic.com: Pregnancy Center: Postpartum Coping: The Blues and Depression: <http://www.mayoclinic.com/>

MedlinePlus: Postpartum Depression: <http://www.nlm.nih.gov/medlineplus/postpartumdepression.html>

HOTLINES

Allergies/Asthma:
1-800-7-ASTHMA
Childhood Immunization Information:
1-800-232-2522
Back to Sleep: Sudden Infant Death Syndrome (SIDS):
1-800-505-CRIB
Depression after Delivery:
1-800-944-4773
Healthy Mothers, Healthy Babies:
1-800-322-2588
La Leche League International:
1-800-525-3243
March of Dimes Birth Defects Foundation:
(888) 663-4637
National Center on Shaken Baby Syndrome:
(888) 273-0071
National Vaccine Information Center:
1-800-909-7468
Prenatal Care:
1-800-311-BABY
Zero to Three: National Center for Infants, Toddlers and Families:
1-800-899-4301

FAQs

Aetna InteliHealth: Babies' Health: Guiding Your Child through the Infant Year: Frequently Asked Questions: Newborn: <http://www.intelihealth.com/IH/ihtIH/WSIHW000/29010/29735/336792.html?d=dmtChild Guide>

American Academy of Pediatrics (AAP): What Parents Should Know About Measles-Mumps-Rubella (MMR) Vaccine and Autism: <http://search.aap.org/aap/CISPframe.html?url=http://www.cispimmunize.org/fam/mmr/a_faq.html>

AskDrSears.com: Sleep Problems: Sleep Problems FAQ (Frequently Asked Questions): <http://www.askdrsears.com/html/7/T071100.asp>

Centers for Disease Control and Prevention (CDC): National Center for Chronic Disease Prevention and Health Promotion: Breastfeeding: Frequently Asked Questions: <http://www.cdc.gov/breastfeeding/faq.htm>

Centers for Disease Control and Prevention (CDC): National Center on Birth Defects and Developmental Disabilities: Early Hearing Detection and Intervention Program (EHDI): Frequently Asked Questions: <http://www.cdc.gov/ncbddd/ehdi/question.htm>

U.S. Food and Drug Administration (FDA): Center for Food Safety and Applied Nutrition: Infant Formula: Frequently Asked Questions: <http://vm.cfsan.fda.gov/~dms/inf-faq.html>

U.S. Department of Agriculture (USDA): Food and Nutrition Service (FNS): Women, Infants, and Children (WIC): Frequently Asked Questions about WIC: <http://www.fns.usda.gov/wic/FAQs/FAQ.HTM>

CHILDREN'S HEALTH PUBLICATIONS ON THE INTERNET

Centers for Disease Control and Prevention (CDC): National Center for Environmental Health: Preventing Lead Poisoning in Young Children: <http://www.cdc.gov/nceh/lead/publications/books/plpyc/contents.htm>

Healthy Child Care America (Winter 2000): Improving Children's Nutrition: Opportunities in Child Care: <http://www.healthychildcare.org/pdf/nutrition.pdf>

National Academies Press (NAP): Institute of Medicine (IOM): *From Neurons to Neighborhoods: The Science of Early Childhood Development* (2000): <http://www.nap.edu/books/0309069882/html/>

U.S. Department of Agriculture (USDA): Food and Nutrition Service (FNS): Feeding Solid Foods: <http://www.fns.usda.gov/tn/Resources/ch7.pdf>

MEDICAL SPECIALTIES

Neonatology; Pediatrics; Perinatology

PROFESSIONAL ORGANIZATIONS

American Academy of Pediatrics (AAP): <http://www.aap.org/>

American College of Obstetrics and Gynecology (ACOG): <http://www.acog.org/>

Ambulatory Pediatric Association: <http://www.ambpeds.org/>

PATIENT SUPPORT ORGANIZATIONS/ DISCUSSIONS GROUPS

BabycareAdvice.com: Useful Links: <http://www.babycareadvice.com/babycare/useful-links.php>

Breastfeeding.com: <http://www.breastfeeding.com/>

drgreene.com: <http://www.drgreene.org/>

keepkidshealthy.com: Ask the Pediatrician: <http://www.keepkidshealthy.com/ask_the_pediatrician.html>

NurtureMom: <http://www.nurturemom.com/>

Physician's Computer Company (PCC): PCC Online: PedTalk: PedTalk FAQ (Frequently Asked Questions): <http://www.pcc.com/lists/pedtalk/faq.html>

Best One-Stop Shops

aHealthyMe!: Children's Health: Development and Behavior: <http://www.ahealthyme.com/topic/child development>

aHealthyMe! Pregnancy and Baby: Baby Health (to Age 1): <http://www.ahealthyme.com/topic/babyshealth>

AskDrSears.com: <http://www.askdrsears.com/>

CNN.com: Health Library: Children's Health: <http://www.cnn.com/HEALTH/library/children/>

New York Online Access to Health (NOAH): Ask NOAH About: Newborns to 2 Years: <http://www.noah-health.org/english/pregnancy/newborn.html>

Keepkidshealthy.com: Infant Health Center: <http://www.keepkidshealthy.com/infant/infant.html>

Keepkidshealthy.com: Newborn Health Center: <http://www.keepkidshealthy.com/newborn/newborn.html>

KidsHealth: Welcome Parents: <http://kidshealth.org/parent/>

MedicineNet.com: Focus on Healthy Kids: Pediatric Medical Information: <http://www.medicinenet.com/healthy_kids/focus.htm>

MedlinePlus: Infant and Newborn Care: <http://www.nlm.nih.gov/medlineplus/infantandnewborncare.html>

MedlinePlus: Infant and Toddler Development: <http://www.nlm.nih.gov/medlineplus/infantandtoddler development.html>

MedlinePlus: Infant and Toddler Health: <http://www.nlm.nih.gov/medlineplus/infantandtoddlerhealth.html>

Part II: Children's Health Issues

Nancy J. Allee

Special Searching Issues for this Topic

This is the second of two parts on searching for health information on the topic of early childhood. Part I focuses on infants and newborns; Part II focuses on children and childhood. Information is readily available on a variety of topics related to children's health. For the younger populations, there are even Web sites targeted specifically to children and teens with information relevant to their health interests and presented in a manner designed to appeal to their age groups. Children visiting these Web sites may discover characters such as Mercy Bear, P.D. Parrot, and Kidd Safety to tell them about visits to the hospital; health, safety, and nutrition; and also about prevention of injury from consumer products and toys.

When you are searching for health information on the Internet, it is always important to carefully evaluate the results of your search efforts. If you are a parent or grandparent searching for information about your child's or grandchild's health, it is even more important to carefully evaluate information found on the Web and to always consult with your family's pediatrician about any questions you might have. Children are a vulnerable population, and they deserve to be protected. If your children or grandchildren are searching the Internet themselves, make sure they feel comfortable about asking questions about the health information they discover. You may want to visit the children's health Web sites together to ensure that this kind of discussion occurs.

What to Ask

Some factors to consider when searching for children's health information are age and developmental level. There may be relevant information in other sections of this book such as "Women's Health Issues" if you are looking for information on infants or in "Adolescents' Health Issues" if you are looking for information on pre-adolescence. Are you looking for information targeted to you, as a parent or grandparent, or Web sites for children themselves to explore? Consider whether you have a question about a specific condition or if you are interested in general health and wellness issues for children. Also, because it may be helpful, as in the case of safety issues, to consider the places that children engage in play and other activities, this topic includes Web sites relevant to both home and school safety.

Where to Start

Many search engines offer special topics that include children's health interests. The names for these special topics can vary. For example, NOAH uses "child health" instead of "children's health," and healthAtoZ uses "happy parenting." The categories of information within the special topics vary by search engine, as well, so it may be helpful to consult more than one Web "General" site below. The Web sites listed under "Professional Organizations" and "Best One Stop Shops" are also good starting points for a variety of information relevant to children's health.

Additional Search Strategies

If you are interested in information about a specific childrens disease or condition, be aware that it may affect individuals across the life span. In these cases it may be helpful to combine the term(s) for the disease or condition with term(s) related to children such as "arthritis" and "children's health."

TOPIC PROFILE

Who

Children, generally defined as individuals between the ages of 2 and 12 years of age. A child between the ages of 2 and 5 is further defined as being of preschool age.

What

A broad category of health topics for parents, grandparents, and other caretakers, as well as Web sites designed for children.

Where

Covers overall health and wellness of children.

When

During the stage of childhood, primarily between infancy and adolescence.

ABBREVIATIONS USED IN THIS SECTION

AAFP = American Academy of Family Physicians
CDC = Centers for Disease Control and Prevention
Hib = Haemophilus Influenzae Type B Bacteria
HRSA = Health Resources and Services Administration
MMR = Measles, Mumps, Rubella
NIAAA = National Institute on Alcohol Abuse and Alcoholism
NOAH = New York Online Access to Health
PTA = Parent Teacher Association

PROCEDURES AND SPECIAL TOPICS

8. GENERAL

Recommended Search Terms

- "Child health"
- Children "school health"
- "Children's health"
- "Children's health" guide

- "Children's health" "health links"
- "Children's health" information
- "Children's health" issues
- "Children's health" prevention
- "Children's health" "risk factors"
- "Children's health" topics
- "Children's health" trends
- "Infants and children"
- "Kids health"
- "Preschool child" health
- School health

Important Sites

Center for Health and Health Care in Schools: <http://www.healthinschools.org/>

Centers for Disease Control and Prevention (CDC): Health Topics: Infants and Children: <http://www.cdc.gov/health/nfantsmenu.htm>

Department of Health and Human Services (DHHS): HHS Pages for Kids: <http://www.hhs.gov/kids/>

Google Directory: Health: Child Health: <http://directory.google.com/Top/Health/Child_Health/>

healthAtoZ: Channels: Parenting: <http://www.healthatoz.com/healthatoz/Atoz/hc/par/parindex.html>

Medem: Medical Library: Children's Health: <http://www.medem.com/>

MedlinePlus: Child and Teen Health Topics: <http://www.nlm.nih.gov/medlineplus/childandteenhealth.html>

MedlinePlus: Children's Health: <http://www.nlm.nih.gov/medlineplus/childrenshealth.html>

New York Online Access to Health (NOAH): Ask NOAH About: Child Health: Kids! <http://www.noah-health.org/english/wellness/healthyliving/childhealth.html>

Stanford Health Library: Health Info: Children's Health: Child and Adolescent Health: <http://healthlibrary.stanford.edu/resources/internet/bodysystems/childrenshealth.html>

WebMDHealth: Pregnancy and Family Center: Parenting and Pregnancy: <http://my.webmd.com/health_and_wellness/pregnancy_family/parenting/default.htm>

Yahoo! Directory: Health: Children's Health: <http://dir.yahoo.com/Health/Children_s_Health/>

9. SITES FOR CHILDREN

Recommended Search Terms

- Children kids health Websites
- Children kids health internet
- "For kids" health Websites
- Kids health Web pages

Important Sites

Bandaids and Blackboards: <http://www.faculty.fairfield.edu/fleitas/contents.html>

Ben's Guide to U.S. Government for Kids: Health and Safety: <http://bensguide.gpo.gov/subject.html#health>

Children's Medical Center of the University of Virginia: Asthma: <http://www.people.virginia.edu/~smb4v/tutorials/asthma/asthma1.html>

Children's Mercy Hospitals and Clinics: Parents and Children: Storybook "Tours": Mercy Bear's Big Adventures: <http://www.childrens-mercy.org/mercybear/index.htm>

Consumer Product Safety Commission (CPSC): Kidd Safety: <http://www.cpsc.gov/kids/kidsafety/index.html>

Department of Health and Human Services (DHHS): Families and Children: Kids' Web Sites: <http://www.hhs.gov/children/index.shtml#kids>

Firstgov for Kids: Health: <http://www.kids.gov/k_health.htm>

Food and Drug Administration (FDA): FDA Kids' Home Page: <http://www.fda.gov/oc/opacom/kids/>

healthfinder: Kids: <http://www.healthfinder.gov/kids/>

Hinkle Creek Elementary, K-4 School in Indiana: Human Body: "Blending In But Staying Special:" <http://library.thinkquest.org/5777/>

Internet Public Library: KidSpace: Health: <http://www.ipl.org/kidspace/browse/hea0000>

KidsHealth For Kids: <http://www.kidshealth.org/kid/index.html>

MedlinePlus: Children's Page: <http://www.nlm.nih.gov/medlineplus/childrenspage.html>

National Jewish Medical and Research Center: Asthma: Asthma Wizard: <http://asthma.nationaljewish.org/about/kids/wizard.php>

P.D. Parrot: <http://www.bmhcc.org/PD_Parrot/>

Sara's Quest (National Institute on Drug Abuse): <http://www.sarasquest.org/>

Yahooligans! Directory: Science and Nature: Health and Safety: <http://www.yahooligans.com/Science_and_Nature/Health_and_Safety/>

10. Advocacy and Healthcare Policy, Research, and Services

Recommended Search Terms

- "Children's health" advocacy
- Children's "health care research"
- Children's "health care services"

Important Sites

Annie E. Casey Foundation (AECF): Kids Count: <http://www.aecf.org/kidscount/>

American Academy of Pediatrics (AAP): AAP Practice Guidelines: <http://www.aap.org/policy/paramtoc.html>

Association of Maternal and Child Health Programs (AMCHP): <http://www.amchp.org/>

Children's Defense Fund: <http://www.childrensdefense.org/>

Connect for Kids: Guidance for Grownups: <http://www.connectforkids.org/homepage1535/index.htm>

Health Resources and Services Administration (HRSA): Maternal and Child Health Bureau: <http://www.mchb.hrsa.gov/>

National Center for Education in Maternal and Child Health (NCEMCH): <http://www.ncemch.org/about/default.html>

11. Child Abuse

Recommended Search Terms

- "Child abuse"
- "Child abuse prevention"
- "Child maltreatment"
- "Child neglect"

Important Sites

Childhelp USA: <http://www.childhelpusa.org/>

Department of Health and Human Services (DHHS): Administration for Children and Families: National Clearinghouse on Child Abuse and Neglect Information: <http://nccanch.acf.hhs.gov/index.cfm>

MedlinePlus: Child Abuse: <http://www.nlm.nih.gov/medlineplus/childabuse.html>

National Council on Child Abuse and Family Violence: Child Abuse Information: <http://www.nccafv.org/child.htm>

12. Child Development

Recommended Search Terms

- "Child development"
- Child "growth and development"
- "Early childhood"
- Parenting "child behavior"
- Parenting "child development"

Important Sites

Familyeducation.com: <http://www.familyeducation.com/home/>

KidSource Online: Early Childhood Growth Chart: <http://www.kidsource.com/kidsource/content4/growth.chart/page1.html>

MedlinePlus: Child Development: <http://www.nlm.nih.gov/medlineplus/childdevelopment.html>

National Parent Information Network: <http://npin.org/>

Zero to Three: Parenting A–Z: <http://www.zerotothree.org/index.html>

13. Child Immunizations
Recommended Search Terms

- Chickenpox child vaccine
- "Childhood immunization"
- "Childhood immunizations"
- Children vaccines
- "Child vaccination"
- "Children's vaccinations"
- Diphtheria child vaccine
- "German measles" child vaccine
- "Haemophilus influenzae type B" child vaccine
- "Hepatitis A" child vaccine
- "Hepatitis B" child vaccine
- Hib Child vaccine
- Lockjaw child vaccine
- MMR child vaccine
- Measles child vaccine
- Mumps child vaccine
- Pertussis child vaccine
- Polio child vaccine
- Rubella child vaccine
- Tetanus child vaccine
- "Vaccine preventable diseases"
- Varicella child vaccine

Important Sites

American Academy of Family Physicians (AAFP): Clinical Care and Research: Immunization Resources: AAFP Clinical Recommendations for Immunizations: Childhood and Adolescent Immunization Schedule: <http://www.aafp.org/x7666.xml>

Centers for Disease Control and Prevention (CDC): National Immunization Program: <http://www.cdc.gov/nip/>

King County (Washington) Public Health: Immunization Program: *Plain Talk About Childhood Immunizations*, 5th Edition: <http://www.metrokc.gov/health/immunization/childimmunity.htm#prevention>

MedlinePlus: Childhood Immunization: <http://www.nlm.nih.gov/medlineplus/childhoodimmunization.html>

14. Child Safety
Recommended Search Terms

- "Bicycle safety"
- "Bike safety"
- "Child safety"
- "Child safety locks"
- "Child safety seats"
- "Childhood injury"
- Children "bike helmets"
- Children "home safety"
- Children "lead poisoning"
- "Children's health and safety"
- "Children's health protection"
- "Infant car seats"
- "Internet filtering" "child safety"
- "Playground safety"
- "School safety"
- "Unintentional childhood injury"

Important Sites

Children's Safety Network (CSN): <http://www.edc.org/HHD/csn/>

Department of Education: ED.gov: Office of Safe and Drug-Free Schools (OSDFS) Program: <http://www.ed.gov/about/offices/list/osdfs/index.html>

Environmental Protection Agency (EPA): Office of Children's Health Protection: <http://yosemite.epa.gov/ochp/ochpWeb.nsf/homepage>

KidSource: The Internet and Young Children: <http://www.kidsource.com/safety/internet.young.html>

MedlinePlus: Child Safety: <http://www.nlm.nih.gov/medlineplus/childsafety.html>

MedlinePlus: Lead Poisoning: <http://www.nlm.nih.gov/medlineplus/leadpoisoning.html>

Centers for Disease Control and Prevention (CDC): National Center for Injury Prevention and Control: Bicycle Related Injuries (National Bicycle Safety Network): <http://www.cdc.gov/ncipc/bike/>

National Highway Traffic Safety Administration (NHTSA): Child Passenger Safety: <http://www.nhtsa.dot.gov/people/injury/childps/>

National PTA (Parent-Teacher Association): Parent Involvement: Health and Safety: <http://www.pta.org/parentinvolvement/healthsafety/index.asp>

National Safe Kids Campaign: <http://www.safekids.org/>

National School Safety Center: <http://www.nssc1.org/>

15. Common Diseases and Illnesses of Childhood
Recommended Search Terms

- Chickenpox
- Ear infections
- German measles
- Head lice
- Measles
- Middle ear infection
- Mumps
- Otitis media
- Pediculosis
- Pertussis
- Rubella
- Scarlet fever
- Strep throat
- Varicella
- Whooping cough

Important Sites

aHealthyme!: Children's Health: Chicken Pox: <http://www.ahealthyme.com/topic/topic13594>

aHealthyMe!: Children's Health: Childhood Illnesses and Conditions: <http://www.ahealthyme.com/topic/childills>

aHealthyme! Children's Health: Lice: <http://www.ahealthyme.com/topic/lice>

aHealthyme! Children's Health: Measles: <http://www.ahealthyme.com/topic/measles>

aHealthyme! Children's Health: Mumps: <http://www.ahealthyme.com/topic/mumps>

aHealthyme! Children's Health: Rubella: <http://www.ahealthyme.com/topic/rubella>

aHealthyme! Children's Health: Scarlet Fever: <http://www.ahealthyme.com/topic/topic13619>

aHealthyme! Children's Health: Strep Throat: <http://www.ahealthyme.com/topic/strepkids>

aHealthyme! Children's Health: Whooping Cough (Pertussis): <http://www.ahealthyme.com/topic/topic13622>

AskDrSears.com: Childhood Illness Index: <http://www.askdrsears.com/html/8/T080100.asp>

Centers for Disease Control and Prevention (CDC): Parasitic Disease Information: Head Lice Infestation (Pediculosis): <http://www.cdc.gov/ncidod/dpd/parasites/headlice/>

KidsHealth: Parents: Infections: <http://kidshealth.org/parent/infections/>

MayoClinic.com: Baby's Health Center: Middle Ear Infection: <http://www.mayoclinic.com/>

MayoClinic.com: Infectious Disease Center: Chickenpox: <http://www.mayoclinic.com/>

MayoClinic.com: Infectious Disease Center: Mumps: <http://www.mayoclinic.com/>

MayoClinic.com: Infectious Disease Center: Rubella: <http://www.mayoclinic.com/>

MayoClinic.com: Infectious Disease Center: Whooping Cough: <http://www.mayoclinic.com/>

MedicineNet.com: Focus on Healthy Kids: Pediatric Medical Information: <http://www.medicinenet.com/healthy_kids/focus.htm>

MedlinePlus: Chickenpox: <http://www.nlm.nih.gov/medlineplus/chickenpox.html>

MedlinePlus: Ear Infections: <http://www.nlm.nih.gov/medlineplus/earinfections.html>

MedlinePlus: Head Lice: <http://www.nlm.nih.gov/medlineplus/headlice.html>

MedlinePlus: Measles: <http://www.nlm.nih.gov/medlineplus/measles.html>

MedlinePlus: Mumps: <http://www.nlm.nih.gov/medlineplus/mumps.html>

MedlinePlus: Rubella: <http://www.nlm.nih.gov/medlineplus/rubella.html>

MedlinePlus: Streptococcal Infections: <http://www.nlm.nih.gov/medlineplus/streptococcalinfections.html>

MedlinePlus: Whooping Cough: <http://www.nlm.nih.gov/medlineplus/whoopingcough.html>

16. Mental Health
Recommended Search Terms

- "Children at risk"
- Children "behavioral concerns"
- Children "behavioral disorders"
- Children "emotional disturbance"
- "Children's mental health"

Important Sites

Child and Family WebGuide: Health/Mental Health: <http://shiva.tcs.tufts.edu/cgi-bin/berger/secondary.pl?category=16&sub_category=143>

Connect for Kids: Children's Mental Health: <http://www.connectforkids.org/content1551/content.htm>

National Mental Health Association (NMHA): Children's Mental Health: What Every Child Needs for Good Mental Health: <http://www.nmha.org/infoctr/factsheets/72.cfm>

Portland State University: Research and Training Center on Family Support and Children's Mental Health: Children's Mental Health Links: <http://www.rtc.pdx.edu/pgChildrensMHLinks.shtml>

Hotlines

Allergies/Asthma:
1-800-7-ASTHMA

Association for Children for Enforcement of Support:
1-800-738-2237

Child Care Aware:
1-800-424-2246

Child Find of America:
1-800-426-5678 or 1-800-I-AM-LOST

Child Health and Human Development:
1-800-370-2943

Childhelp:
1-800-4-A-CHILD1-800-422-4453

Children's Defense Fund:
1-800-233-1200

Children's Health Insurance:
1-877-KIDS-NOW

Children's Hospice International:
1-800-242-4453

Girls and Boys Town National Hotline:
1-800-448-3000

Kidsrights:
1-800-892-5437

Lead Poisoning:
1-800-424-LEAD

National Association for Children of Alcoholics (NACoA):
1-888-554-2627

National Association for the Education of Young Children (NAEYC):
1-800-424-2460

National Center for Missing and Exploited Children:
1-800-843-5678

National Child Abuse Hotline:
1-800-422-4453

National Child Care Information Center (NCCIC):
1-800-616-2242

National Child Safety Council Childwatch:
1-800-222-1464

National Institute of Child Health and Human Development (NICHD) Information Resource Center:
1-800-370-2943

School Health Education:
1-800-311-3435

Shriners Hospital Referral Line:
1-800-237-5055

Toxic Substances:
1-888-422-8737

Zero to Three: National Center for Infants, Toddlers and Families:
1-800-899-4301

FAQs

Educational Resources Information Center (ERIC) Clearinghouse on Disabilities and Gifted Education: Frequently Asked Questions (FAQs): <http://ericec.org/faqs.html>

Environmental Protection Agency (EPA): Asthma and Indoor Environments: Asthma Frequent Questions: <http://www.epa.gov/asthma/introduction.html>

Maternal and Child Health Library: Frequently Asked Questions (FAQs): <http://www.mchlibrary.info/faqs.html>

Nemours.org: Frequently Asked Questions: <http://www.nemours.org/no/faq/index.html>

CHILDREN'S HEALTH PUBLICATIONS ON THE INTERNET

BioMed Central (BMC) Pediatrics: <http://www.biomedcentral.com/1471-2431/>

Children's Memorial Hospital (Chicago): The Child's Doctor: <http://www.childsdoc.org/>

Early Childhood Research and Practice (ECRP): <http://ecrp.uiuc.edu/>

David and Lucile Packard Foundation: The Future of Children: <http://www.futureofchildren.org/>

Federal Interagency Forum on Child and Family Statistics: Child Stats: America's Children: Key National Indicators of Well-Being 2003: <http://www.childstats.gov/ac2003/pdf/ac2003.pdf>

National Academies Press (NAP): Board on Health Sciences Policy and Institute of Medicine: *When Children Die: Improving Palliative and End-of-Life Care for Children and Their Families* (2003): <http://www.nap.edu/books/0309084377/html/index.html>

National Academies Press (NAP): Institute of Medicine (IOM): *Schools and Health: Our Nation's Investment* (1997): <http://books.nap.edu/books/0309054354/html/index.html>

National Institute of Child Health & Human Development (NICHD): Health Information and Media: Publications: *America's Children: Key National Indicators of Well-Being 2002*: <http://www.nichd.nih.gov/publications/pubs/childstats/americas.htm>

National Institute on Alcohol Abuse and Alcoholism (NIAAA): Keep Kids Alcohol Free: Strategies for Action: (2001): <http://www.alcoholfreechildren.org/gs/pubs/pdf/prevention.pdf>

National Institute on Alcohol Abuse and Alcoholism (NIAAA) and the Robert Wood Johnson Foundation: *How Does Alcohol Affect the World of a Child* (2003): <http://www.alcoholfreechildren.org/gs/pubs/pdf/statbooklet.pdf>

MEDICAL SPECIALTIES

Child psychology; Family practice; Pediatrics

PROFESSIONAL ORGANIZATIONS

American Academy of Allergy Asthma and Immunology (AAAAI): <http://www.aaaai.org/>

American Academy of Child and Adolescent Psychiatry (AACAP): <http://www.aacap.org/>

American Academy of Pediatric Dentistry (AAPD): <http://www.aapd.org/>

American Academy of Pediatrics (AAP): <http://www.aap.org/>

American Professional Society on the Abuse of Children (APSAC): <http://www.apsac.org/>

American School Health Association (ASHA): <http://www.ashaWeb.org/>

American SIDS (Sudden Infant Death Syndrome) Institute: <http://www.sids.org/>

Asthma and Allergy Foundation of America: <http://www.aafa.org/>

Patient Support Organizations/ Discussions Groups

AsthmaMoms: <http://www.asthmamoms.com/>

BellaOnline: Sons: <http://www.bellaonline.com/site.asp?name=Sons>

Brave Kids: Help for Children with Chronic, Life-Threatening Illnesses or Disabilities: <http://www.bravekids.org/>

Contemporary Moms: <http://www.contemporarymoms.com/>

Contemporary Moms: Positive Websites for Girls: <http://www.contemporarymoms.com/sitesforgirls.htm>

Early Childhood Links: Motherhood: <http://www.earlychildhoodlinks.com/parents/motherhood.htm>

Early Childhood Links: Fatherhood: <http://www.earlychildhoodlinks.com/parents/fatherhood.htm>

Fathering Magazine: <http://www.fathermag.com/>

Physician's Computer Company (PCC): PCC Online: PedTalk: <http://www.pcc.com/lists/pedtalk/faq.html>

Shykids.com: Kids-Tweens: <http://www.shykids.com/kids direction.htm>

Best One-Stop Shops

aHealthyMe!: Children's Health: <http://www.ahealthyme.com/topic/childrens>

CNN.com: Health Library: Children's Health: <http://www.cnn.com/HEALTH/library/children/>

Consumer and Patient Health Information Section (CAPHIS): Specific Conditions in Children: <http://www.caphis.mlanet.org/consumer/consumerKidscon.html>

Keepkidshealthy.com: <http://www.keepkidshealthy.com/>

KidsHealth: <http://www.kidshealth.org/index_noflash.html>

KidSource Online: Healthcare: <http://www.kidsource.com/kidsource/pages/Health.html>

MedlinePlus: Children's Health: <http://www.nlm.nih.gov/medlineplus/childrenshealth.html>

National Education Association (NEA) Health Information Network (HIN): <http://www.neahin.org/>

New York Online Access to Health (NOAH): Ask NOAH About: Child Health, Kids! <http://www.noah-health.org/english/wellness/healthyliving/childhealth.html>

Part III: Adolescents' Health Issues

Nancy J. Allee

Special Searching Issues for this Topic

The period of adolescence covers many significant moments and developmental stages between the end of childhood and the beginning of adulthood. Teenagers as a special population are well-represented on the Internet, and the topics included below are representative of those found within the category of "adolescents health" in Web directories. These topics reflect the "growing pains" and special challenges of the teen years and efforts to forge one's individual identity.

What to Ask

Some issues to consider in your search for adolescents' health information are age and developmental level. Depending on what you are looking for, you could find the information in the special topic section of "teen health" or under "child and adolescent health," "men's health" or "women's health," depending on these factors. Also consider whether you are looking for general health and wellness information or a specific disease or condition. Volume 1 covers many diseases and conditions in more detail.

Where to Start

If you are a parent, a good place to start the search for health information for adolescents is the "General" section listed below. Many search engines include young adults' health as a special topic under the category of "teenagers," "teens," or "adolescents health." Each of these sites includes different categories of information, so you will want to visit more than one. Additional Web sites worth reviewing are located under "Professional Organizations" and "Best One-Stop Shops." If you are a teen looking for information for yourself, you may want to begin with the "Site for Adolescents" listings before exploring other topics and Web sites.

Additional Search Strategies

If you are interested in information about a specific disease or condition that can affect individuals across the life span, it may be helpful to combine the term or terms for the disease or condition with terms related to adolescents, such as "heart disease" and "adolescents' health" or "teen health." You will also want to consult your physician with any questions or concerns about the information you discover.

TOPIC PROFILE

Who

Adolescents, generally defined as individuals between the ages of 13 and 18.

What

A broad category of health topics for parents and caretakers as well as Web sites designed for teens.

Where

Covers overall health and wellness of adolescents.

When

During the stage of adolescence, primarily between puberty and young adulthood.

ABBREVIATIONS USED IN THIS SECTION

CDC = Centers for Disease Control and Prevention
NAMI = National Alliance for the Mentally Ill
NIAMS = National Institute of Arthritis and Musculoskeletal and Skin Diseases
NIDA = National Institute of Drug Abuse
NIMH = National Institute of Mental Health
SAMHSA = Substance Abuse and Mental Health Services Administration

PROCEDURES AND SPECIAL TOPICS

17. GENERAL

Recommended Search Terms

- "Adolescent health" boys
- "Adolescent health" girls
- "Teen health"
- "Teenagers health"
- "Teen health" guide
- "Teen health" "health links"
- "Teen health" information
- "Teen health" issues
- "Teen health" prevention

- "Teen health" risk factors
- "Teen health" topics
- "Teen health" trends
- "Teens health"

Important Sites

Aetna InteliHealth: Teens' Health: Guiding Your Child through the Adolescent Years: Early Adolescence 11–14 Years: <http://www.intelihealth.com/IH/ihtIH/WSIHW000/34970/34989.html>

Aetna InteliHealth: Teens' Health: Guiding Your Child through the Adolescent Years: Middle Adolescence 15–17 Years: <http://www.intelihealth.com/IH/ihtIH/WSIHW000/34970/34990.html>

Aetna InteliHealth: Teens' Health: Guiding Your Child through the Adolescent Years: Late Adolescence 18–21 Years: <http://www.intelihealth.com/IH/ihtIH/WSIHW000/34970/34991.html>

AltaVista Directory: Health: Teen Health: <http://www.overture.com/d/search/p/altavista/odp/us/?c=directory&s=teen+health&topic=Top%2fHealth%2fTeen_Health>

The Aware Foundation: Teens: <http://www.awarefoundation.org/aware/teens.asp>

Centers for Disease Control and Prevention (CDC): Health Topic: Adolescents and Teens: <http://www.cdc.gov/health/adolescent.htm>

Centers for Disease Control and Prevention (CDC): National Center for Chronic Disease Prevention and Health Promotion: Adolescent and School Health: Health Topics: <http://www.cdc.gov/nccdphp/dash/healthtopics/>

Google Directory: Health: Teen Health: <http://directory.google.com/Top/Health/Teen_Health/>

Focus on Your Family's Health: Teens: <http://health.family.org/teens/articles/>

healthfinder: Just for You: Teenagers: <http://www.healthfinder.gov/justforyou/justforyou.asp?KeyWordID=169&branch=1>

Keepkidshealthy.com: Adolescent Health Center: <http://www.keepkidshealthy.com/adolescent/adolescent.html>

MedlinePlus: Teen Health: <http://www.nlm.nih.gov/medlineplus/teenhealth.html>

National Institute of Diabetes and Digestive and Kidney Diseases (NIDDK): *Take Charge of Your Health: A Teenager's Guide to Better Health*: <http://www.niddk.nih.gov/health/nutrit/pubs/winteen/>

NetWellness: Health Topics: Teen Health: <http://www.netwellness.org/healthtopics/25.cfm>

Stanford Health Library: Health Info: Children's Health: Child and Adolescent Health: <http://healthlibrary.stanford.edu/resources/internet/bodysystems/childrenshealth.html>

Yahoo! Directory: Health: Teen Health: <http://dir.yahoo.com/Health/Teen_Health/>

18. SITES FOR ADOLESCENTS
Recommended Search Terms

* "Teenagers Web sites"
* Web sites health teenagers
* Web sites teens health
* Web sites "teens health"
* "Web sites for teens"

Important Sites
Centers for Disease Control and Prevention (CDC): Powerful Girls Have Powerful Bones: <http://www.cdc.gov/powerfulbones/>

Cool Nurse: <http://www.coolnurse.com/>

Department of Health and Human Services (DHHS): Girl Power: <http://www.girlpower.gov/>

Department of Health and Human Services (DHHS): Office of Women's Health: 4 Girls Health: <http://www.4girls.gov/index2.htm>

Indiana University: School of Education: Center for Adolescent and Family Studies (CAFS): Adolescent Directory Online: Teens Only! <http://education.indiana.edu/cas/adol/teen.html>

Internet Public Library: TeenSpace: Health: <http://www.ipl.org/div/teen/browse/he0000/>

LifeBytes (Wired for Health): <http://www.lifebytes.gov.uk/indexmenu.html>

Mind, Body & Soul (Wired for Health) (UK): <http://www.mindbodysoul.gov.uk/>

Red Spot: <http://onewoman.com/redspot/>

Sex, Etc.: A Web Site by Teens for Teens: <http://www.sxetc.org/>

TeenGrowth.com: All about Your Health: <http://www.teengrowth.com/>

Teen Health Website (Canada): <http://www.chebucto.ns.ca/Health/TeenHealth/>

TeensHealth: <http://www.teenshealth.org/teen/index2.html>

Teen-Matters: <http://www.teen-matters.com/home.htm>

19. ADVOCACY AND HEALTHCARE POLICY, RESEARCH AND SERVICES
Recommended Search Terms

* Adolescents health advocacy
* Teenagers "health care research"
* Teens "health care services"

Important Sites
National Adolescent Health Information Center (NAHIC): <http://youth.ucsf.edu/nahic/>

National Alliance for the Mentally Ill (NAMI): Inform Yourself: About Public Policy: Child and Adolescent Action Center: <http://www.nami.org/youth/>

Pacific Institute for Research and Evaluation: Center for Adolescent and Child Health Research (CACHR): <http://www.pire.org/PRC/cachr/>

RAND Health: Maternal, Child, and Adolescent Health: <http://www.rand.org/health/researchareas/maternal.html>

The Society for Adolescent Medicine (SAM): <http://www.adolescenthealth.org/>

Society for Research on Adolescence (SRA): <http://www.s-r-a.org/>

20. BODY PIERCING AND TATTOOS
Recommended Search Terms

* "Body piercing" teens
* "Tattoo artists" teens
* Tattoos teens
* Tattoing teenagers

Important Sites
Immunization Action Coalition (IAC): Tattooing and Body Piercing Information: <http://www.immunize.org/tattoos/>

MedlinePlus: Piercing and Tattoos: <http://www.nlm.nih.gov/medlineplus/piercingandtattoos.html>

Virtual Children's Hospital: For Patients: Health Topics A–Z: Piercing and Tattoos: Tattooing and Body Piercing: Decision Making for Teens: <http://www.vh.org/Patients/IHB/Derm/Tattoo/>

21. EATING DISORDERS
Recommended Search Terms

* "Anorexia nervosa"
* "Binge eating disorder"
* Bulimia
* "Compulsive overeating"
* "Eating disorders" teenagers
* "Healthy body image" teens

Important Sites
Eating Disorder Referral and Information Center (EDReferral.com): <http://www.edreferral.com/>

MedlinePlus: Eating Disorders: <http://ww.nlm.nih.gov/medlineplus/eatingdisorders.html>

National Association of Anorexia Nervosa and Associated Disorders (ANAD): <http://www.anad.org/>

National Eating Disorders Association: <http://www.nationaleatingdisorders.org>

Something Fishy: Website on Eating Disorders: <http://www.something-fishy.org/>

22. MENTAL HEALTH

Recommended Search Terms

- "Adolescents' mental health"
- "At-risk teens"
- "Teenage anxiety disorder"
- "Teenage depression"
- Teenagers "emotional health"
- Teenagers "behavioral concerns"
- "Teens at risk"
- Teens "behavioral disorders"
- Teens "emotional disturbance"
- Teens "self esteem"

Important Sites

American Medical Association (AMA): Public Health: Adolescent Health Links: <http://www.ama-assn.org/ama/pub/category/1979.html>

Children's Hospitals and Clinics (Minneapolis/St. Paul, Minnesota): Clinics and Departments: National Mental Health and Education Center: Mental Health and Adolescents: <http://www.naspcenter.org/parents/parents_mental.htm>

Children's Hospitals and Clinics (Minneapolis/St. Paul, Minnesota): Clinics and Departments: Psychological Services: Teenage Depression: What Parents Can Do: <http://xpedio02.childrenshc.org/stellent/groups/public/@xcp/@Web/@mentalhealth/documents/policyreferenceprocedure/Web010841.asp>

Stanford University Medical Center: Lucile Packard Children's Hospital: Child and Adolescent Mental Health: <http://www.lpch.org/DiseaseHealthInfo/HealthLibrary/mentalhealth/index.html>

23. SEXUAL BEHAVIORS AND CHOICES

Recommended Search Terms

- "Sex education"
- "Teenage pregnancy"
- Teenage "sexual behavior"
- "Teen sexuality"
- Teens "abstinence education"
- Teens "sexual choices"
- Teens "sexual health"

Important Sites

American Social Health Association (ASHA): <http://www.iwannaknow.org/>

MedlinePlus: Teen Sexual Health: <http://www.nlm.nih.gov/medlineplus/teensexualhealth.html>

MedlinePlus: Teenage Pregnancy: <http://www.nlm.nih.gov/medlineplus/teenagepregnancy.html>

Planned Parenthood Federation of America, Inc: Teens: Teen Issues: <http://www.plannedparenthood.org/teens/>

Sexuality Information and Education Council of the United States (SIECUS): <http://www.siecus.org/>

Teen Sexuality: In a Culture of Confusion: A Documentary Study by Dan Habib: <http://www.intac.com/~jdeck/habib/>

Teenwire: <http://www.teenwire.com/index.asp>

24. SUBSTANCE ABUSE

Recommended Search Terms

- Cocaine
- Crack-cocaine
- "Drug education" prevention
- Ecstasy
- GHB
- Heroin
- Inhalants
- LSD tablets
- Marijuana
- Methamphetamine
- Teens alcohol
- Teens "alcohol and drugs"
- Teens "drug abuse"
- Teens "substance abuse"

Important Sites

Department of Health and Human Services and SAMHSA's (Substance Abuse and Mental Health Services Administration) National Clearinghouse for Alcohol and Drug Information: Publications: Tips for Teens: The Truth about Cocaine: <http://www.health.org/govpubs/phd640i/>

Drug Abuse Resistance Education (DARE): <http://www.dare.com/>

healthfinder: Just for You: Teenagers: Alcohol Abuse: <http://www.healthfinder.gov/>

healthfinder: Just for You: Teenagers: Drug Abuse: <http://www.healthfinder.gov/>

MedlinePlus: Alcohol and Youth: <http://www.nlm.nih.gov/medlineplus/alcoholandyouth.html>

MedlinePlus: Drug Abuse: <http://www.nlm.nih.gov/medlineplus/drugabuse.html>

MedlinePlus: Smoking and Youth: <http://www.nlm.nih .gov/medlineplus/smokingandyouth.html>

National Institute on Drug Abuse (NIDA): Information on Common Drugs of Abuse: <http://www.drugabuse .gov/DrugPages/>

Partnership for a Drug-Free America: <http://www.drug freeamerica.org/>

Partnership for a Drug-Free America: Help for Teens: Are Drugs Really That Bad For You?: <http://www.drugfree america.org/>

25. VIOLENCE

Recommended Search Terms

- "Gang violence"
- "Hate crimes"
- "Violence prevention"
- "Youth violence"

Important Sites

American Psychological Association: Warning Signs: <http://helping.apa.org/warningsigns/about.html>

MedlinePlus: Teen Violence: <http://www.nlm.nih.gov/ medlineplus/teenviolence.html>

National Youth Gang Center (NYGC): <http://www.iir .com/nygc/>

National Youth Violence Prevention Resource Center (NYVPRC): <http://www.safeyouth.org/home.htm>

U.S. Public Health Service: Office of the Surgeon General: *Youth Violence: A Report of the Surgeon General*: <http:// www.surgeongeneral.gov/library/youthviolence/>

HOTLINES

Alateen Family Group Meeting Information Line:
(888) 425-2666

Alcohol and Drug Abuse Crisis Line:
1-800-234-0420

Bureau for At-Risk Youth:
1-800-999-6884

Covenant House:
1-800-999-9999

Eating Disorders Help Line:
1-800-383-2832

National Runaway Hotline:
1-800-621-4000

National STD/AIDS Hotline:
1-800-342-2437

Rape Crisis Hotline:
1-800-656-HOPE

Sexually Transmitted Diseases Helpline:
1-800-227-8922

Suicide Prevention:
1-800-SUICIDE/1-800-784-2433

Youth Crisis Line:
1-800-448-4663

FAQs

Aetna InteliHealth: Frequently Asked Questions: Early Adolescence (11 through 14 Years): <http://www.inteli health.com/IH/ihtIH/WSIHW000/34970/34993/363 119.html>

Aetna InteliHealth: Frequently Asked Questions: Middle Adolescence (15 through 17 Years): <http://www.inteli health.com/IH/ihtIH/WSIHW000/34970/34995/363 121.html>

Aetna InteliHealth: Frequently Asked Questions: Late Adolescence (18 through 21 Years): <http://www.inteli health.com/IH/ihtIH/WSIHW000/34970/34997/363 122.html>

BracesInfo.com: Frequently Asked Questions: Teenage Orthodontic Patients: <http://www.bracesinfo.com/ teenage.html>

National Cancer Institute (NCI): Questions and Answers about Care for Children and Adolescents with Cancer: <http://cis.nci.nih.gov/fact/1_21.htm>

National Institute of Arthritis and Musculoskeletal and Skin Diseases (NIAMS): Health Topics: Questions and Answers about Acne: <http://www.niams.nih.gov/ hi/topics/acne/acne.htm>

National Institute of Arthritis and Musculoskeletal and Skin Diseases (NIAMS): Questions and Answers about Growth Plate Injuries: <http://www.niams.nih .gov/hi/topics/growth_plate/growth.htm>

National Institute of Child Health and Human Development (NICHD): Health Research: Fact Sheet for Health Professionals: Why Milk Matters: Questions and Answers for Professionals: <http://www.nichd.nih .gov/milk/healthresearch/fact_sheet.cfm>

National Institute on Alcohol Abuse and Alcoholism (NI AAA): Frequently Asked Questions: <http://www .niaaa.nih.gov/faq/faq.htm>

National Institute on Drug Abuse (NIDA): Publications: Principles of Drug Addiction Treatment: Frequently Asked Questions: <http://www.nida.nih.gov/PODAT/ PODAT4.html>

TeensHealth (Nemours Foundation): Q&A: <http://www .kidshealth.org/teen/question/>

ADOLESCENTS' HEALTH PUBLICATIONS ON THE INTERNET

Focus Adolescent Services: <http://focusas.com/index .html>

National Center for Health Statistics (NCHS): Adolescent Health Chartbook: Health, United States, 2000: <http://www.cdc.gov/nchs/data/hus/hus00cht.pdf>

National Heart, Lung, and Blood Institute (NHLBI): Awake at the Wheel : Top 5 Reasons to Get Enough Sleep : <http://www.nhlbi.nih.gov/health/public/sleep/aaw/brochure.pdf>

National Institute of Arthritis and Musculoskeletal and Skin Diseases (NIAMS): Questions and Answers about Scoliosis in Children and Adolescents (2001): <http://www.niams.nih.gov/hi/topics/scoliosis/Scoliosis RP.pdf>

National Institute of Mental Health (NIMH): Child and Adolescent Violence Research (2000): <http://www.nimh.nih.gov/publicat/violenceresfact.pdf>

National Institute of Mental Health (NIMH): *Helping Children and Adolescents Cope with Violence and Disasters* (2001): <http://www.nimh.nih.gov/publicat/violence.pdf>

National Institute on Alcohol Abuse and Alcoholism (NIAAA): *Changing the Culture of Campus Drinking* (2002): <http://www.niaaa.nih.gov/publications/AA58.pdf>

National Institute on Drug Abuse (NIDA): Marijuana : Facts for Teens (Revised, 2003): <http://www.drugabuse.gov/PDF/TEENS_Marijuana_brochure.pdf>

MEDICAL SPECIALTIES

Adolescent medicine; Pediatrics

PROFESSIONAL ORGANIZATIONS

American Academy of Child and Adolescent Psychiatry (AACAP): <http://www.aacap.org/>

American Academy of Pediatrics (AAP): <http://www.aap.org/>

National Education Association (NEA): Health Information Network: <http://www.neahin.org/>

Society for Adolescent Medicine (SAM): <http://www.adolescenthealth.org/>

PATIENT SUPPORT ORGANIZATIONS/ DISCUSSIONS GROUPS

Self-Injury: You are NOT the Only One: <http://www.palace.net/~llama/psych/intro.html>

Shykids.com: Teens: <http://www.shykids.com/teensdirection.htm>

Teen Advice Online: <http://www.teenadviceonline.org/>

Teen-Anon: <http://www.teen-anon.com/home.htm>

Teen Help: <http://www.vpp.com/teenhelp/>

BEST ONE-STOP SHOPS

Go Ask Alice! <http://www.goaskalice.columbia.edu/>

Keepkidshealthy.com: Adolescent Health Center: <http://www.keepkidshealthy.com/adolescent/adolescent.html>

TeensHealth: <http://www.teenshealth.org/teen/index2.html>

MedlinePlus: Teen Development: <http://www.nlm.nih.gov/medlineplus/teendevelopment.html>

MedlinePlus: Teen Health: <http://www.nlm.nih.gov/medlineplus/teenhealth.html>

National Institutes of Health (NIH): Child and Teen Health: <http://health.nih.gov/search.asp?category_id=24>

TeensHealth (Nemours Foundation): <http://www.kidshealth.org/teen/>

University of Michigan Health System: Child and Adolescent Health Topics A–Z: <http://www.med.umich.edu/1libr/pa/pa_index.htm>

Part IV: Adults' Health Issues (Men)

Nancy J. Allee

[*See also* "Prostate Disorders," p. 171; "Reproductive Cancers (Men); "Sexual Health Issues," p. 178.]

SPECIAL SEARCHING ISSUES FOR THIS TOPIC

Topics in "Men's Health Issues" cover general health and wellness as well as issues specific to men and the male reproductive organs. Information is selective, not comprehensive, so the listings of Web sites should be considered a starting point for information. There are several references to other sections with more detailed coverage of topics related to men's health as duplication of information has been avoided as much as possible.

What to Ask

One of the first questions to consider is whether the health issue of concern is uniquely relevant to men? Is a particular part or organ of the anatomy involved? Is the interest in overall health and wellness, that is, men's health in general, or on a specific topic or disease condition?

Where to Start

If you are interested in general health and wellness, one of the best places to start is a health search engine such as healthAtoZ, NOAH, or MedlinePlus that includes a special topic on "men's health." It is important to consult more than one special topics section because the categories and quantity of information varies. If men's health is not in a separate health topics section, or if you do not find the particular aspect of men's health for which you are searching, then identify the keywords or concepts and search these terms separately in the health search engine or in your preferred general search engine.

Additional Search Strategies

Some diseases or conditions uniquely affect men, such as prostate cancer. For these diseases or conditions, searching with the particular keywords or terms is sufficient to locate the information. For other diseases and conditions that affect both men and women such as coronary heart disease, it may be helpful to combine terms for the disease or condition with "men's health."

TOPIC PROFILE

Who

Men, generally defined as human males over the age of 18.

What

A broad category of health topics of primary interest to men.

Where

Covers overall health and wellness of men and issues specific to the male anatomy.

When

During the stage of adulthood.

ABBREVIATIONS USED IN THIS SECTION

AAFP = American Academy of Family Physicians

AIDS = Acquired Immune Deficiency Syndrome

AUA = American Urological Association

CDC = Centers for Disease Control and Prevention

HPV = Human Papillomavirus

MHN = Men's Health Network

PTSD = Post-Traumatic Stress Disorder

STD = Sexually Transmitted Disease

VD = Venereal Diseases

PROCEDURES AND SPECIAL TOPICS

26. GENERAL

Recommended Search Terms

- Male health
- "Men's health"
- "Men's health" guide
- "Men's health" "health links"
- "Men's health" information
- "Men's health" issues
- "Men's health" prevention
- "Men's health" risk factors
- "Men's health" topics
- "Men's health" trends

Important Sites

American Academy of Family Physicians (AAFP): Family Doctor: Men's Health: <http://www.familydoctor.org/men.xml>

Centers for Disease Control and Prevention (CDC): Health Topic: Men's Health: <http://www.cdc.gov/health/mens_health.htm>

British Broadcasting Corporation (BBCi): Your Health: Men's Health: <http://www.bbc.co.uk/health/mens/>

Google Directory: Health: Men's Health: <http://directory.google.com/Top/Health/Men%27s_Health/>

HealthandAge: Men's Health Center: <http://www.healthandage.de/Home/gc=28>

healthAtoZ.com: Health Channels: Men's Health: <http://www.healthatoz.com/atoz/centers/menshealth/mensindex.html>

healthfinder: Just for You: Men: <http://www.healthfinder.gov/>

MayoClinic.com: Healthy Living: Men's Health Center: <http://www.mayoclinic.com/>

Medem: Medical Library: Men's Health: <http://www.medem.com/medlb/sub_detaillb.cfm?parent_id=55&act=disp>

MedlinePlus: Men's Health Issues: <http://www.nlm.nih.gov/medlineplus/menshealthgeneral.html>

National Women's Health Information Center: 4woman.gov: What Do You Know about Men's Health? <http://www.4woman.gov/mens/>

NetWellness: Men's Health: <http://www.netwellness.org/healthtopics/20.cfm>

New York Online Access to Health (NOAH): Ask NOAH About: Men's Health: <http://www.noah-health.org/english/wellness/healthyliving/menshealth.html>

Stanford Health Library: Diseases and Disorders: Men's Health: <http://healthlibrary.stanford.edu/resources/internet/bodysystems/genital.html>

WebMDHealth: Health and Wellness: Women, Men, Lifestyle: Healthy Men: <http://my.webmd.com/living_better/him>

Yahoo! Directory: Health: Men's Health: <http://dir.yahoo.com/Health/Men_s_Health/>

27. Advocacy and Healthcare Policy, Research, and Services

Recommended Search Terms

- "Men's health" advocacy
- "Men's health care research"
- "Men's health care services"
- Men's health study
- Men's health studies
- Men's health initiative
- Men's health initiatives

Important Sites

Men's Health Network (MHN): <http://www.menshealth network.org/>

Men's Health Network (MHN): Office of Men's Health: Resource Center: <http://www.menshealthnetwork .org/omh_talkpoints.html>

National Men's Health Week: <http://www.menshealth week.org/>

Prostate.org: <http://www.prostatitis.org/prostateorg/>

28. Baldness

Recommended Search Terms

- Alopecia areata
- Baldness
- "Hair loss" men
- "Hair replacement" men
- "Hair restoration" treatment
- Male baldness
- "Male pattern hair loss"

Important Sites

American Academy of Family Physicians (AAFP): Family Doctor: Men's Health: Hair Loss: Hair Loss and Its Causes: <http://familydoctor.org/handouts/081.html>

American Society for Dermatologic Surgery: Patients: Fact Sheets: Hair Restoration Treatments: <http://www .asds-net.org/FactSheets/hair_restoration.html>

Family Doctor: Men's Health: Hair Loss: Hair Loss and Its Causes: <http://familydoctor.org/handouts/081.html>

Medem: Medical Library: American Medical Association: Male Pattern Baldness: <http://www.medem.com/>

MedlinePlus: Hair Diseases and Hair Loss: <http://www .nlm.nih.gov/medlineplus/hairdiseasesandhairloss .html>

29. Fatherhood and Parenting

Recommended Search Terms

- "Custodial fathers"
- "Expectant fathers"
- "Just for dads"
- "New fathers"
- "Single fathers"

Important Sites

BabyCenter: Pregnancy: Work and Family: Paternity Leave: What are the options for dads? <http://www .babycenter.com/>

Boot Camp for New Dads: <http://www.newdads.com/>

Father Resource Network: <http://www.father.com/links .php?op=MostPopular>

Fathers' Forum Online: <http://www.fathersforum.com/>

Fathers Resource Center: Parenting: <http://fathers resourcecenter.org/parenting.htm>

National Center on Fathers and Families (NCOFF): <http://www.ncoff.gse.upenn.edu/>

National Fatherhood Initiative: <http://www.fatherhood .org/>

Paternity Angel: Men and Pregnancy: <http://www .paternityangel.com/Preg_info_zone/MenPregnancy .htm>

Responsible Single Fathers: <http://www.singlefather.org/ #rdads>

30. Genital Disorders

Recommended Search Terms

- "Male genital disorders"
- Men genital problems
- Male reproductive system disorders
- "Penile cancer"
- "Penile disorders"
- "Peyronie's disease"
- "Prostate cancer"
- "Scrotal masses"
- "Testicular cancer"
- "Testicular disorders"
- "Undescended testicles"
- Urinary tract infections men

Important Sites

Aetna InteliHealth: Women's Health: Urinary Tract Infection in Men: <http://www.intelihealth.com/>

American Academy of Family Physicians (AAFP): Family Doctor: Health Tools: Search by Symptom: Genital

Problems in Men: <http://familydoctor.org/flowcharts/539.html>

MedlinePlus: Male Genital Disorders: <http://www.nlm.nih.gov/medlineplus/malegenitaldisorders.html>

National Cancer Institute (NCI): cancer.gov: Testicular Cancer Home Page: <http://www.cancer.gov/cancerinfo/types/testicular>

National Institute of Diabetes and Diagestive and Kidney Diseases (NIDDK): National Kidney and Urologic Diseases Information Clearinghouse (NKUDIC): Peyronie's Disease: <http://www.niddk.nih.gov/health/urolog/pubs/peyronie/peyronie.htm>

31. IMPOTENCE

Recommended Search Terms

- "Erectile dysfunction"
- Impotence
- Impotence causes
- Impotence "clinical trials"
- "Male infertility"
- "Sexual dysfunction" men
- "Sexual dysfunction" treatment

Important Sites

American Academy of Family Physicians (AAFP): Family Doctor: Erectile Dysfunction: <http://familydoctor.org/109.xml>

American Foundation for Urologic Disease: Diseases and Conditions: Sexual Function: Confronting Erectile Dysfunction as a Team: <http://www.afud.org/education/sexualfunction/impotence.asp>

Erectile Dysfunction Institute: <http://www.erectile-dysfunction-impotence.org/>

Impotence.org: <http://www.impotence.org/>

MedlinePlus: Impotence: <http://www.nlm.nih.gov/medlineplus/impotence.html>

National Institutes of Health: ClinicalTrials.gov: Browse: By Condition: Alphabetically: Impotence: Effects of Yohimbine and Naltrexone on Sexual Function: <http://clinicaltrials.gov/>

32. MENTAL HEALTH

Recommended Search Terms

- Male depression
- "Mental health" men
- Men depression
- Men psychological distress
- Men psychosocial health
- "Men's health" psychosocial
- Men stress
- "Post-traumatic stress disorder"

Important Sites

Cleveland Clinic Health System: Health Information: Depression: Special Populations: Depression in Men: <http://www.cchs.net/health/health-info/docs/2200/2286.asp?index=9307>

National Center for PTSD (Post Traumatic Stress Disorder): Fact Sheet: What Is Posttraumatic Stress Disorder? <http://www.ncptsd.org/facts/general/fs_what_is_ptsd.html>

National Institute of Mental Health (NIMH): Depression: <http://www.nimh.nih.gov/publicat/depression.cfm#ptdep1>

National Mental Health Association (NMHA): Mental Health Information: Fact Sheets: Depression Screening: National Screening for Depression: <http://www.nmha.org/ccd/support/screening.cfm>

National Women's Health Information Center: 4woman.gov: Mental Health in Men: <http://www.4woman.gov/mens/men.cfm?page=118&mtitle=mental%20health>

33. SCREENING TESTS

Recommended Search Terms

- "Colorectal cancer screening"
- "Digital rectal exam"
- Males "screening tests"
- Men "screening tests"
- "Prostate-specific antigen testing"
- "PSA testing"
- "Testicular exam"

Important Sites

Centers for Disease Control and Prevention (CDC): Cancer Prevention and Control: Colorectal Cancer Information: <http://www.cdc.gov/cancer/screenforlife/info.htm>

Memorial Sloan-Kettering Cancer Center: Cancer Information: Prevention and Screening: Screening Guidelines and Resources: Screening Checklist—Men: <http://www.mskcc.org/mskcc/html/8241.cfm>

MayoClinic.com: Men's Health Center: Men's Screening Tests: What, Why, and How Often? <http://www.mayoclinic.com/>

Palo Alto Medical Foundation: Health Information: Preventive Health Guidelines: Guidelines for Prostate Cancer

Testing/Prostate Specific Antigen Testing (PSA): <http://www.pamf.org/health/guidelines/psa.html>

Testicular Cancer Resource Center (TCRC): How to Do a Testicular Self Examination: <http://tcrc.acor.org/tcexam.html>

34. SEXUALLY TRANSMITTED DISEASES

[*See also*: "Sexual Safety," p. 23; "Sexual Health Issues," p. 178.]

Recommended Search Terms

- AIDS
- Chlamydia
- Gonorrhea
- Herpes
- HPV
- Human papillomavirus
- "Safe sex" men
- "Sexually Transmitted Diseases" men
- STDs
- Syphilis
- VD
- Venereal diseases
- [Name of STD] "clinical trials"
- [Name of STD] diagnosis
- [Name of STD] "patient information"
- [Name of STD] prevention
- [Name of STD] research
- [Name of STD] "risk factors"
- [Name of STD] treatment

Important Sites

American Academy of Family Physicians (AAFP): Family Doctor: STDs: Common Symptoms & Tips on Prevention: <http://www.familydoctor.org/x5170.xml>

American Social Health Association: Facts and Answers about STDs: STD Glossary: <http://www.ashastd.org/stdfaqs/glossaryindex.html>

Centers for Disease Control and Prevention (CDC): National Center for HIV, STD and TB Prevention: Fact Sheet for Public Health Personnel: Male Latex Condoms and Sexually Transmitted Diseases: <http://www.cdc.gov/nchstp/od/latex.htm>

MayoClinic.com: Infectious Disease Center: STD Quiz: Are You Taking Proper, Preventive Steps? <http://www.mayoclinic.com/>

MedlinePlus: Sexually Transmitted Diseases: <http://www.nlm.nih.gov/medlineplus/sexuallytransmitteddiseases.html>

New York City Department of Health and Mental Hygiene: Sexually Transmitted Diseases: Prevent the Spread of STDs: <http://www.ci.nyc.ny.us/html/doh/html/std/std4.html>

New York Online Access to Health (NOAH): Ask NOAH About: Sexually Transmitted Diseases: <http://www.noah-health.org/english/illness/stds/stds.html>

35. UROLOGY

[See: "Kidney Diseases and Bladder Disorders," p. 109, vol. 2.]

Recommended Search Terms

- "Bladder infection" men
- "Genital tract" diseases
- "Male infertility"
- "Urinary Incontinence" men
- Urinary tract diseases males
- "Urinary tract" diseases men
- Urogenital neoplasms
- "Urogenital system"
- Urologic diseases
- Urologic "patient care"
- Urology

Important Sites

MedlinePlus: Bladder Diseases: <http://www.nlm.nih.gov/medlineplus/bladderdiseases.html>

MedlinePlus: Urinary Incontinence: <http://www.nlm.nih.gov/medlineplus/urinaryincontinence.html>

MedlinePlus: Urinary Tract Infections: <http://www.nlm.nih.gov/medlineplus/urinarytractinfections.html>

National Kidney and Urologic Diseases Information Clearinghouse (NKUDIC): What I Need to Know about Urinary Tract Infections: <http://kidney.niddk.nih.gov/kudiseases/pubs/uti_ez/>

Urology Channel: Overactive Bladder: <http://www.urologychannel.com/bladdercontrol/index.shtml>

Urology Channel: Urinary Tract Infections: <http://www.urologychannel.com/uti/>

Urology Channel: Urological Emergencies: <http://www.urologychannel.com/emergencies/>

WebMD: Boxers or Briefs: Myths and Facts about Men's Infertility: <http://my.webmd.com/>

36. VASECTOMY

Recommended Search Terms

- "Male birth control"
- Vasectomy
- "Vasectomy reversal"

Important Sites

Planned Parenthood Federation of America Birth Control: Permanent Methods (Sterilization): All about Vasectomy: <http://www.plannedparenthood.org/BIRTH-CONTROL/allaboutvas.htm>

National Cancer Institute (NCI): Cancer Facts: Questions and Answers about the Prostate-Specific Antigen (PSA) Test: <http://cis.nci.nih.gov/fact/5_29.htm>

National Cancer Institute (NCI): Cancer Facts: Testicular Cancer: Questions and Answers: <http://cis.nci.nih.gov/fact/6_34.htm>

Resolve: National Infertility Association: Frequently Asked Questions about Infertility: <http://www.resolve.org/main/national/trying/whatis/faq.jsp?name=trying&tag=whatis>

Vasectomy.com: <http://www.vasectomy.com/main.asp>

Vasectomymedical.com: Vasectomy Reversal: <http://www.vasectomymedical.com/vasectomy-reversal.html>

HOTLINES

Alcohol and Drug Abuse Hotline:
1-800-ALCOHOL
American Foundation for Urologic Disease: Patient Information:
1-800-242-2383
Cocaine Helpline:
1-800-262-2463
Erectile Dysfunction Institute:
1-866-563-2432
Impotence Information Center:
1-800-843-4315
National Crisis Helpline:
1-800-999-9999
National Suicide Hotline:
1-800-SUICIDE

FAQs

Impotence.org: Frequently Asked Questions: <http://www.impotence.org/FAQ/index.asp>

National Alopecia Areata Foundation: Frequently Asked Questions: <http://www.alopeciaareata.com/request info/faq.asp#1>

MEN'S HEALTH PUBLICATIONS ON THE INTERNET

Agency for Healthcare Research and Quality (AHRQ): *Focus on Research*: Issues in Men's Health Care (2002): <http://www.ahrq.gov/news/focus/menshc.pdf>

Agency for Healthcare Research and Quality (AHRQ): *Focus on Research*: Men: Stay Healthy at Any Age: Checklist for Your Next Checkup (2003): <http://www.ahrq.gov/news/focus/menshc.pdf>

Centers for Disease Control and Prevention (CDC): National Center for Chronic Disease Prevention and Health Promotion: Cardiovascular Health: Men and Heart Disease: An Atlas of Racial and Ethnic Disparities in Mortality: <http://www.cdc.gov/cvh/maps/cvdatlas/atlas_mens/mens_download.htm>

Commonwealth Fund: *Out of Touch: American Men and the Health Care System* (2000): <http://www.cmwf.org/programs/women/sandman_outoftouch_374.pdf>

Guttmacher Institute: *In Their Own Right: Addressing the Sexual and Reproductive Health Needs of American Men*: <http://www.guttmacher.org/us_men/us_men.pdf>

Harvard Men's Health Watch: <http://www.health.harvard.edu/hhp/publication/view.do;jsessionid=701BB12902396DCA74BFF2B6AA196358?name=N> [NOTE: Subscription required]

International Journal of Men's Health: <http://www.mensstudies.com/mspjournals.html> [NOTE: Subscription required]

Men's Health Journal: <http://www.menshealthforum.org.uk/default.asp?goto=resources/resources> [NOTE: Subscription required]

Men's Health Network (MHN): Healthy E-Male Weekly Electronic Newsletter: <http://www.menshealthnetwork.org/addlist-mensissues.htm> [NOTE: Registration required]

MenWeb: Men's Health: <http://www.vix.com/menmag/mensheal.htm>

National Cancer Institute (NCI): *Understanding Prostate Changes: A Health Guide for All Men* (1999): <http://www.nci.nih.gov/images/Documents/50985f62-b2eb-48f4-b325-8a20123b60eb/prostate_booklet.pdf>

National Kidney and Urologic Diseases Information Clearinghouse (NKUDIC): *What I Need to Know about Prostate Problems* (2002): <http://kidney.niddk.nih.gov/kudiseases/pubs/pdf/prostate_ez.pdf>

MEDICAL SPECIALTIES

Andrology; Dermatology; Family practice; Internal medicine; Neurology; Plastic surgery; Psychiatry; Reproductive medicine; Sports medicine; Urology; Venereology

PROFESSIONAL ORGANIZATIONS

American Academy of Family Physicians (AAFP): <http://www.aafp.org/>

American Cancer Society (ACS): <http://www.cancer.org/>

American Heart Association: <http://www.american-heart.org/>

American Medical Association (AMA): <http://www.ama-assn.org/>

American Psychiatric Association: <http://www.psych.org/>

American Society for Reproductive Medicine (ASRM): <http://www.asrm.org/>

American Stroke Association: <http://www.strokeassociation.org/>

American Urological Association (AUA): <http://www.auanet.org/index_hi.cfm>

Association of Reproductive Health Professionals (ARHP): <http://www.arhp.org/>

National Kidney Foundation: <http://www.kidney.org/>

PATIENT SUPPORT ORGANIZATIONS/ DISCUSSIONS GROUPS

Children, Youth, and Family Consortium: Father to Father: <http://www.cyfc.umn.edu/communities/programs/ftf.html>

Dads and Daughters: <http://www.dadsanddaughters.org/>

Fathers' Network: <http://www.fathersnetwork.org/page.php>

Men Stopping Violence: <http://www.menstoppingviolence.org/>

Men'sHealth: <http://www.menshealth.com/cda/home/0,6922,s1-0-0-0-0,00.html>

Men's Sexual Health Center: <http://www.mens-sexual-health.org/wwboard/>

Men's Health Network (MHN): HealthZone: <http://www.menshealthnetwork.org/healthzone/> [NOTE: Registration required]

Vasectomy Decisions: Are You Considering a Vasectomy? <http://www.geocities.com/fl_cheshire/>

BEST ONE-STOP SHOPS

CNN.com: Health Library: Men's Health: <http://www.cnn.com/HEALTH/library/men/>

Health-Nexus: Men's Health: <http://www.health-nexus.com/mens_health.htm>

MedlinePlus: Men's Health Topics: <http://www.nlm.nih.gov/medlineplus/menshealth.html>

National Institutes of Health (NIH): Men's Health: <http://health.nih.gov/search.asp?category_id=25>

New York Online Access to Health (NOAH): Ask NOAH About: Men's Health: <http://www.noah-health.org/english/wellness/healthyliving/menshealth.html>

WebMDHealth: Diseases and Conditions: Men's Conditions Health Center: <http://my.webmd.com/condition_center_hub/mhp>

Part V: Adults' Health Issues (Women)

Nancy J. Allee

[See also "Reproductive Cancer (Women)," p. 15, vol. 2; "Sexual Health Issues" p. 178.]

SPECIAL SEARCHING ISSUES FOR THIS TOPIC

In the past, women's health has sometimes been referred to as "navel to knees" health because often the focus in defining this area of specialization has been on reproductive health issues and diseases specific to the female reproductive organs. There may be certain logic to this approach since it is true that some diseases or health conditions do uniquely involve the female anatomy—such as uterine cancer, ovarian cysts, or pregnancy. But as any woman will attest, they are more than the sum of their female parts, and their interest in their own personal health has many dimensions, ranging from A to Z. This limited perspective has changed and expanded, and there is greater understanding of the need for a holistic point of view with attention to diverse issues such as diet and nutrition, psychosocial health, and heart disease, among many others. Newer definitions of women's health, such as that of the National Academy on Women's Health Medical Education, focus on issues such as "preservation of wellness" and "prevention of illness in women," including conditions that "are unique to women, are more common in women, are more serious in women, or have manifestations, risk factors, or interventions that are different in women."[1]

Bridging the past and present, "Women's Health Issues" includes Web sites related to reproductive health issues as well as overall health and wellness for women. The information is selective rather than comprehensive, so the Web sites listed should be considered only the beginning of the journey for finding resources on the topic of women's health. Also, in reading this section note that it attempts not to duplicate information in other parts of the book, so there are several "see" and "see also" references to other chapters that will cover related topics in more detail.

What to Ask

Women's health, like most subject areas, is multidimensional, and it can be somewhat difficult to locate reliable information on the Web. It is important, therefore, to ask some initial questions. First, is the health issue uniquely relevant to women? Is a particular part or organ of the anatomy involved? Is the interest in overall health and wellness, that is, women's health in general, or in a specific topic or disease condition? Is the health issue a single topic or a combination of interests, such as pregnancy and exercise or hormone replacement therapy and osteoporosis? Is the health topic one that can affect males as well but the interest is primarily in aspects relevant to females, such as women and coronary heart disease? Is age a factor? Some issues are more relevant to women at particular stages of their life, such as menstruation, osteoporosis, and menopause, and it may be helpful to look for information on these topics not only in women's health categories but in areas that are somewhat overlapping, such as young women's or senior's health. All of these decisions make a difference in the search process. Once they are made, you are ready to begin searching for information.

Where to Start

If you are looking for women's health in general, the best place to start is with a health search engine such as healthAtoZ, healthfinder, NOAH, or MedlinePlus rather than a general search engine, which could produce more than a million hits on the subject. Also, because women's health is an established area of research and is of interest to at least half the population of the U.S., many health search engines include this category as one of their special categories of health topics. So, begin by looking for health topics within the health search engine, then in the "W" section for women's health. Within the women's health section, you will find a variety of resources, including information on specific diseases and health conditions. If women's health is not a separate health topics section, or if you do not find the particular aspect of women's health for which you are searching, then identify the keywords or concepts and search these terms in the health search engine or in a general search engine. Some illnesses predominately or singularly affect women, such as Sjögren's syndrome or interstitial cystitis. The terms for these conditions can be searched individually. Other conditions, such as lupus or coronary heart disease, can affect both men and women, so it may be helpful to combine terms for these conditions with "women's health" or "women" to ensure you are finding information targeted to the female gender.

Additional Search Strategies

In searching for information in this category, grammar can be important. If you include an apostrophe—for example, "women's health"—you will retrieve different results from what you will retrieve if you search "womens health." You will also retrieve different results with searches using "women" or "female" or spelling variations such as "womyn." Since women's health covers a wide amount of territory and since each of the health search engines may define it differently or include different categories, it may

be helpful to consult more than one. For instance, you may find uterine diseases in MedlinePlus but not diseases of the fallopian tubes, so you would need to consult another health search engine or conduct a search in a general search engine using keywords such as "fallopian tubes" and "diseases." It is also important to think of synonyms and alternate phrases to describe a topic since information may be found under a variety of subject headings. For instance, contraceptive information may be found under "birth control," "family planning," "reproductive health," or simply "the pill."

Volume 1 covers how to evaluate health information on the Web, so you may want to become familiar with those criteria and approaches to help you to evaluate the Web sites you retrieve with the "Recommended Search Term." These searches will result in vast amounts of information from many sources. The "Important Sites" that follow primarily represent professional organizations, associations, and government resources, considered to be among the most reliable sources of information on the Web. Also, some of the sites have been drawn from Web sites such as those of the Consumer and Patient Health Information Section (CAPHIS) of the Medical Library Association and the American Accreditation HealthCare Commission (URAC), offering the quality assurance that they have been selected by health sciences information and health professionals.

TOPIC PROFILE

Who

Women, generally defined as adult females over the age of 18.

What

A broad category of health topics of primary interest to women.

Where

Covers overall health and wellness of women and issues specific to the female anatomy.

When

During the stage of adulthood.

ABBREVIATIONS USED IN THIS SECTION

AHRQ = Agency for Healthcare Research and Quality
AIDS = Acquired Immune Deficiency Syndrome
AAFP = American Academy of Family Physicians

BSE = Breast Self-Examination

CAPHIS = Consumer and Patient Health Information Section of the Medical Library Association

CPR = National Center for Policy Research for Women and Families

HPV = Human Papillomavirus

HRT = Hormone Replacement Therapy

IUD = Intrauterine device

NCI = National Cancer Institute

NOAH = New York Online Access to Health

PCOS = Polycystic ovarian syndrome

PDQ = Physician Data Query

PMDD = Premenstrual Dysphoric Disorder

PMS = Premenstrual syndrome

STD = Sexually Transmitted Disease

URAC = American Accreditation HealthCare Commission

VD = Venereal Diseases

PROCEDURES AND SPECIAL TOPICS

37. GENERAL

Recommended Search Terms

- Female health
- Women healthcare
- "Women's health"
- "Women's health" guide
- "Women's health" "health links"
- "Women's health" information
- "Women's health" issues
- "Women's health" policy
- "Women's health" prevention
- "Women's health" risk factors
- "Women's health" topics
- "Women's health" trends
- "Womyn's health"

Important Sites

American Academy of Family Physicians (AAFP): Family Doctor: Women: <http://www.familydoctor.org/women.xml>

Boston Women's Health Book Collective: Our Bodies, Our Selves: <http://www.ourbodiesourselves.org/specific.htm>

British Broadcasting Corporation (BBCi): Your Health: Women's Health: <http://www.bbc.co.uk/health/womens/>

Centers for Disease Control and Prevention (CDC): National Center for Chronic Disease Prevention and Health Promotion: Wisewoman: Facts and Tools Every Woman Can Use: <http://www.cdc.gov/wisewoman/factsandtools.htm>

Estronaut: A Forum for Women's Health: <http://www.womenshealth.org/>

Food and Drug Administration (FDA): Women's Health Topics: <http://www.fda.gov/womens/informat.html>

Google Directory: Health: Women's Health: <http://directory.google.com/Top/Health/Women%27s_Health/>

HealthandAge: Women's Health Center: <http://www.healthandage.de/Home/gc=29>

healthAtoZ.com: Channels: Women's Health: <http://www.healthatoz.com/atoz/centers/womenshealth/womindex.html>

healthfinder: Just for You: Women: <http://www.healthfinder.gov/>

Health Resources and Services Administration (HRSA): Women's Health: <http://www.hrsa.gov/WomensHealth>

Medem: Medical Library: Women's Health: <http://www.medem.com/medlb/sub_detaillb.cfm?parent_id=1&act=disp>

MedlinePlus: Women's Health Issues: <http://www.nlm.nih.gov/medlineplus/womenshealthgeneral.html>

MedlinePlus: Women's Health Topics: <http://www.nlm.nih.gov/medlineplus/womenshealth.html>

National Center for Policy Research (CPR) for Women and Families: Women's Health: <http://www.cpr4womenandfamilies.org/womenhlth1.html>

National Institutes of Health (NIH): Women's Health (General): <http://health.nih.gov/search.asp?category_id=28>

NetWellness: Health Topics: Women's Health: <http://www.netwellness.com/healthtopics/27.cfm>

New York Online Access to Health (NOAH): Ask NOAH About: Women's Health: <http://www.noah-health.org/english/wellness/healthyliving/womenshealth.html>

Stanford Health Library: Health Info: Women's Health: <http://healthlibrary.stanford.edu/resources/internet/bodysystems/womenshealth.html>

University of Pennsylvania Health System: Press Releases: America's Health Policies are Failing Women, Finds Most Comprehensive Women's Health Study Ever: <http://www.uphs.upenn.edu/news/News_Releases/aug00/womenshealth.shtml>

WebMDHealth: Health and Wellness: Women, Men, Lifestyle: Healthy Women: <http://my.webmd.com/living_better/her>

Yahoo! Directory: Health: Women's Health: <http://dir.yahoo.com/Health/Women_s_Health>

38. Advocacy and Healthcare Policy, Research, and Services

Recommended Search Terms

- "Women's health" advocacy
- "Women's health care research"
- "Women's health care services"
- Women's health study
- Women's health studies
- Women's health initiative
- Women's health initiatives

Important Sites

Agency for Healthcare Research and Quality (AHRQ): Women's Health: <http://www.ahrq.gov/research/womenix.htm>

American Medical Women's Association (AMWA): <http://www.amwa-doc.org>

National Center for Policy Research (CPR) for Women and Families: Women's Health: <http://www.center4policy.org/womenhlth1.html>

National Women's Health Network: <http://www.womenshealthnetwork.org>

National Women's Law Center: Health: <http://www.nwlc.org/display.cfm?section=health>

Society for Women's Health Research: <http://www.womens-health.org>

Women's Health Initiative: <http://www.nhlbi.nih.gov/whi/>

39. Birth Control and Contraception

Recommended Search Terms

- "Assistive reproductive technology"
- "Birth control"
- Contraception
- "Emergency contraception"
- "Family planning"
- "Female condom"
- "Female contraception"
- IUD
- I.U.D.
- "Intrauterine device"
- "Reproductive health"
- "The pill"
- "Tubal ligation"
- Women contraceptives

Important Sites

Ann Rose's Ultimate Birth Control Links: <http://www.ultimatebirthcontrol.com>

Association of Reproductive Health Professionals (ARHP): <http://www.arhp.org>

Feminist Women's Health Center: <http://www.fwhc.org/index.htm>

MedlinePlus: Birth Control/Contraception: <http://www.nlm.nih.gov/medlineplus/birthcontrolcontraception.html>

NOT-2-LATE.com: The Emergency Contraception Web Site: <http://ec.princeton.edu>

Planned Parenthood Federation of America: Emergency Contraception: <http://www.plannedparenthood.org/ec>

Planned Parenthood Federation of America: Women's Health: <http://www.plannedparenthood.org/WOMENSHEALTH/index.html>

40. Breast and Cervical Cancer

[*See also* "Cancers," p. 12, vol. 2.]

Recommended Search Terms

- Breast cancer
- "Breast cancer"
- Cervical cancer
- "Cervical cancer"
- [Type of cancer] "clinical trials"
- Type of cancer] "early detection"
- [Type of cancer] diagnosis
- [Type of cancer] genetics
- [Type of cancer] patient info
- [Type of cancer] "patient information"
- [Type of cancer] prevention
- [Type of cancer] research
- [Type of cancer] risk
- [Type of cancer] "risk factors"
- [Type of cancer] screening
- [Type of cancer] symptoms
- [Type of cancer] treatment

Important Sites

The Avon Foundation Breast Center at Johns Hopkins: Breast Cancer: Making the Right Choices for You: <http://www.hopkinsmedicine.org/breastcenter/library/diagnosis_treatment/choices.html>

BreastCancer.Net: Web Sites: <http://www.breastcancer.net/bcn.html>

Centers for Disease Control and Prevention (CDC): Cancer Prevention and Control: The National Breast and Cervical Cancer Early Detection Program: <http://www.cdc.gov/cancer/nbccedp/>

MedlinePlus: Breast Cancer: <http://www.nlm.nih.gov/medlineplus/breastcancer.html>

MedlinePlus: Cervical Cancer: <http://www.nlm.nih.gov/medlineplus/cervicalcancer.html>

National Cancer Institute (NCI): cancer.gov: Breast Cancer (PDQ) Treatment: <http://www.cancer.gov/cancerinfo/pdq/treatment/breast/patient/>

National Cancer Institute (NCI): cancer.gov: Cervical Cancer (PDQ) Treatment: <http://www.cancer.gov/cancerinfo/pdq/treatment/cervical/patient/>

National Cancer Institute (NCI): cancer.gov: What You Need to Know about Cancer of the Cervix: <http://www.cancer.gov/cancerinfo/wyntk/cervix>

National Cervical Cancer Coalition (NCCC): Research and Treatment: <http://www.nccc-online.org/>

Netwellness: Breast Cancer: <http://www.netwellness.org/healthtopics/breastcancer/>

WebMDHealth: Breast Cancer Health Center: <http://my.webmd.com/medical_information/condition_centers/breast_cancer/default.htm>

University of Massachusetts Medical School: The Lamar Soutter Library: Cancer Prevention Sites: <http://library.umassmed.edu/cancerprev.cfm>

41. Cosmetics, Cosmetic Issues, and Surgeries

Recommended Search Terms

- "Botox injections"
- "Breast implants"
- "Breast enlargement"
- "Breast prosthesis reconstruction"
- "Breast reduction"
- Cosmetics
- Cosmetics "consumer health"
- Cosmetics "women's health"
- "Face lift"
- "Permanent makeup"
- "Plastic surgery"

Important Sites

American Academy of Cosmetic Surgery (AACS): <http://www.cosmeticsurgery.org>

American Academy of Facial Plastic and Reconstructive Surgery: <http://www.facial-plastic-surgery.org>

American Board of Plastic Surgery (ABPS): <http://www.abplsurg.org>

American Society of Plastic Surgeons: <http://www.plasticsurgery.org>

Food and Drug Administration (FDA): Center for Food Safety and Applied Nutrition: Cosmetics: <http://www.cfsan.fda.gov/~dms/cos-toc.html>

MedlinePlus: Breast Implants/Breast Reconstruction: <http://www.nlm.nih.gov/medlineplus/breastimplantsbreastreconstruction.html>

MedlinePlus: Cosmetics: <http://www.nlm.nih.gov/medlineplus/cosmetics.html>

MedlinePlus: Plastic and Cosmetic Surgery: <http://www.nlm.nih.gov/medlineplus/plasticcosmeticsurgery.html>

42. Diet, Nutrition, and Exercise

Recommended Search Terms

- Diet "women's health"
- Nutrition "women's health"
- Women balanced diet
- Women "dietary habits"
- Women "healthy diet"
- "Women's health" "body image"
- "Women's health" exercise
- "Women's health" "exercise and fitness"
- "Women's health" "weight gain"
- "Women's health" "weight loss"

Important Sites

American Dietetic Association: <http://www.eatright.org>

American Heart Association: Delicious Decisions: <http://www.deliciousdecisions.org>

American Heart Association: Dietary Guidelines: <http://www.amhrt.org/>

Cyberdiet: <http://www.cyberdiet.com/reg/index.html>

Food and Drug Administration (FDA): Center for Food Safety and Applied Nutrition: Information for Women on Food Safety, Nutrition, and Cosmetics: <http://www.cfsan.fda.gov/~dms/wh-toc.html>

MedlinePlus: Nutrition: <http://www.nlm.nih.gov/medlineplus/nutrition.html>

National Heart, Lung, and Blood Institute (NHLBI): Interactive Meal Planner: <http://hin.nhlbi.nih.gov/menuplanner>

Nutrition.gov: Lifecycle Issues: Women: <http://www.nutrition.gov/framesets/frameset.php3?topic=lifecycle%20issues&subtopic=women>

Tufts University: Gerald J. and Dorothy R. Friedman School of Nutrition Services and Policy: Nutrition Navigator: <http://navigator.tufts.edu>

43. General Women's Anatomy

[*See also* "Cancers: Breast, Cervical and Other Reproductive Cancers (Women)," p. 15, vol. 2.]

Recommended Search Terms

- "Female reproductive anatomy"
- "Female perineal anatomy"
- "Normal female anatomy"

Important Sites

KidsHealth: Parents: General Health: Body Basics: Female Reproductive System: <http://kidshealth.org/parent/general/body_basics/female_reproductive_system.html>

MedlinePlus: Anatomy: <http://www.nlm.nih.gov/medlineplus/anatomy.html>

44. BLADDER

Recommended Search Terms

- Cystocele
- "Fallen bladder"
- "Interstitial cystitis"
- "Urinary tract infections"

Important Sites

Aetna InteliHealth: Women's Health: Urinary-Tract Infection in Women: <http://www.intelihealth.com/IH/ihtIH?t=9554&p=~br,IHW|~st,9103|~r,WSIHW000|~b,*|>

International Interstitial Cystitis Patient Network: <http://www.interstitial-cystitis.org/>

Interstitial Cystitis Network: <http://www.ic-network.com/>

MedlinePlus: Bladder Diseases: <http://www.nlm.nih.gov/medlineplus/bladderdiseases.html>

MedlinePlus: Urinary Tract Infections: <http://www.nlm.nih.gov/medlineplus/urinarytractinfections.html>

National Institute of Diabetes and Digestive and Kidney Diseases (NIDDK): National Kidney and Urologic Diseases Information Clearinghouse (NKUDIC): Kidney & Urologic Diseases Topics List: Cystocele (Fallen Bladder): <http://www.niddk.nih.gov/health/urolog/summary/cystocel/index.htm>

National Institute of Diabetes and Digestive and Kidney Diseases (NIDDK): National Kidney and Urologic Diseases Information Clearinghouse (NKUDIC): Urinary Incontinence in Women: <http://kidney.niddk.nih.gov/kudiseases/pubs/uiwomen/>

45. BREASTS

Recommended Search Terms

- "Breast changes"
- "Breast lumps"
- "Fibrocystic breast disease"

Important Sites

About: Women's Health: Fibrocystic Breast Lumps-Bumps-Pain: <http://womenshealth.about.com/library/weekly/aa031799.htm>

MedlinePlus: Breast Diseases: <http://www.nlm.nih.gov/medlineplus/breastdiseases.html>

National Cancer Institute: cancer.gov: Understanding Breast Changes: A Health Guide for All Women: <http://www.cancer.gov/cancerinfo/understanding-breast-changes>

46. OVARIES

Recommended Search Terms

- "Ovarian cysts"
- "Polycystic ovary disease"
- "Polycystic ovarian syndrome"
- PCOS

Important Sites

Aetna InteliHealth: Women's Health: Polycystic Ovary Syndrome: <http://www.intelihealth.com/>

MayoClinic.com: Women's Health Center: Ovarian Cysts: <http://www.mayoclinic.com/>

MedlinePlus: Ovarian Cysts: <http://www.nlm.nih.gov/medlineplus/ovariancysts.html>

47. UTERUS

Recommended Search Terms

- "Dysfunctional uterine bleeding"
- Endometriosis
- Fibroids
- Hysterectomy
- "Pelvic inflammatory disease"
- "Uterine and bladder prolapse"
- "Uterine conditions"
- "Uterine diseases"
- "Uterine fibroids"

Important Sites

Aetna InteliHealth: Sexual and Reproductive Health: Dysfunctional Uterine Bleeding: <http://www.intelihealth.com>

Food and Drug Administration (FDA): Alternatives to Hysterectomy: New Technologies, More Options: <http://www.fda.gov/fdac/features/2001/601_tech.html>

MedlinePlus: Endometriosis: <http://www.nlm.nih.gov/medlineplus/endometriosis.html>

MedlinePlus: Hysterectomy: <http://www.nlm.nih.gov/medlineplus/hysterectomy.html>

MedlinePlus: Uterine Diseases: <http://www.nlm.nih.gov/medlineplus/uterinediseases.html>

MedlinePlus: Uterine Fibroids: <http://www.nlm.nih.gov/medlineplus/uterinefibroids.html>

National Institute of Child Health and Human Development (NICHD): Health Information and Media: Publications: Endometriosis: Fast Facts about Endometriosis: <http://www.nichd.nih.gov/publications/pubs/endometriosis/index.htm>

48. VAGINA
Recommended Search Terms

- "Bacterial vaginosis"
- "Bartholin's gland cyst"
- Candidiasis
- "Chronic vulvar pain"
- Dyspareunia
- "Painful sexual intercourse"
- "Vaginal atrophy"
- "Vaginal discharge"
- "Vaginal infections"
- Vaginismus
- Vaginitis
- Vulvodynia

Important Sites

Aetna InteliHealth: Women's Health: Bartholin's Gland Cyst: <http://www.intelihealth.com/>

MayoClinic.com: Women's Health Center: Valvodynia: <http://www.mayoclinic.com/>

MedlinePlus: Candidiasis: <http://www.nlm.nih.gov/medlineplus/candidiasis.html>

MedlinePlus: Vaginal Diseases: <http://www.nlm.nih.gov/medlineplus/vaginaldiseases.html>

National Institute of Child Health and Human Development (NICHD): Health Information and Media: Publications: Vaginitis: <http://www.nichd.nih.gov/publications/pubs/vagtoc.htm>

49. DOMESTIC VIOLENCE
Recommended Search Terms

- Abuse
- "Battered spouse"
- "Domestic abuse"
- "Domestic violence"
- "Gender-based violence"
- "Intimate partner violence"
- "Physical abuse" women
- Rape
- "Sexual abuse"
- "Sexual assault" women
- "Spouse abuse"
- "Violence against women"

Important Sites

MedlinePlus: Domestic Violence: <http://www.nlm.nih.gov/medlineplus/domesticviolence.html>

Department of Justice: Office on Violence against Women: <http://www.ojp.usdoj.gov/vawo/>

The National Women's Health Information Center: 4woman.gov: Violence against Women: State Resources: <http://www.4woman.gov/violence/state.cfm>

50. HEART DISEASE

[*See also* "Heart and Circulatory Disease," p. 86, vol. 2.]

Recommended Search Terms

- Female "heart attack"
- Female "heart disease"
- Female heart health
- Female heart prevention
- Women "acute myocardial infarction"
- Women "cardiac arrhythmias"
- Women "cardiovascular health"
- Women "coronary heart disease"
- Women "electrolyte disturbances"
- Women "heart disease"
- Women "heart failure"
- Women heart prevention
- Women "heart problems"
- Women's heart health

Important Sites

American College of Cardiology Foundation: Clinical Statements/Guidelines: AHA (American Heart Association)/ACC (American College of Cardiology) Scientific Statement: Consensus Statement—Guide to Preventive Cardiology for Women: <http://www.acc.org/clinical/consensus/women/may99a/jac2673fla1.htm>

American Heart Association (AHA): Women, Heart Disease and Stroke: <http://www.americanheart.org/presenter.jhtml?identifier=4786>

MedlinePlus: Heart Diseases—Prevention: <http://www.nlm.nih.gov/medlineplus/heartdiseasesprevention.html>

The National Coalition for Women with Heart Disease: WomenHeart: <http://www.womenheart.org/>

National Heart, Lung, and Blood Institute (NHLBI): Information for Patients and the Public: Heart and Vascular Information: <http://www.nhlbi.nih.gov/health/public/heart/index.htm>

51. Hormone Replacement Therapy

Recommended Search Terms

- "Estrogen replacement therapy"
- "Hormone replacement therapy"
- "Hormone replacement therapy" benefits
- "Hormone replacement therapy" risks
- "Hormone replacement therapy" screening
- "Hot flashes"
- "Perimenopause"
- "Women's health" HRT

Important Sites

Agency for Healthcare Research and Quality (AHRQ): Clinical Information: U.S. Preventive Services Task Force: Chemoprevention: Hormone Replacement Therapy: <http://www.ahrq.gov/clinic/3rduspstf/hrt/>

The Hormone Foundation: <http://www.hormone.org/index.php3>

MedlinePlus: Hormone Replacement Therapy: <http://www.nlm.nih.gov/medlineplus/hormonereplacement therapy.html>

52. Menopause

Recommended Search Terms

- "Change of life" women
- "Climacteric symptoms"
- Menopausal symptoms
- Menopause
- Menopause "clinical trials"
- Menopause "dry eye"
- Menopause "hot flashes"
- Menopause research
- Menopause "signs and symptoms"
- Menopause treatment
- Perimenopause
- Postmenopause

Important Sites

Medem: Midlife Transitions: A Guide to Approaching Menopause: <http://www.medem.com/>

MedlinePlus: Menopause: <http://www.nlm.nih.gov/medlineplus/menopause.html>

Menopause Online: <http://menopause-online.com>

North American Menopause Society (NAMS): <http://www.menopause.org>

Planned Parenthood: Women's Health: Menopause: Another Change in Life: <http://www.plannedparent hood.org/WOMENSHEALTH/menopause.htm>

Power Surge: <http://hometown.aol.com/dearest/intro.htm>

Women's Health Access: Perimenopause: Preparing for the Change of Life: <http://www.womenshealth.com/patientinfo/menonewsletter/perimenochange.html>

53. Menstruation

Recommended Search Terms

- Amenorrhea
- "Chronic pelvic pain"
- Dysmenorrhea
- Dyspareunia
- Menorrhagia
- "Menstrual cycles"
- "Menstrual disorders"
- Menstruation
- "Premenstrual dysphoric disorder"
- "Premenstrual syndrome"
- PMDD
- PMS
- "Toxic shock syndrome"

Important Sites

American Academy of Family Physicians (AAFP): Family Doctor: Health Tools: Search by Symptom: Menstrual Cycle Problems: <http://www.familydoctor.org/flow charts/538.html>

MayoClinic.com: Women's Health Center: Amenorrhea: When Menstruation Goes Away: <http://www.mayo clinic.com/invoke.cfm?id=HQ00224>

MedlinePlus: Menstruation and Premenstrual Syndrome: <http://www.nlm.nih.gov/medlineplus/menstruation andpremenstrualsyndrome.html>

Museum of Menstruation and Women's Health: <http://www.mum.org>

Women's Health America: Premenstrual Syndrome FAQ (Frequently Asked Questions): What Is PMS (Premenstrual Syndrome)? <http://www.womenshealth.com/wha.html#pmsfaq>

54. Mental Health

Recommended Search Terms

- Female depression
- "Mental health" women
- Postpartum depression
- Women depression
- Women psychological distress
- Women psychosocial health
- "Women's health" psychosocial

Important Sites

MedlinePlus: Depression: <http://www.nlm.nih.gov/medlineplus/depression.html>

MedlinePlus: Mental Health: <http://www.nlm.nih.gov/medlineplus/mentalhealth.html>

National Institute of Mental Health (NIMH): <http://www.nimh.nih.gov>

National Institute of Mental Health (NIMH): Stories of Depression: Does This Sound Like You? <http://www.nimh.nih.gov/publicat/depstory01.cfm>

National Mental Health Association (NMHA): Clinical Depression in Women: <http://www.nmha.org/ccd/support/women.cfm>

Substance Abuse and Mental Health Services Administration (SAMHSA): National Mental Health Information Center: Women and Depression Fast Facts: <http://www.mentalhealth.org/publications/allpubs/fastfact6/>

55. OSTEOPOROSIS

[*See also* "Osteoporosis," p. 124, vol. 2.]

Recommended Search Terms

- "Bone diseases" men
- "Bone diseases" women
- "Bone health" "vitamin A"
- Osteoporosis
- Osteoporosis "bone density"
- Osteoporosis "calcium supplements"
- Osteoporosis "clinical trials"
- Osteoporosis diagnosis
- Osteoporosis exercise
- Osteoporosis "fashion tips"
- Osteoporosis medications
- Osteoporosis men
- Osteoporosis nutrition
- Osteoporosis "patient info"
- Osteoporosis "patient information"
- Osteoporosis prevention
- Osteoporosis research
- Osteoporosis signs
- Osteoporosis tests
- Osteoporosis treatment
- Osteoporosis "vitamin D"

Important Sites

MayoClinic.com: Health Tools: Slide Shows: Exercises for Osteoporosis: <http://www.mayoclinic.com/programsandtools/slideshows.cfm>

MayoClinic.com: Men's Health Center: Osteoporosis in Men: Bone Up on the Facts: <http://www.mayoclinic.com/>

MayoClinic.com: Women's Health Center: Bone Density Testing: Measure Your Risk of Broken Bones: <http://www.mayoclinic.com/>

MedlinePlus: Osteoporosis: <http://www.nlm.nih.gov/medlineplus/osteoporosis.html>

National Institutes of Health (NIH): Osteoporosis and Related Bone Diseases: National Resource Center: Vitamin A and Bone Health: <http://www.osteo.org/>

National Institutes of Health (NIH): Osteoporosis and Related Bone Diseases: National Resource Center: Osteoporosis Overview: <http://www.osteo.org/>

National Osteoporosis Foundation: Prevention: How Can I Prevent Osteoporosis?: <http://www.nof.org/prevention/>

National Osteoporosis Foundation: Medications to Prevent and Treat Osteoporosis: <http://www.nof.org/patientinfo/medications.htm>

Osteoporosis: Patient Information: Fashion Tips: <http://www.nof.org/patientinfo/fashion_tips.htm>

56. PREGNANCY AND CHILDBIRTH

[*See also* "Pregnancy Problems and Complications," p. 164.]

Recommended Search Terms

- "Baby formula"
- Breastfeeding
- "Breast milk"
- Caesarean
- "C-section"
- "Caesarean section"
- Childbirth
- "Childbirth education"
- Doulas
- "Expectant Fathers"
- "Expectant mothers"
- "Expectant parents"
- "Giving birth"
- "Infant care"
- "Infant feeding"
- "Infant formula"
- "Infant nutrition"
- "Labor & delivery"
- Midwifery
- Miscarriage
- Motherhood
- "Natural childbirth"
- "New mothers"
- Pregnancy

- "Pregnancy and childbirth"
- "Pregnancy and childbirth"
- "Prenatal care"

Important Sites

BabyCenter: <http://www.babycenter.com/>

ePregnancy: <http://www.epregnancy.com/>

La Leche League: Frequently Asked Questions: <http://www.lalecheleague.org/FAQ/FAQMain.html>

March of Dimes: Pregnancy and Newborn Health Education Center: Prenatal Care: <http://www.marchofdimes.com/pnhec/159_513.asp>

MedlinePlus: Labor and Delivery: <http://www.nlm.nih.gov/medlineplus/laboranddelivery.html>

MedlinePlus: Pregnancy: <http://www.nlm.nih.gov/medlineplus/pregnancy.html>

MedlinePlus: Prenatal Care: <http://www.nlm.nih.gov/medlineplus/prenatalcare.html>

National Health Information Women's Center: 4woman.gov: Healthy Pregnancy: <http://www.4woman.gov/pregnancy/>

New York Online Access to Health (NOAH): Ask NOAH About: Pregnancy: <http://www.noah-health.org/english/pregnancy/pregnancy.html>

57. Screening Tests
Recommended Search Terms

- BSE "women's health"
- "Breast imaging"
- "Breast self-examination"
- Mammogram
- Mammography
- "Pap smear"
- "Pelvic examination"

Important Sites

American Academy of Family Physicians (AAFP): Family Doctor: Parents and Kids: For Teens: How to Perform a Breast Self-Examination: <http://www.kidshealth.org/PageManager.jsp?dn=familydoctor&lic=44&article_set=22459>

American Society for Clinical Pathology (ASCP): Should I Have a Pap Smear?: <http://www.ascp.org/general/pub_resources/pap/>

Food and Drug Administration (FDA): Mammography Today: <http://www.fda.gov/cdrh/mammography/mmwebbro/mambrochure.html>

MedlinePlus: Medical Encyclopedia: Mammography: <http://www.nlm.nih.gov/medlineplus/ency/article/003380.htm>

National Cancer Institute (NCI): Cancer Facts: Screening Mammograms: Questions and Answers: <http://cis.nci.nih.gov/fact/5_28.htm>

National Cancer Institute (NCI): Get a Mammogram: Do It for Yourself, Do It for Your Family: <http://www.nci.nih.gov/cancerinfo/breasthealth>

National Cancer Institute (NCI): cancer.gov: Pap Tests for Older Women: A Healthy Habit for Life: <http://www.cancer.gov/cancer_information/doc.aspx?viewid=10ac5067-8217-47b4-a009-570bb4961eae>

The Susan G. Komen Breast Cancer Foundation: How to Do Breast Self-Exams (BSE): <http://www.komen.org/bse/>

58. Sexually Transmitted Diseases

[See: "Sexual Safety," p. 23; "Sexual Health Issues," p. 178.]

Recommended Search Terms

- AIDS
- Chlamydia
- Gonorrhea
- Herpes
- HPV
- Human papillomavirus
- "Safe sex" women
- "Sexually transmitted diseases" women
- "Sexually transmitted diseases" pregnancy
- "Sexually transmitted infections"
- STDs
- Syphilis
- VD
- Venereal diseases
- [Name of STD] "clinical trials"
- [Name of STD] diagnosis
- [Name of STD] "patient information"
- [Name of STD] prevention
- [Name of STD] research
- [Name of STD] "risk factors"
- [Name of STD] treatment

Important Sites

About Women's Health: STDs and Pregnancy: What You Need to Know about Sexually Transmitted Diseases during Pregnancy: <http://womenshealth.about.com/cs/pregnancy/l/aastdpregnancya.htm>

Aetna InteliHealth: Sexually Transmitted Diseases: Know the Symptoms of Sexually Transmitted Diseases: <http://www.intelihealth.com/>

healthAtoZ: Sexually Transmitted Diseases: <http://www.healthatoz.com/healthatoz/Atoz/dc/caz/repr/stds/stdindex.html>

HealthGate: STD's Center: <http://community.healthgate.com/GetContent.asp?siteid=geisinger&docid=/hic/std/index>

Healthy People 2010: Sexually Transmitted Diseases: <http://www.healthypeople.gov/document/HTML/Volume2/25STDs.htm>

MedlinePlus: Sexually Transmitted Diseases: <http://www.nlm.nih.gov/medlineplus/sexuallytransmitteddiseases.html>

National Institutes of Health (NIH): Sexually Transmitted Diseases: <http://health.nih.gov/result.asp?disease_id=588>

Planned Parenthood: Sexually Transmitted Infections: <http://www.plannedparenthood.org/sti/>

HOTLINES

AIDS Treatment:
1-800-448-0440
Alcohol and Drug Abuse:
1-800-222-2225
American Dietetic Association:
1-800-366-1655
American Heart Association:
1-800-242-8721
Bladder Control for Women:
1-800-891-5388
Emergency Contraception Hotline:
(888) NOT-2-LATE
Endometriosis Association:
1-800-992-3636
National Cancer Institute:
1-800-422-6237)
National Domestic Violence Hotline:
1-800-799-SAFE
National Drug and Alcohol Treatment Referral Routing Service:
1-800-662-4357
National Women's Health Information Center:
1-800-994-9662
National Women's Health Resource Center:
1-877-986-9472
Ovulation Research:
1-888-644-8891
PMS Access:
1-800-222-4767
SHARE: Self-Help for Women with Breast or Ovarian Cancer:
1-866-891-2392

Weight Control:
1-877-946-4627
Women's Sports Foundation Information and Referral Service:
1-800-227-3988

FAQs

National Heart, Lung, and Blood Institute: Postmenopausal Hormone Therapy: Information for the Public: Questions and Answers: <http://www.nhlbi.nih.gov/health/women/q_a.htm>

National Institute of Arthritis and Musculoskeletal and Skin Diseases (NIAMS): Health Topics: Questions and Answers on the Use of Hormones After Menopause for Osteoporosis and Recent Findings from the Women's Health Initiative: <http://www.niams.nih.gov/hi/topics/osteoporosis/hormones.htm>

National Mental Health Information Center: Mental Health and Mental Health Services: Frequently Asked Questions: <http://www.mentalhealth.samhsa.gov/publications/allpubs/government/>

National Women's Health Information Center: 4woman.gov: Breast Cancer (2003): <http://www.4woman.gov/faq/cbreast.htm>

National Women's Health Information Center: 4woman.gov: Breast Self-Exam (2003): <http://www.4woman.gov/faq/bsefaq.htm>

National Women's Health Information Center: 4woman.gov: Frequently Asked Questions About Women's Health: <http://www.4women.gov/faq>

National Women's Health Information Center: 4woman.gov: A Healthy Diet (2003): <http://www.4woman.gov/faq/diet.htm>

National Women's Health Information Center: 4woman.gov: Lupus (2003): <http://www.4woman.gov/faq/lupus.htm>

National Women's Health Information Center: 4woman.gov: Menopause (2003): <http://www.4woman.gov/faq/menopaus.htm>

National Women's Health Information Center: 4woman.gov: Physical Activity (Exercise) (2003): <http://www.4woman.gov/faq/exercise.htm>

National Women's Health Information Center: 4woman.gov: Smoking (2003): <http://www.4woman.gov/faq/smoking.htm>

National Women's Health Information Center: 4woman.gov: Uterine Fibroids (2003): <http://www.4woman.gov/faq/fibroids.htm>

Planned Parenthood Federation of America: Women's Health: <http://www.plannedparenthood.org/WOMENSHEALTH/>

PubMed Central: The Women's Health Questionnaire (WHQ): Frequently Asked Questions (FAQ): <http://www.pubmedcentral.nih.gov/>

WOMEN'S HEALTH PUBLICATIONS ON THE INTERNET

American Psychological Association: *Summit on Women and Depression* (2002): <http://www.apa.org/pi/wpo/women&depression.pdf>

Harvard Women's Health Watch: <http://www.health.harvard.edu/> [NOTE: Subscription required]

Journal of the American Medical Women's Association (JAMWA): <http://jamwa.amwa-doc.org>

Journal Watch: Women's Health: <http://women.jwatch.org>

National Academies Press (NAP): Institute of Medicine (IOM): *Dietary Risk Assessment in the WIC Program* (2002): <http://www.nap.edu/catalog/10342.html>

National Heart, Lung, and Blood Institute (NHLBI): *The Healthy Heart Handbook for Women* (2003): <http://www.nhlbi.nih.gov/health/public/heart/other/hhw/hdbk_wmn.pdf>

National Heart, Lung, and Blood Institute (NHLBI): *Women's Health and Menopause: A Comprehensive Approach*: <http://www.nhlbi.nih.gov/health/prof/heart/other/menopaus/index.htm>

National Institute of Allergy and Infectious Diseases (NIAID): *Women's Health in the U.S.: Research on Health Issues Affecting Women* (2002): <http://www.niaid.nih.gov/publications/womenshealth/womenshealth.pdf>

National Institute of Diabetes and Digestive and Kidney Diseases (NIDDKD): Bladder Control for Women (2003): <http://kidney.niddk.nih.gov/kudiseases/pubs/pdf/bcw.pdf>

National Institute of Mental Health (NIMH): *Depression: What Every Woman Should Know* (2000): <http://www.nimh.nih.gov/publicat/depwomenknows.pdf>

National Institute on Alcohol Abuse and Alcoholism (NIAAA): Publications: *Alcohol: A Women's Health Issue* (2003): <http://www.niaaa.nih.gov/publications/brochurewomen/women.htm>

National Women's Health Information Center: 4woman.gov: *Women's Health for the Homefront 2003 Daybook: Including a State-by-State Guide to Women's Health Resources*: <http://www.4woman.gov/faq/2003daybook.pdf>

National Women's Law Center: *Women's Health Report Card 2001: Making the Grade on Women's Health: A National and State-by-State Report Card*: <http://www.nwlc.org/display.cfm?section=health#(Women's%20Health%20Report%20Card%202001)>

Society for Women's Health Research: Quarterly Newsletter: *Sexx Matters* (Fall 2003): <http://www.womens-health.org/about/newsletter_fall_03.pdf>

MEDICAL SPECIALTIES

Dermatology; Gynecology; Family practice; Internal medicine; Neurology; Obstetrics; Plastic surgery; Psychiatry; Reproductive medicine; Sports medicine; Venereology

PROFESSIONAL ORGANIZATIONS

American College of Obstetricians and Gynecologists (ACOG): <http://www.acog.org>

American Heart Association: Go Red for Women: <http://www.americanheart.org/presenter.jhtml?identifier=3017091>

American Medical Women's Association: <http://www.amwa-doc.org/>

Society for Women's Health Research: <http://www.womens-health.org/>

Susan G. Komen Breast Cancer Foundation: <http://www.komen.org/>

Women's Heart Foundation: <http://www.womensheartfoundation.org/>

PATIENT SUPPORT ORGANIZATIONS/ DISCUSSIONS GROUPS

Obgyn.net: Women's Health: A Forum for Women: <http://forums.obgyn.net/womens-health/>

PCOS.net: <http://www.pcos.net/>

BEST ONE-STOP SHOPS

aHealthyMe! Women's Health: <http://www.ahealthyme.com/>

Association of College and Research Libraries: Women's Studies Section: Women's Health Sites: <http://cc.usu.edu/~fshrode/wss_health.htm>

American Academy of Family Physicians (AAFP): Family Doctor: Women: <http://www.familydoctor.org/cgi-bin/familydoc.pl?op=search&query=Women>

CNN.com: Health Library: Women's Health: <http://www.cnn.com/HEALTH/library/women/>

Consumer and Patient Health Information Section (CAPHIS): Women's Health Web Sites: <http://caphis.mlanet.org/consumer/consumerWomen.html>

MedlinePlus: Women's Health Topics: <http://www.nlm.nih.gov/medlineplus/womenshealth.html>

National Institutes of Health (NIH): Women's Health: <http://health.nih.gov/>

National Women's Health Information Center: 4woman.gov: <http://www.4women.gov>

National Women's Health Resource Center (NWHRC) Healthy Women: <http://www.healthywomen.org>

New York Online Access to Health (NOAH): Ask NOAH About: Women's Health: <http://www.noah-health .org/english/wellness/healthyliving/womenshealth .html>

OBGYN.net: Women's Pavilion: <http://www.obgyn.net/ women/women.asp>

REFERENCE

1. Goldman, M. B., and M. C. Hatch. "An Overview of Women and Health." In *Women and Health*, edited by Marlene B. Goldman and Maureen C. Hatch. San Diego, Calif.: Academic Press, 2000.

Part VI: Seniors' Health Issues

Nancy J. Allee

SPECIAL SEARCHING ISSUES FOR THIS TOPIC

This is the last of the sections devoted to age- and gender-related health information. As with the previous sections, this gives an overview of issues pertaining to individuals of a certain life stage. It includes topics particularly relevant to older adults, such as assisted living, prescription drugs, and Medicare, as well as coverage of resources for seniors' general health information. In keeping with other sections, it takes a holistic view of health and includes information on mental health issues, exercise, and nutrition. There is also information for caregivers and health advocates.

What to Ask

Here are some questions to help focus your search for health information on the Internet: Are you looking for organizations and associations that address a wide array of topics for seniors? In this case, it would be most useful to begin searching sites listed in the "Seniors' Health—General," "Seniors' Health Advocacy and Healthcare Policy, Research, and Services," or "Best One-Stop Shops" sections below. Or, are you looking for information about a specific disease or condition? Is it a disease or condition that is gender specific, such as prostatitis or vaginitis? In this case, it may also be beneficial to consult the sections for either "Men's Health Issues" (p. 130) or "Women's Health Issues," (p. 136).

Where to Start

Often search engines have a special topics section devoted to seniors' health information.

Remember that the names for these special topics can vary, so information may be found under "seniors' health," "aging," or "older adults," among others. The information within the special topics sections vary by category as well as quantity of links, so it may be helpful to consult more than one of the Web sites listed under "Seniors' Health – General" below.

Additional Search Strategies

If you are interested in information about a specific disease or condition that may affect older adults as well as individuals at other life stages, it may be helpful to combine the term or terms for the disease or condition with terms related to seniors, for example, "diabetes" and "seniors' health" or "older adults." Since this section attempts not to duplicate information in other sections, try exploring other topics in this guide for information on diseases or conditions that particularly affect older adults, such as osteoporosis, arthritis, Alzheimer's, and others.

TOPIC PROFILE

Who

Seniors, generally defined as individuals over the age of 65.

What

A broad category of health topics of primary interest to older adults.

Where

Overall health and wellness of seniors.

When

During the stage of older adulthood, often defined as beginning at age 65.

ABBREVIATIONS USED IN THIS SECTION

AARP = American Association of Retired Persons

ABA = American Bar Association

AGS = American Geriatrics Society

NCOA = National Council on the Aging

UCLA = University of California Los Angeles

PROCEDURES AND SPECIAL TOPICS

59. GENERAL

Recommended Search Terms

- Aged health
- "Aging and health"
- Elderly health
- Elderly parents health
- "Older adults health"
- "Senior health"
- "Seniors' health"
- Seniors "health and wellness"
- "Seniors' health" guide
- "Seniors' health" "health links"
- "Seniors' health" information
- "Seniors' health" issues
- "Seniors' health" prevention
- "Seniors' health" risk factors
- "Seniors' health" topics
- "Seniors' health" trends

Important Sites

American Academy of Family Physician (AAFP): Family Doctor: Seniors: <http://www.familydoctor.org/seniors.xml>

British Broadcasting Corporation (BBCi): Your Health: Health at 50+: <http://www.bbc.co.uk/health/50plus/>

Centers for Disease Control and Prevention (CDC): Healthy Aging for Older Adults: <http://www.cdc.gov/aging/>

ElderWeb: Organizations: <http://www.elderweb.com/default.php?PageID=1091>

Google Directory: Health: Senior Health: <http://directory.google.com/Top/Health/Senior_Health/>

HealthandAge: Positive Aging Center: <http://www.healthandage.de/Home?gm=20&gc=37&select.x=33&select.y=11>

healthAtoZ: Channels: Seniors' Health: <http://www.healthatoz.com/healthatoz/Atoz/hc/sen/sixtyplus.html>

healthfinder: Just for You: Seniors: <http://www.healthfinder.gov/justforyou/justforyou.asp?KeyWordID=172&branch=1>

Medem: Medical Library: Senior Health: <http://www.medem.com/medlb/sub_detaillb.cfm?parent_id=60&act=disp>

MedlinePlus: Seniors' Health Issues: <http://www.nlm.nih.gov/medlineplus/seniorshealthgeneral.html>

MedlinePlus: Seniors' Health Topics: <http://www.nlm.nih.gov/medlineplus/seniorshealth.html>

National Academy on an Aging Society: Links to Selected Online Resources: Aging Related Web Sites: <http://www.agingsociety.org/agingsociety/links/links_aging.html>

NetWellness: Health Topics: Aging: <http://www.netwellness.org/healthtopics/2.cfm>

New York Online Access to Health (NOAH): Ask NOAH About: Aging: <http:/www.noah-health.org/english/aging/aging.html>

Senior Health Care: <http://www.seniorhealthcare.org/>

Stanford Health Library: Health Topics: Senior Health: <http://healthlibrary.stanford.edu/resources/internet/bodysystems/seniors.html>

WebMDHealth: Health and Wellness: Women, Men, Lifestyle: Healthy Seniors: <http://my.webmd.com/living_better/age>

Yahoo! Directory: Health: Senior Health: <http://dir.yahoo.com/Health/Senior_Health/>

60. ADVOCACY AND HEALTHCARE POLICY, RESEARCH, AND SERVICES

Recommended Search Terms

- Aged healthcare services
- Elderly health advocacy
- "Seniors' health" advocacy
- "Seniors' health care research"
- "Seniors' health care services"

Important Sites

American Association of Retired Persons (AARP): <http://www.aarp.org/>

American Bar Association (ABA): Commission on Law and Aging: <http://www.abanet.org/aging/>

American Geriatrics Society (AGS): <http://www.americangeriatrics.org/>

American Geriatrics Society (AGS): Foundation for Health in Aging (FHA): <http://www.healthinaging.org/>

American Society on Aging (ASA): <http://www.asaging.org/>

National Association of Area Agencies on Aging: <http://www.n4a.org/default.cfm>

National Council on the Aging (NCOA): <http://www.ncoa.org/>

National Institute on Aging: <http://www.nia.nih.gov/>

61. CAREGIVERS

Recommended Search Terms

- "Aging parents" caregiving
- Caregivers aged

- Caregivers elderly
- Caregivers elderly "home modifications"
- "Caregivers resources"

Important Sites

American Association for Marriage and Family Therapy (AAMFT): Public Update: Families and Health: Caregiving for the Elderly: <http://www.aamft.org/families/Consumer_Updates/Caregiving_Elderly.asp>

Caregivers-USA.org: <http://www.caregivers-usa.org/>

Caregivers, Inc.: <http://www.caregiversnh.org/>

Caregiving.com: <http://www.caregiving.com/>

Children of Aging Parents: <http://www.caps4caregivers.org/index.htm>

Family Caregiver Alliance (FCA): <http://www.caregiver.org/index.html>

HealthandAge.com (Novartis Foundation for Gerontology): Ageing and Its Implications: An Online Primer for Healthcare Professionals and Carers: <http://www.healthandage.com/html/res/primer/>

National Academy on an Aging Society: Caregiving: Helping the Elderly with Activity Limitations: <http://www.agingsociety.org/agingsociety/pdf/Caregiving.pdf>

National Resource Center on Supportive Housing and Home Modification: homemods.org: <http://www.homemods.org/>

Open Directory Project (DMOZ): Health: Senior Health: Caregivers Resources: <http://dmoz.org/Health/Senior_Health/Caregivers_Resources/>

62. DRUGS AND MEDICATION

Recommended Search Terms

- Aged "medication management"
- Elderly medication use
- Elderly pharmaceuticals
- "Older adults" "medication misuse"
- "Prescription drug" "cost comparisons"
- Seniors "long-term illnesses" medication
- Seniors "over-the-counter drugs"
- Seniors "pain management"
- Seniors pills
- Seniors "prescription drug" education
- Seniors "prescription drug" information
- Seniors "prescription drugs"

Important Sites

Food and Drug Administration (FDA): Center for Drug Evaluation and Research (CDER): Drug Information <http://www.fda.gov/cder/drug/default.htm>

Food and Drug Administration (FDA): FDA Information for Older People: <http://www.fda.gov/oc/olderpersons/>

Families USA: Issues: Prescription Drugs: <http://www.familiesusa.org/html/drugs/drugs_medicare.htm>

New York Online Access to Health (NOAH): Ask NOAH About: Pharmacy: Drugs and Medications: <http://www.noah-health.org/english/pharmacy/pharmacy.html>

MedlinePlus: About Your Medicines: <http://www.nlm.nih.gov/medlineplus/aboutyourmedicines.html>

PillBot.com: <http://www.pillbot.com/Frameset.asp>

63. ELDER ABUSE

Recommended Search Terms

- "Elder abuse"
- "Elder abuse" prevention
- Seniors "domestic violence"

Important Sites

Administration on Aging: Elders and Families: Elder Rights and Resources: Elder Abuse: <http://www.aoa.gov/eldfam/Elder_Rights/Elder_Abuse/Elder_Abuse.asp>

American Psychological Association (APA) Online: Public Interest: Aging Issues: Elder Abuse and Neglect: In Search of Solutions: <http://www.apa.org/pi/aging/eldabuse.html>

MedlinePlus: Elder Abuse: <http://www.nlm.nih.gov/medlineplus/elderabuse.html>

National Center on Elder Abuse (NCEA): <http://www.elderabusecenter.org/>

National Committee for the Prevention of Elder Abuse (NCPEA): <http://www.preventelderabuse.org/about/about.html>

64. EXERCISE AND NUTRITION

Recommended Search Terms

- Aged "exercise and fitness"
- Aging "exercise and fitness"
- Elderly nutrition
- Older adults exercise benefits
- Older adults "physical activity"
- Seniors exercise
- Seniors "health and wellness"
- Seniors "good nutrition"
- Seniors "healthy diet"

Important Sites

Administration on Aging: Promoting Healthy Lifestyles: Physical Activity and Nutrition: <http://www.aoa.gov/eldfam/Healthy_Lifestyles/Phy_Act_Nut/Phy_Act_Nut.asp>

American Public Health Association: Aging: <http://www.apha.org/public_health/aging.htm>

MedlinePlus: Exercise for Seniors: <http://www.nlm.nih.gov/medlineplus/exerciseforseniors.html>

MedlinePlus: Nutrition for Seniors: <http://www.nlm.nih.gov/medlineplus/nutritionforseniors.html>

National Institute on Aging: Exercise: A Guide from the National Institute on Aging: <http://nia.nih.gov/exercisebook/toc.htm>

New York State: Office for the Aging: Aging Well: A Health and Wellness Village for Mature Adults: <http://agingwell.state.ny.us/>

Nutrition.gov: Lifecycle Issues: Seniors: <http://www.nutrition.gov/>

65. LIVING ARRANGEMENTS

Recommended Search Terms

- Affordable senior housing
- Aging "assisted living"
- Continuing care retirement communities
- Elderly residential care facility
- "Older adults" long-term care
- Nursing home care
- Senior care retirement communities
- Senior residential care
- Seniors independent housing
- Seniors skilled nursing facility

Important Sites

American Association of Homes and Services for the Aging (AAHSA): Consumer and Family Caregiver Information: <http://www.aahsa.org/public/consumer.htm>

American Health Care Association (AHCA): Long Term Care News and Information: <http://www.ahca.org/news/index.html>

American Seniors Housing Association (ASHA): <http://www.seniorshousing.org/>

Assisted Living Federation of America (ALFA): Consumer Information Center: <http://www.alfa.org/>

ElderWeb: <http://www.elderWeb.com/>

ElderWeb: Senior Housing Organizations: <http://www.elderweb.com/>

National Center for Assisted Living (NCAL): <http://www.ncal.org/>

A Place for Mom: <http://www.aplaceformom.com/index.html>

Seniors on the Move: Assisted Later Life Relocation Services: <http://www.seniorsonthemove.us/ourservices.htm>

66. MEDICARE

Recommended Search Terms

- Medicare
- Medicare benefits

Important Sites

Centers for Medicare and Medicaid Services (CMS): <http://cms.hhs.gov/default.asp?fromhcfadotgov=true>

Century Foundation: Medicare Watch: <http://www.medicarewatch.org/>

Consumers Union: Health Care: Medicare: <http://www.consumersunion.org/i/Health_Care/Medicare/index.html>

Families USA: Issues: Medicare: <http://www.familiesusa.org/>

Medicare: The Official U.S. Government Site for People with Medicare: <http://www.medicare.gov/>

Medicare Rights Center: Links: <http://www.medicarerights.org/linksframeset.html>

MedlinePlus: Medicare: <http://www.nlm.nih.gov/medlineplus/medicare.html>

67. MENTAL HEALTH

Recommended Search Terms

- Aged depression
- Elderly depression
- Elderly psychological disorders
- Geriatric psychiatry
- "Mental health" seniors
- Seniors depression
- Seniors psychosocial health

Important Sites

American Academy of Family Physicians (AAFP): Family Doctor: Depression and Older Adults: What It Is and How to Get Help: <http://familydoctor.org/handouts/588.html>

American Association for Geriatric Psychiatry (AAGP): Patients and Caregivers: Depression in Late Life: Not a Natural Part of Aging: <http://www.aagponline.org/p_c/depression2.asp>

American Association for Geriatric Psychiatry (AAGP): The Expert Consensus Guideline Series: *Depression in Older Adults: A Guide for Patients and Families*: <http://www.aagponline.org/p_c/GerPtFamHandout.pdf>

American Psychological Association (APA): Help Center: Family and Relationships: Elder Care More than "Parenting a Parent": <http://helping.apa.org/family/elderly.html>

Mental Health and Aging (MHandA): <http://www.mhaging.org/>

68. SEXUALITY AND AGING

[*See also* "Sexual Health Issues," p. 178]

Recommended Search Terms

- Sexuality aging midlife
- Sexuality seniors
- Intimacy aging
- Intimacy seniors

Important Sites

aHealthyMe!: Health After 60: The 70-Year Itch: Seniors and Sexuality <http://www.ahealthyme.com/topic/srsex>

Aetna InteliHealth: Sexual and Reproductive Health: Sexuality & Aging: <http://www.intelihealth.com/IH/ihtIH/WSIHW000/23414/11127.html>

American Association of Retired Persons(AARP): Modern Maturity Sexuality Survey: Summary of Findings: <http://research.aarp.org/health/mmsexsurvey_1.html>

American Psychological Association (APA): APA Online: Aging and Human Sexuality Resource Guide: <http://www.apa.org/pi/aging/sexuality.html#F>

MayoClinic.com: Senior Health Center: Intimacy and Aging: Tips for Sexual Health and Happiness: <http://www.mayoclinic.com/>

MedlinePlus: Sexual Health Issues: <http://www.nlm.nih.gov/medlineplus/sexualhealthissues.html>

National Institute on Aging: AgePage: Sexuality in Later Life: <http://www.niapublications.org/engagepages/sexuality.asp>

SeniorSex.org: Sex Tips for Older Adults: <http://instruct1.cit.cornell.edu/courses/psych431/student2000/dp51/sex_tips.html>

Sexuality Information and Education Council of the United States (SIECUS): Fact Sheet: Sexuality in Middle and Later Life: <http://63.73.227.69/pubs/fact/FS_middle_laterlife.pdf>

University of Washington: Orthopaedics and Sports Medicine: Living with Arthritis: Sex and Arthritis: <http://www.orthop.washington.edu/arthritis/living/sex/05?faq#b>

Men
Recommended Search Terms

- "Men's health" intimacy "over 50"
- "Men's health" sexuality aging
- "Men's health" sexuality senior

Important Sites

Health and Age: Health Centers: Men's Health Center: Sexual Problems in Men: <http://healthandage.com/PHome/gm=0!gc=28!gid2=737>

ICanOnline: Relationships: Dating and Romance: Men's Sexual Health: The Aging Male: <http://www.ican.com/>

MerckSource: Men's Health Center: Sexual Health and STDs: Aging Changes in the Male Reproductive System: <http://www.mercksource.com/>

Women
Recommended Search Terms

- "Women's health" sexuality aging
- "Women's health" sexuality midlife
- "Women's health" intimacy senior
- "Women's health" intimacy midlife
- "Women's health" intimacy menopause

Important Sites

Engenderhealth: Sexuality and Sexual Health: Sexual Response and Sexual Practices: Sexual Response and Aging: <http://www.engenderhealth.org/res/onc/sexuality/response/pg3.html>

Health and Age: Sexual Problems in Women: <http://healthandage.com/>

MayoClinic.com: Women's Health Center: Midlife Sexuality and Women: Getting Better with Age: <http://www.mayoclinic.com/>

HOTLINES

American Association of Retired Persons(AARP): 1-800-424-2277

Children of Aging Parents: 1-800-227-7294

Citizens for Better Care:
1-800-833-9548
Community Transportation Association of America:
1-800-527-8279
Eldercare Locator:
1-800-677-1116
Hearing Aid Helpline:
1-800-521-5247
Medicare Hotline:
1-800-638-6833
National Aging Information Center:
1-800-877-8339
National Institutes of Health: Aging Information:
1-800-222-2225
National Institute on Aging:
1-800-222-2225
Senior's Eye Care Program:
1-800-222-3937

FAQs

Centers for Medicare and Medicaid Services: Frequently Asked Questions: <http://questions.cms.hhs.gov/>

Massachusetts General Hospital: Senior Health: FAQs (Frequently Asked Questions): <http://www.massgeneral.org/depts/seniorhealthweb/seniorhealth_faq.htm>

Medicare: The Official U.S. Government Site for People with Medicare: Frequently Asked Questions: <http://medicare.custhelp.com/cgi-bin/medicare.cfg/php/enduser/std_alp.php>

National Institutes of Health (NIH): NIH Senior Health: Exercise for Older Adults: Frequently Asked Questions: <http://nihseniorhealth.gov/exercise/faq/faqlist.html>

Today's Seniors: Health Care: Senior Health: Health FAQs: <http://www.a-guide-for-seniors.com/Pages/Seniors_Health.html#Seniors%20Health%20FAQs>

SENIORS' HEALTH PUBLICATIONS ON THE INTERNET

AARP (American Association of Retired Persons): *AARP The Magazine*: <http://www.aarpmagazine.org/>

American Geriatrics Society: *Geriatrics at Your Fingertips* (Online Edition, 2003): <http://www.geriatricsatyourfingertips.org/> [NOTE: Registration required.]

American Society on Aging (ASA): *Aging Today*: <http://www.asaging.org/at/index.cfm>

Assisted Living Success: <http://www.alsuccess.com/>

Center for Strategic and International Studies and Watson Wyatt Worldwide: 2003 *Aging Vulnerability Index: An Assessment of the Capacity of Twelve Developed Countries to Meet the Aging Challenge* (2003): <http://www.csis.org/gai/aging_index.pdf>

Centers for Medicare and Medicaid Services (CMS): *Guide to Choosing a Nursing Home* (2003): <http://www.medicare.gov/Publications/Pubs/pdf/02174.pdf>

Department of Justice and Department of Health and Human Services: Office of Justice Programs Issues and Practices Report: *Our Aging Population: Promoting Empowerment, Preventing Victimization, and Implementing Coordinated Interventions* (2000): <http://www.ojp.usdoj.gov/docs/ncj_186256.pdf>

Generations: Journal of the American Society on Aging: <http://www.generationsjournal.org/genhome.cfm>

Grandtimes.com: <http://www.grandtimes.com/>

National Academy on an Aging Society (Gerontological Society of America) and Merck Institute of Aging and Health: *State of Aging and Health in America* (2003): <http://www.agingsociety.org/agingsociety/pdf/state_of_aging_report.pdf>

National Academies Press (NAP): Institute of Medicine (IOM): *Approaching Death: Improving Care at the End of Life* (1997): <http://www.nap.edu/books/0309063728/html/index.html>

National Academies Press (NAP): Institute of Medicine (IOM): *The Role of Nutrition in Maintaining Health in the Nation's Elderly: Evaluating Coverage of Nutrition Services for the Medicare Population* (2000): <http://www.nap.edu/books/0309068460/html/>

National Academies Press (NAP): Institute of Medicine (IOM): *Testosterone and Aging: Clinical Research Directions* (2003): <http://www.nap.edu/books/0309090636/html/>

University of California, Los Angeles (UCLA): UCLA Center on Aging: Newsletters: <http://www.aging.ucla.edu/newsletters.html>

MEDICAL SPECIALTIES

Geriatric psychiatry; Geriatrics

PROFESSIONAL ORGANIZATIONS

American Association for Geriatric Psychiatry (AAGP): <http://www.aagponline.org/default.asp>

American Geriatrics Society (AGS): <http://www.americangeriatrics.org/>

American Society on Aging (ASA): <http://www.asaging.org/>

Gerontological Society of America (GSA): <http://www.geron.org/>

National Council on the Aging (NCOA): <http://www.ncoa.org/>

PATIENT SUPPORT ORGANIZATIONS/ DISCUSSIONS GROUPS

American Association of Retired Persons (AARP): <http://www.aarp.org/>

American Association of Retired Persons (AARP) Online Community: <http://www.aarp.org/community/>

American College of Health Care Administrators (ACHCA): ACHCA Discussion Forum: Assisted Living Forum: <http://www.achca.org/>

American Federation for Aging Research (AFAR): <http://www.afar.org/>

Elder Care Online: <http://www.ec-online.net/>

Empowering Caregivers: <http://www.care-givers.com/>

SeniorNet: <http://www.seniornet.org/php/>

Well Spouse Foundation: Support Groups: <http://www.wellspouse.org/support.html>

SeniorNet: <http://www.seniornet.org/php/>

BEST ONE-STOP SHOPS

CNN.com: Health Library: Seniors' Health: <http://www.cnn.com/HEALTH/library/seniors/>

FirstGov for Seniors: Health: <http://www.seniors.gov/health.html>

MedlinePlus: Seniors' Health Topics: <http://www.nlm.nih.gov/medlineplus/seniorshealth.html>

National Institute on Aging: Health Information: Resource Directory for Older People: <http://www.nia.nih.gov/resource/>

National Institutes of Health (NIH): Seniors' Health: <http://health.nih.gov/>

New York Online Access to Health (NOAH): Ask NOAH About: Aging: <http://www.noah-health.org/english/aging/aging.html>

Part VII: Birth Defects

Deborah L. Lauseng

Each year about 150,000 children (1 in 28 births) are born with birth defects. Birth defects range from minor to serious; many can be treated and some cured while others cannot be treated at all. During the first year of life, birth defects are the leading cause of death.[1] Many children with birth defects live with physical or mental disabilities throughout their lives.

The primary known causes of birth defects are genetic and environmental factors. Genetic causes are either inherited or a result of malformed genes. Environmental factors can be: harmful habits by the mother (smoking, drinking, or illegal drug use), maternal infections (rubella, syphilis, or toxoplasmosis), or external agents (mercury, lead, or pesticides) that can affect both mother and child. A number of birth defects are considered multifactorial, that is both the genetic and environmental factors contribute to the disorder. Examples include cleft lip or cleft palate, clubfoot, and some heart defects. Unfortunately, as many as 70 percent of all defects have no known cause.

There are a number of things women can do to have a healthy pregnancy and to reduce the risk of birth defects. But there are no guarantees; even with a healthy pregnancy, infants can still be born with congenital defects.

SPECIAL SEARCHING ISSUES FOR THIS TOPIC

While there are a number of Web sites specifically on birth defects, consider searching for Web sites geared toward expectant mothers. Information about birth-disorder prevention and prenatal testing for defects are typically covered on pregnancy-related Web sites.

Finding Web sites that present general information on birth defects can be a challenge when there are so many Web pages that cover one particular birth defect. Be aware of Web sites that discuss one specific case of a congenital disorder or one specific individual and his or her disorder. Reading about an individual case, usually from a professional's perspective, may or may not be helpful. Each individual with a birth defect responds differently to his or her environment; therefore, be cautious about generalizing from one case.

What to Ask

Sometimes the presence of a birth defect is known prior to birth through prenatal screening. In other cases the birth defect is detected at the time of birth. Still in other cases, it is not diagnosed until the child is almost school age. Then comes a flood of questions: how? Why? When? Not all the questions can be answered, but learning about what is known can help you to cope with a specific birth defect.

What is the specific name of the birth defect? What kind of birth defect is it (for example, genetic, metabolic)? Is there a way to correct or treat it? What will life be like for the child with a specific defect? What is the child's life expectancy? Is there a known cause for this specific birth defect? Are there ways to prevent birth defects?

Along with all the questions comes the need to carefully review the Internet resources found on any given birth disorder. Check whether the information is coming from research or from a personal narrative. Are there references and links to other Web sites, or is the information personal experience or opinion?

Where to Start

With such a large body of information concerning birth defects available, searching can seem overwhelming. If you are looking for general overview material, start searching for frequently asked questions (FAQs) by using "birth defects" with "questions," or use "birth disorders" with "FAQs." Another place to start is directly at the March of Dimes Web site <http://www.marchofdimes.com/>.

If you are searching for a specific birth defect or disorder, use the formal name or words describing the defect. An example would be "spina bifida" or "malformed spine" to search for the condition in which the backbone does not develop properly around the spinal cord.

MedlinePlus <http://medlineplus.gov> provides extensive information in an overview of birth defects, as well as information on specific birth defects. healthfinder <http://healthfinder.gov> also provides extensive lists of Internet resources according to specific birth defects or issues.

Additional Strategies

Alternative broad search terms to consider are those used by the medical community, including "congenital defect(s)," "congenital abnormality," or "congenital abnormalities." Using the broader general terms of "deformities" or "abnormalities'" could retrieve a large number of Web sites referring to amphibians, and specifically frogs. To eliminate these references use a "NOT" in the search, for example: "deformities –frogs" (where a dash or a minus sign and in Google represents searching without the particular term). Also look at the search engine's advance search options for specifics on how to exclude the search term "frogs."

TOPIC PROFILE

Who

Birth defects are usually diagnosed in newborns but may not be apparent until later in life. Three percent of birth defects are seen at birth. Six to seven percent of children with birth defects are diagnosed by age one, and between 12-14 percent are diagnosed by school age.[2]

What

There are several types of abnormalities:

- Structural: a missing or malformed part, either external or internal. Examples include heart defects spina bifida (malformed spine), and urinary tract defects (including missing kidneys).

- Metabolic: related to abnormal or missing enzymes or protein to help the body chemistry function properly, usually inherited. Examples include Tay-Sachs disease (accumulation of a harmful fatty substance in the brain nerve cells) and phenylketonuria (PKU-deficiency of a liver enzyme contributing to mental disabilities, behavior abnormalities, and other symptoms).

- Chromosomal [*See also*: "Genetic Diseases," p. 159]: abnormal number or pairing of chromosomes. Examples include Down syndrome (presence of additional third chromosome 21), Klinefelter syndrome (males with extra sex chromosome XXY), or Turner syndrome (female missing or partially missing an X chromosome). [*See also* "Turner Syndrome," p. 170, vol. 2.]

- Perinatal: related to infections or environmental exposures during pregnancy or at birth. Examples include fetal alcohol syndrome (results of drinking, usually heavily, during pregnancy), low birth weight, Rh disease (incompatiabilty between the blood of the mother and the fetus).

Where

Each type birth defect affects development and functioning of the body differently. Symptoms or outcomes of a specific birth defect are not always apparent to the general public. Some birth defects are visible, as in the case of malformations of external body parts; others may not be discovered for years, as in the case of some congenital heart defects. Metabolic birth defects affect the normal functioning of a particular chemical in the body and, in turn, causes external symptoms of mental disabilities starting in the brain. Chromosomal abnormalities usually affect the whole body because of the change in genetic code that determines the development of the fetus and ultimately the child/adult. Environmental or perinatal causes of birth disorders may or may not show external physical symptoms but will influence behavior and mental development.

When

During fetal development or during birth (passage through the birth canal).

ABBREVIATIONS USED IN THIS SECTION

AFP = Alpha fetoprotein
CERHR = Center for the Evaluation of Risks to Human Reproduction

CHD = Congenital heart disease
CVS = Chorionic villus sampling
NBDPN = National Birth Defects Prevention Network
NCBDDD = National Center on Birth Defects and Developmental Disabilities
NINDS = National Institute of Neurological Disorders and Stroke
NTD = Neural tube defect(s)
PCRM = Physicians Committee for Responsible Medicine
SBAA = Spina Bifida Association of America

PROCEDURES AND SPECIAL TOPICS

69. GENERAL

[*See also*: "Genetic Diseases," p. 159, particularly for recommended search terms related to "chromosomal abnormalities."]

Recommended Search Terms

- "Birth defect"
- "Birth defects"
- "Birth disorders"
- "Chromosomal abnormalities"
- "Chromosome abnormality"
- "Congenital abnormalities"
- "Congenital abnormality"
- "Congenital defect"
- Abnormalities
- Abnormality
- Deformities

Important Sites

Centers for Disease Control and Prevention (CDC): National Center on Birth Defects and Developmental Disorders (NCBDDD): <http://www.cdc.gov/ncbddd/>

Health on the Net (HON) Foundation: HON Dossier: Mother and Child Glossary: Birth: Birth Defects: <http://www.hon.ch/Dossier/MotherChild/birth_disorders/birth_defects.html>

KidsHealth: Parents: Doctors and Hospitals: Caring for a Seriously or Chronically Ill Child: Birth Defects: <http://kidshealth.org/parent/system/ill/birth_defects.html>

March of Dimes Home Page: <http://www.marchofdimes.com/>

March of Dimes: Professionals and Researchers: Quick Reference and Fact Sheets: Chromosomal Abnormalities: <http://www.marchofdimes.com/professionals/681_1209.asp>

MedlinePlus: Birth Defects: <http://www.nlm.nih.gov/medlineplus/birthdefects.html>

National Birth Defects Prevention Network (NBDPN): <http://www.nbdpn.org/>

70. DIAGNOSIS

Recommended Search Terms

- "Birth defects" "alpha fetoprotein"
- "Birth defects" "chorionic villus sampling"
- "Birth defects" "diagnostic tests"
- "Birth defects" AFP
- "Birth defects" amniocentesis
- "Birth defects" CVS
- "Birth defects" diagnosis
- "Birth disorder" detection
- "Birth disorders" "maternal serum screening"
- "Birth disorders" screening
- "Chorionic villus sampling"
- "Chromosomal abnormalities" "screening tests"
- "Congenital abnormalities" "blood tests"
- "Congenital abnormalities" ultrasound
- "Congenital defects" ultrasound
- "Fetal blood test"
- "Genetic screening"
- "Maternal serum"
- "Newborn screening"
- "Prenatal testing"
- Amniocentesis
- Cordocentesis

Important Sites

American Academy of Family Physicians (AAFP): Family Doctor: Women: Pregnancy and Childbirth: Amniocentesis and CVS: <http://familydoctor.org/handouts/144.html>

Health on the Net (HON) Foundation: HON Dossier Mother and Child Glossary: Birth: Genetic Screening: <http://www.hon.ch/Dossier/MotherChild/birth_disorders/genetic_screening.html>

KidsHealth: Parents: Doctors and Hospitals: Medical Test and Exams: Prenatal Tests: <http://www.kidshealth.org/parent/system/medical/prenatal_tests.html>

March of Dimes: Pregnancy and Newborn Health Education Center: Chorionic Villus Sampling: <http://www.marchofdimes.com/pnhec/159_521.asp>

March of Dimes: Professionals and Researchers: Quick Reference and Fact Sheets: Maternal Blood Screening for Down Syndrome and Neural Tube Defects: <http://www.marchofdimes.com/professionals/681_1166.asp>

March of Dimes: Professionals and Researchers: Quick Reference and Fact Sheets: Newborn Screening Tests: <http://www.marchofdimes.com/professionals/681_1200.asp>

71. Congenital Heart Defects

Recommended Search Terms

- "Congenital heart defects"
- "Heart defects" congenital
- CHD birth
- "Heart malformation"

Important Sites

Congenital Heart Defects (CHD): <http://www.congenitalheartdefects.com/>

The Congenital Heart Information Network (TCHIN): <http://www.tchin.org/>

KidsHealth: Parents: Medical Problems: Heart and Blood Vessels: Congenital Heart Defects: <http://kidshealth.org/parent/medical/heart/congenital_heart_defects.html>

March of Dimes: Professionals and Researchers: Quick Reference and Fact Sheets: Congenital Heart Defects: <http://www.marchofdimes.com/professionals/681_1212.asp>

New York Online Access to Health (NOAH): Ask NOAH About: Congenital Heart Defects: <http://www.noah-health.org/english/illness/genetic_diseases/chd.html>

72. Neural Tube Defects

Recommended Search Terms

- "Chiari malformation"
- "Folic acid"
- "Neural tube defects"
- "Spina bifida"
- Anencephaly
- Encephalocele
- Hydrocephalus
- Meningocele
- NTD birth
- NTD pregnancy

Important Sites

Duke University Medical Center: Center for Human Genetics: For Patients and Families: Neural Tube Defects (NTD): <http://www.chg.duke.edu/patients/neural.html>

KidsHealth: Parents: Doctors and Hospitals: Caring for a Seriously or Chronically Ill Child: Spina Bifida: <http://www.kidshealth.org/parent/system/ill/spina_bifida.html>

MedlinePlus: Neural Tube Defects: <http://www.nlm.nih.gov/medlineplus/neuraltubedefects.html>

National Institute of Neurological Disorders and Stroke (NINDS): Anencephaly Information Page: <http://www.ninds.nih.gov/health_and_medical/disorders/anencephaly_doc.htm>

Northwestern Memorial Hospital: Health Library: Illnesses and Conditions: Encephalocele: <http://health_info.nmh.org/Library/HealthGuide/IllnessConditions/topic.asp?hwid=nord867#nord867-general-discussion>

March of Dimes: Pregnancy and Newborn Health Education Center: Folic Acid: <http://www.marchofdimes.com/pnhec/887.asp>

March of Dimes: Professionals and Researchers: Quick Reference and Facts Sheets: Spina Bifida: <http://www.marchofdimes.com/professionals/681_1224.asp>

Spina Bifida Association of America (SB): Facts about Spina Bifida: <http://www.sbaa.org/html/sbaa_facts.html>

Spina Bifida Association of America (SB): Folic Acid Information: <http://www.sbaa.org/html/sbaa_folic.html>

73. Accutane

Recommended Search Terms

- "Birth defects" "vitamin A"
- "Birth defects" accutane
- "Birth defects" isotretinoin
- Pregnancy accutane
- Pregnancy retinoids

Important Sites

Center for the Evaluation of Risks to Human Reproductions (CERHR): Vitamin A (5/20/02): <http://cerhr.niehs.nih.gov/genpub/topics/vitamin_a-ccae.html>

Centers for Disease Control and Prevention (CDC): National Center on Birth Defects and Developmental Disabilities (NCBDDD): Birth Defects: Accutane-Exposed Pregnancies: <http://www.cdc.gov/ncbddd/bd/accutane.htm>

March of Dimes: Professionals and Researchers: Quick Reference and Fact Sheets: Accutane and Other Retinoids: <http://www.marchofdimes.com/professionals/681_1168.asp>

74. THALIDOMIDE

Recommended Search Terms

- Thalidomide
- Thalomid

Important Sites

Food and Drug Administration (FDA) : Center for Drug Evaluation and Research: Thalidomide Important Patient Information: <http://www.fda.gov/cder/news/thalidomide.htm>

March of Dimes: Professionals and Researchers: Quick Reference and Facts Sheets: Thalidomide: <http://www.marchofdimes.com/professionals/681_1172.asp>

MedlinePlus Drug Information: Thalidomide: <http://www.nlm.nih.gov/medlineplus/druginfo/medmaster/a699032.html>

75. PREVENTION AND SURVEILLANCE

Recommended Search Terms

- "Birth defects" prevention
- "Birth defects" surveillance

Important Sites

Centers for Disease Control and Prevention (CDC): National Center on Birth Defects and Developmental Disorders (NCBDDD): Birth Defects Surveillance: <http://www.cdc.gov/ncbddd/bd/bdsurv.htm>

Citizens' Council on Health (CCH): Medical Privacy: Birth Defects Prevention Act of 1998 (Public Law 105-168): <http://www.cchconline.org/privacy/bdact.php3>

U.S. Food and Drug Administration (FDA): *FDA Consumer Magazine*: Decreasing the Chance of Birth Defects: <http://www.fda.gov/fdac/features/996_bd.html>

Healthnotes: Health Concerns: Birth Defects Prevention: <http://www.gnc.com/health_notes/Concern/Birth_Defects.htm>

National Birth Defects Prevention Network (NBDPN): <http://www.nbdpn.org/>

HOTLINES

National Birth Defects Center:
1-800-332-5014; (781) 466-8474; (781) 466-9555

March of Dimes: The Pregnancy and Newborn Health Education Center:
1-800-663 4637 (English); 1-800-925-1855 (Spanish)

FAQs

Centers for Disease Control and Prevention (CDC): National Center on Birth Defects and Developmental Disorders (NCBDDD): Birth Defects: Frequently Asked Questions: <http://www.cdc.gov/ncbddd/bd/faq1.htm>

KidsHealth: Parents: Doctors and Hospitals: Caring for a Seriously or Chronically Ill Child: Birth Defects: <http://kidshealth.org/parent/system/ill/birth_defects.html>

March of Dimes: Professionals and Researchers: Quick Reference and Fact Sheets: Birth Defects: <http://www.marchofdimes.com/professionals/681_1206.asp>

Physicians Committee for Responsible Medicine (PCRM): Research Controversies and Issues: Ethics in Human Research: Birth Defect Statistics: <http://www.pcrm.org/issues/Ethics_in_Human_Research/ethics_human_birthdefects.html>

BIRTH DEFECTS PUBLICATIONS ON THE INTERNET

Centers for Disease Control and Prevention (CDC): National Center on Birth Defects and Developmental Disorders (NCBDDD): *Preventing Neural Tube Birth Defects: A Prevention Model and Resources*: <http://www.cdc.gov/ncbddd/folicacid/ntd/cover.htm>

National Library of Medicine (NLM): Library Services: Medical Subject Headings (MeSH): *Online Multiple Congenital Anomaly/Mental Retardation (MCA/MR) Syndromes* by Stanley Jablonski: <http://www.nlm.nih.gov/mesh/jablonski/syndrome_title.html>

MEDICAL SPECIALTIES

Medical genetics; Clinical genetics; Genetic counseling; Pediatrics; Neonatal-perinatal medicine; Neonatology; Perinatology

PROFESSIONAL ORGANIZATIONS

American Academy of Pediatrics: <http://www.aap.org/>

American College of Medical Genetics: <http://www.acmg.net/>

National Society of Genetic Counselors (NSGC): <http://www.nsgc.org/>

Patient Support Organizations/ Discussion Group

Birth Defect Research Children (BDRC): <http://www .birthdefects.org/>

Centers for Disease Control and Prevention (CDC): National Center on Birth Defects and Developmental Disorders (NCBDDD): <http://www.cdc.gov/ncb ddd/>

March of Dimes: <http://www.marchofdimes.com/>

Best One-Stop Shops

healthfinder: Health Library: Birth Defects: <http://health finder.gov/scripts/SearchContext.asp?topic=107>

March of Dimes: <http://www.marchofdimes.com/>

MedlinePlus: Birth Defects: <http://www.nlm.nih.gov/ medlineplus/birthdefects.html>

Merck Manual, 2nd Home edition: Section 23. Children's Health Issues: Chapter 265 Birth Defects: <http://www.merck.com/mrkshared/mmanual_home2 /sec23/ch265/ch265a.jsp >

References

1. March of Dimes: Quick Reference and Fact Sheets: Birth Defects. (2003, March) Retrieved December 13, 2003, from <http://www.marchofdimes.com/ professionals/681_1206.asp>.

2. Physicians Committee for Responsible Medicine: *Birth Defects Statistics:* (1999, May 25) Retrieved November 21, 2002, from <http://www.pcrm.org/ issues/Ethics_in_Human_Research/ethics_human _birthdefects.html>.

Part VIII: Genetic Diseases

Susan K. Kendall

[*See also* "Birth Defects" and "Turner Syndrome"]

Special Searching Issues for This Topic

Our understanding of genetic diseases has been changing in recent years. It now seems clear that almost every disease has a genetic component. Take, for instance, an infectious disease like AIDS. It appears that some people, because of their genetic makeup, may be more resistant to the HIV virus. A combination of environmental and lifestyle components mixed with genetic susceptibility is responsible for Western society's most common diseases, including heart disease and cancer. Rather than tackle all of these diseases (which are discussed in other sections), this section will focus on some of the more traditionally defined genetic diseases and genetic issues you may be searching for. It is important to keep in mind that genetic diseases have in common the fact that they result from one or more gene defects, but the organ(s) affected and the symptoms of these diseases are greatly varied. You will probably want to search for your genetic disease of interest using some of the ideas in this section but also refer to the section in this book that discusses the disease by its symptoms. For instance, hereditary hemochromatosis is discussed in "Iron Overload" (p. 106, vol. 2).

What to Ask

Genes are codes for the making of proteins. They consist of long, double-helixed molecules called DNA (deoxyribonucleic acid). DNA contains four chemicals called bases, and the exact sequence of these four bases serves as a code that cells can read to make a protein. Many genes, encoding many different proteins, can be found on one long DNA molecule that is packaged up into a chromosome. Humans have 23 pairs of these chromosomes, and one set is inherited from each parent. The matched pairs contain copies of the same genes except for the sex chromosomes X and Y. Two X chromosomes are found in females, and an X plus a Y chromosome are found in males. As you encounter unfamiliar genetic terms in your searches, you may want to consult an online glossary, such as the *Talking Glossary of Genetic Terms* <http:// www.genome.gov/glossary.cfm> (National Human Genome Research Institute) or a primer such as *DNA from the Beginning* <http://www.dnaftb.org/dnaftb/> listed in the "Genetic Diseases Publications on the Internet" (p. 163).

The importance of genes lies in the proteins for which they encode. Proteins do the work of the body—building muscle or skin and acting as hormones, enzymes, or messengers of crucial signals in all systems of the body, from the immune system to the nervous system, growth, and metabolism. Genetic diseases occur when a mistake (a mutation) in the code causes a faulty protein to be made. Faulty proteins can wreak havoc on the system in which that protein was supposed to be functioning. There are basically three types of genetic diseases:

- simple genetic diseases caused by a mutation in a single gene (examples: cystic fibrosis and sickle cell anemia);
- complex genetic diseases (called multifactorial diseases) caused by mutations in several genes (examples include many cancers); and

- complex genetic diseases caused by chromosomal abnormalities in which a piece of chromosome may be deleted or mislocated or a whole chromosome may be missing altogether, which affects many genes all at once (such as Down syndrome and Turner syndrome).

One of the first things you may read about your genetic disease of interest may be whether it is caused by one or more genes. If several genes are involved, variations in which genes are affected can cause variations in disease symptoms from person to person. If a disease has many different symptoms because more than one gene is involved, it is usually called a syndrome. Even if only a single gene is involved, the location of and type of mutation may be different for different people, producing a more or less faulty protein.

As you read about the genetic basis for your disease of interest, you will find that the gene culprit may or may not be known. If it is unknown, you might be interested in finding out who is researching this area or sponsoring the research. You will no doubt be interested in finding out whether or how the disease is inherited. One myth often encountered is that a genetic disease must "run in the family." Some genetic diseases result from mutations or chromosomal breaks that happen during development of the embryo; these are not inherited from either parent. Many genetic diseases are inherited, however, but even then there are different kinds of inheritance. As mentioned above, each person inherits two copies of each gene. It could be that one inherited copy (say, from the father) is normal and the other (say, from the mother) is mutated. Autosomal dominant inheritance means that the gene(s) affected are on non-sex chromosomes (autosomes), and that only one copy of the gene needs to be mutated to cause the disease (dominant). If both copies of the gene need to be mutated to cause the disease, the inheritance is called recessive. A person carrying a single mutated copy of such a genes is called a "carrier" and can pass on the gene defect to offspring although he or she does not have the disease.

Finally, there are sex-linked diseases which are usually caused by mutations on the X chromosome. Since females have two X chromosomes, carrying a single mutated gene for a recessive sex-linked disease will not affect them. Males, who have only one X chromosome, will be affected by those diseases if their only copy of the gene involved is mutated. Finding out the mode of inheritance of your genetic disease of interest will be very important in determining the likelihood that others in your family will inherit the same disease. These issues are addressed in genetic counseling.

Genetic testing is another issue you may encounter in your searches. Tests have been developed for several genetic diseases for which the exact genes and mutations are known. Many ethical and legal issues surround genetic testing, whether it is done on fetuses, newborns, or adults. There is really no "cure" right now for genetic diseases, as a cure would involve fixing the mutation(s) in the gene(s) themselves. This is a goal of gene therapy researchers, who hope someday to be able to correct gene defects. Recently, gene therapy research has had some limited successes but also some setbacks. Meanwhile, today's usual treatment for these diseases focuses on the symptoms. Suggestions on how to search for treatment information is covered in the appropriate section of this book for your particular disease symptoms.

Where to Start

The amount of information available usually depends on the prevalence of your disease of interest. If your disease is rare, refer also to "Rare Diseases" (pp, 140, vol. 2) for search strategies. It would be best to start with some of the Web sites listed in "Best One-Stop Shops." Most of these have extensive lists of genetic diseases, and you will want to check to see if yours is listed. Try also doing a search of these sites with your disease name to check what other information is available.

Because of the sheer number of genetic diseases, only a few of the more prevalent are given as examples. By starting with the terms you know for your disease and learning alternative terms to try as you go along, you should be able to apply similar search strategies for your disease of interest. After gaining all the information you can from these sites, you might want to search one of the health-related search engines. Finally, you might want to proceed to the Internet at large, performing a Google search, for instance, using your disease name and other aspects that interest you, using the "Recommended Search Terms" under "Procedures and Special Topics." If you are looking for a very specific fact about a disease—the "needle in the haystack," so to speak—this broader search may be necessary and helpful. Of course, always check to see who is responsible for any information that you find. Using this search strategy sequence, you should at least be able to come up with an association or fact sheet dealing with your disease of interest.

Additional Search Strategies

You may want to supplement information you gain from health-related Web sites with first-hand information from others who have experience with your disease. Check for your disease in the directory listings of support groups for genetic diseases. Support groups can be excellent sources of disease-related information. The Genetic Alliance InfoNetwork Resource Center Helpline (listed in "Hotlines"), which is staffed by genetic counselors and interns, also provides referrals to support groups, research studies, and organizations. You may also want to seek out the advice and knowledge of a genetic counselor trained to help you understand the issues and options surrounding genetic diseases. The search strategy sample shown below for "genetic counseling" leads to several Web sites that can help you locate a counselor in your area.

TOPIC PROFILE

Who

Anyone can have a genetic disease. Different diseases are more prevalent among different ethnic groups. In the United States, for instance, cystic fibrosis is more prevalent among Caucasians, and sickle cell anemia is found mostly among African Americans. Genetic diseases affecting the sex chromosomes may be found solely or primarily in one sex—for instance, X-linked recessive genetic diseases are much more likely to affect males than females.

What

Genetic diseases can be caused by abnormalities in a single gene, several genes, a cluster of genes, or whole chromosomes. These abnormalities can be inherited from one or both parents or can occur in the developing egg, sperm, or embryo.

Where

Any part of the body can be affected depending on the particular disease.

When

Genetic diseases range from birth defects to those that have later or adult-stage onset.

ABBREVIATIONS USED IN THIS SECTION

ACMG = American College of Medical Genetics
ASHG = American Society of Human Genetics
CF = Cystic fibrosis
DNA = Deoxyribonucleic acid
GSA = Genetics Society of America
HGP = Human Genome Project
NHGRI = National Human Genome Research Institute
NICHHD = National Institute of Child Health and Human Development
NORD = National Organization of Rare Disorders
NSGC = National Society of Genetic Counselors

PROCEDURES AND SPECIAL TOPICS

76. GENERAL

Recommended Search Terms

- "Chromosomal abnormalities"
- "Genetic diseases"
- "Genetic disorders"
- "Genetic mutations"
- "Genetic abnormalities"
- "Medical genetics"
- "Paediatric genetics"
- "Pediatric genetics"

Important Sites

Dolan DNA Learning Center: Cold Spring Harbor Laboratory: Your Genes Your Health: <http://www.ygyh.org/>
MedlinePlus: Genetic Disorders: <http://www.nlm.nih.gov/medlineplus/geneticdisorders.html>
New York Online Access to Health (NOAH): Ask NOAH About: Genetic Disorders: <http://www.noah-health.org/english/illness/genetic_diseases/geneticdis.html>
University of Kansas Medical Center: Medical Genetics: Genetic and Rare Conditions Site: <http://www.kumc.edu/gec/support/groups.html>

77. CYSTIC FIBROSIS

Recommended Search Terms

- "Cystic fibrosis"
- "Cystic fibrosis" diagnosis
- "Cystic fibrosis" testing
- "Cystic fibrosis" "clinical trials"
- "Cystic fibrosis" research
- "Cystic fibrosis" treatment
- "CF" disease
- "CF" respiratory

Important Sites

Clinical Trials.gov: Cystic Fibrosis: <http://clinicaltrials.gov/>
Cystic Fibrosis (CF) Foundation: <http://www.cff.org/>
Medem: Medical Library: American College of Obstetricians and Gynecologists: Cystic Fibrosis Testing: The Decision Is Yours: <http://www.medem.com/>
MedlinePlus: Cystic Fibrosis: <http://www.nlm.nih.gov/medlineplus/cysticfibrosis.html>

MedlinePlus: Medical Encyclopedia: Cystic Fibrosis: <http://www.nlm.nih.gov/medlineplus/ency/article/000107.htm>

Merck Manual of Diagnosis and Therapy: Section 19. Pediatrics: Chapter 267. Cystic Fibrosis: <http://www.merck.com/pubs/mmanual/section19/chapter267/267a.htm>

National Heart, Lung, and Blood Institute (NHLBI): Information for Patients and the Public: Publications: Facts about Cystic Fibrosis: <http://www.nhlbi.nih.gov/health/public/lung/other/cf.htm>

New York Online Access to Health (NOAH): Ask NOAH About: Cystic Fibrosis: <http://www.noah-health.org/english/illness/respiratory/cystic.html>

78. SICKLE CELL ANEMIA
Recommended Search Terms

- "Sickle cell anemia"
- "Sickle cell disease"
- "Sickle cell trait"
- "Sickle cell" testing
- "Sickle cell" screening
- "Sickle cell" pain
- "Sickle cell" treatment
- "Sickle cell" research
- "Sickle cell" "clinical trials"

Important Sites

American Sickle Cell Anemia Association: <http://www.ascaa.org/>

ClinicalTrials.gov: Anemia, Sickle Cell: <http://clinicaltrials.gov/>

KidsHealth: Kids: Kids' Health Problems: Blood: Do You Know about Sickle Cell Disease? <http://kidshealth.org/kid/health_problems/blood/sickle_cell.html>

MedlinePlus: Sickle Cell Anemia: <http://www.nlm.nih.gov/medlineplus/sicklecellanemia.html>

New York Online Access to Health (NOAH): Ask NOAH About: Sickle Cell Disease: <http://www.noah-health.org/english/illness/genetic_diseases/sickle.html>

Sickle Cell Disease Association of America (SCDAA): <http://www.sicklecelldisease.org/>

79. DOWN SYNDROME
Recommended Search Terms

- "Down syndrome"
- "Down's syndrome"
- "Trisomy 21"
- "Down syndrome" screening
- "Down syndrome" research
- "Down syndrome" complications
- "Down syndrome" management
- "Down syndrome" prenatal testing

Important Sites

March of Dimes: Professionals and Researchers: Quick Reference and Fact Sheets: Down Syndrome: <http://www.marchofdimes.com/professionals/681_1214.asp>

MedlinePlus: Down Syndrome: <http://www.nlm.nih.gov/medlineplus/downsyndrome.html>

National Down Syndrome Society (NDSS): <http://www.ndss.org/>

MedlinePlus: Medical Encyclopedia: Down Syndrome: <http://www.nlm.nih.gov/medlineplus/ency/article/000997.htm#altNames>

National Institute of Child Health and Human Development (NICHD): Health Information and Media: Publications: Facts about Down Syndrome: <http://www.nichd.nih.gov/publications/pubs/downsyndrome/down.htm>

New York Online Access to Health (NOAH): Ask NOAH About: Genetic Diseases: Down Syndrome: <http://www.noah-health.org/english/illness/genetic_diseases/downs.html>

80. GENETIC COUNSELING
Recommended Search Terms

- "Genetic counseling"
- "Genetic counselors"
- Prenatal "genetic counseling"
- Locating "genetic counselors"

Important Sites

Baby Center: Pregnancy: Prenatal Health: Prenatal Genetic Counseling: <http://www.babycenter.com/refcap/pregnancy/prenatalhealth/1607.html>

Eccles Institute of Human Genetics: Genetic Science Learning Center: Genetic Disorders Corner: Genetic Counselors: <http://gslc.genetics.utah.edu/units/disorders/counselors/>

Human Genome Project (HGP) Information: Genetic Counseling: <http://www.ornl.gov/hgmis/medicine/genecounseling.html>

National Society of Genetic Counselors (NSGC): Consumer Information: Genetic Counseling and You: <http://www.nsgc.org/consumer/index.asp>

New York Online Access to Health (NOAH): Ask NOAH About: Genetic Disorders: Genetic Testing and Counseling: <http://www.noah-health.org/english/illness/genetic_diseases/geneticdis.html#DIAGNOSING>

University of Kansas Medical Center: Genetics Education Center: Genetic Counseling Resources: <http://www.kumc.edu/gec/prof/gc.html>

81. GENETIC TESTING

Recommended Search Terms

- "Genetic testing"
- "Gene testing"
- "Genetic screening"
- "Prenatal testing"
- "Fetal testing"

Important Sites

Department of Health and Human Services: Access Excellence: Resource Center: Understanding Gene Testing: <http://www.accessexcellence.org/AE/AEPC/NIH/>

Human Genome Project (HGP) Information: Medicine and the New Genetics: Gene Testing: <http://www.ornl.gov/hgmis/medicine/genetest.html>

Lawrence Berkeley National Laboratory: Ethical, Legal, and Social Issues in Science (ELSI): What is Genetic Testing? <http://www.lbl.gov/Education/ELSI/genetic-testing.html>

MayoClinic.com: Diseases and Conditions: Cancer Center: Genetic Testing: Weighing Its benefits and risks: <http://www.mayoclinic.com/>

MedlinePlus: Genetic Testing/Counseling: <http://www.nlm.nih.gov/medlineplus/genetictestingcounseling.html>

HOTLINES

Genetic Alliance InfoNetwork Resource Center Helpline: 1-800-336-GENE/1-800-336-4363

National Organization of Rare Disorders (NORD): (203) 744-0100

FAQs

Human Genome Project (HGP) Information: Medicine and the New Genetics: Gene Testing: <http://www.ornl.gov/hgmis/medicine/genetest.html>

Human Genome Project (HGP) Information: Medicine and the New Genetics: Genetic Disease Information: <http://www.ornl.gov/hgmis/medicine/assist.html>

National Human Genome Research Institute: Learning about Genetics: Frequently Asked Questions about Genetics: <http://www.genome.gov/page.cfm?pageID=10001191>

GENETIC DISEASES PUBLICATIONS ON THE INTERNET

Department of Health and Human Services: Access Excellence: Resource Center: Understanding Gene Testing: <http://www.accessexcellence.org/AE/AEPC/NIH/>

National Human Genome Resource Institute: Educational Resources: Talking Glossary of Genetic Terms: <http://www.genome.gov/glossary.cfm>

DNA from the Beginning: <http://www.dnaftb.org/dnaftb/>

Howard Hughes Medical Institute: Blazing a Genetic Trail: <http://www.hhmi.org/genetictrail/>

TeensHealth: Your Body: Health Basics: The Basics on Genes and Genetic Disorders: <http://kidshealth.org/teen/your_body/health_basics/genes_genetic_disorders.html>

MEDICAL SPECIALTY

Medical genetics

PROFESSIONAL ORGANIZATIONS

NOTE: The following organizations deal with all genetic diseases. You may also want to do a search for specific organizations pertaining to your particular disease of interest.

American Board of Genetic Counseling (ABGC): <http://www.abgc.net/>

American Board of Medical Genetics: <http://www.abmg.org/>

American College of Medical Genetics: <http://www.acmg.net>

American Society of Gene Therapy: <http://www.asgt/org>

American Society of Human Genetics (ASHG): <http://www.ashg.org/>

Association of Genetic Technologists (AGT): <http://www.agt-info.org/>

Canadian Association of Genetic Counsellors: <http://www.cagc-accg.ca/>

Canadian College of Medical Geneticists: <http://ccmg.medical.org/>

Genetics Society of America (GSA): <http://www.genetics-gsa.org/>

National Society for Genetic Counselors (NSGC): <http://www.nsgc.org/>

PATIENT SUPPORT ORGANIZATIONS/ DISCUSSION GROUPS

NOTE: The following directories list support and advocacy groups for many different genetic diseases. Look for a listing under your disease of interest.

Directory of Online Genetic Support Groups: <http://www.mostgene.org/support/>

University of Kansas Medical Center: Medical Genetics: Genetic and Rare Conditions Site: Lay Advocacy Groups, Support Groups: <http://www.kumc.edu/gec/support/>

Best One-Stop Shops

Genetic Alliance: http://www.geneticalliance.org/

Genetic Health: <http://www.genetichealth.com/>

MedlinePlus: Genetic Disorders: <http://www.nlm.nih.gov/medlineplus/geneticdisorders.html>

MedlinePlus: Genetic Testing/Counseling: <http://www.nlm.nih.gov/medlineplus/genetictestingcounseling.html>

National Human Genome Research Institute: Health: <http://www.genome.gov/Health/>

New York Online Access to Health (NOAH): Ask NOAH About: Genetic Disorders: <http://www.noah-health.org/english/illness/genetic_diseases/geneticdis.html>

Part IX: Pregnancy Problems and Complications

Deborah L. Lauseng

Special Searching Issues for This Topic

For the nine months of pregnancy, the focus of a woman's life is changed. Physical and chemical changes are taking place daily in her body—all aspects of a woman's health are affected as the pregnancy advances. This is all the more true when pregnancy risk factors or health problems pre-exist, or a pregnancy complication is assessed. Then pregnancy problems cross a variety of health topics. To be thorough in investigating pregnancy-related health concerns also consider reviewing the following sections: "Women's Health" (p. 136) "Adolescent Health" (p. 125), "Sexual Health Issues" (p. 178), "Birth Defects" (p. 154), and any other sections covering the specific health disease or condition that may be involved.

Generally, risk factors in pregnancy include pre-existing health issues, such as a smoking habit, alcohol or drug use, diabetes, or hypertension. The term "complications" usually refers to health issues that arise during the course of the pregnancy, such as gestational diabetes, uterine fibroids, or maternal infections. "Risk factors," "high-risk," "complications," and "problems" are sometimes used interchangeably to describe additional health conditions or issues in an otherwise healthy pregnancy.

The significance of understanding and working toward prevention of complications in pregnancy goes beyond just the benefit in health to the pregnant woman. Efforts to reduce risks and complications can also benefit the baby before, during, and after childbirth.

What to Ask

What is the diagnosis? What are the symptoms? Are there alternative names for the diagnosis?

What is the specific pregnancy complication or problem? Is there a name for the condition? What is the cause? Is there a way to correct or treat the problem? What lifestyle changes may be necessary? How will the complication or problem affect the baby? Is the complication or problem related only to the present pregnancy? Are there ways to prevent the same problems occurring in the next pregnancy?

Along with all the questions comes the need to carefully review the Internet resources found on any given birth disorder. Understand whether the information is coming from research or from a personal narrative. Are there references and links to other Web sites or is the information personal experience or opinion?

Where to Start

Using general search engines such as Google <http://www.google.com/> or AlltheWeb <http://www.alltheweb.com/> for searching "pregnancy problems" or "pregnancy complications" retrieves many Web sites. Some relevant Web sites are maintained by support organizations or health-related organizations. Even some of the Web sites by individuals can be of value. In some cases, the search retrieval may include non-health-related sites.

Since there is such a wide range of issues and information relating to pregnancy problems and complications, the best starting place for reliable information is through one of the Web sites in "Best One-Stop Shops." Good starting strategies include searching MedlinePlus or Ask NOAH About under the topic "pregnancy complications."

Additional Strategies

Recognizing that there is more than one way to describe pregnancy-related health topics, try more than one search term to find relevant information. To find the difference between normal pregnancy events and those related to problems in pregnancy add the word "complications" to the search. Sometimes "pregnancy" Web sites also provide information related to complications, problems, and risks.

Searching for information on pregnancy in later life or at a later age can be challenging because there is no consistent term for searching. Some Web sites discuss increases in complications during pregnancy for women older than 35 years of age, while others list the age as 40 plus years and older.

Topic Profile

Who

Pregnancy, and therefore the possibility of complications in pregnancy, can occur as early as the start of menstruation in adolescent girls and as late as a women going through menopause.

What

Normal pregnancy involves many changes in a woman's body. Complications or problems in pregnancy can occur as responses to these normal changes of pregnancy or to pre-existing health or chronic conditions. External factors, such as smoking, alcohol or drug use, or STDs, also contribute to high risks in pregnancy. Additional environmental factors can influence the outcome of the pregnancy.

Where

Since pregnancy involves physical and metabolic changes throughout a woman's body, complications can affect almost any aspect of a woman's health and any part of a woman's body.

When

Complications and problems in pregnancy can start at conception and continue on through labor and delivery, and potentially into the postpartum period.

Abbreviations Used in This Section

HON = Health on the Net
NWHIC = National Women's Health Information Center
STDs = Sexually transmitted diseases

Procedures and Special Topics

82. General

[*See also* "Women's Health Issues," p. 136.]

Recommended Search Terms

- "High risk pregnancy"
- "Pregnancy complication"
- "Pregnancy complications"
- Pregnancy "high risks"
- Pregnancy "risk factors"
- Pregnancy problems
- Pregnancy risks

Important Sites

All about Moms: High Risk Pregnancy and Pregnancy Complications: <http://www.allaboutmoms.com/hih risk.htm>

Baby-Parenting: Pregnancy: Pregnancy Complaints: <http://www.baby-parenting.com/pregnancy/pregnancy_probs.html>

Childbirth.org: Complications: Complications of Pregnancy: <http://www.childbirth.org/articles/pregnancy/pcomp.html>

Health on the Net (HON) Foundation: HON Dossier: Mother and Child Glossary: During Pregnancy: Pregnancy Problems and Complications: <http://www.hon.ch/Dossier/MotherChild/complications/problems.html>

Sidelines National Support Network Resources: <http://www.sidelines.org/resource.htm>

83. Teen Pregnancy

[*See also* "Adolescent Health," p. 125.]

Recommended Search Terms

- "Pregnancy complications" "young women"
- "Pregnancy complications" teenage
- "Pregnancy problems" teen
- "Pregnancy risks" adolescents
- "Pregnancy risks" teens
- Pregnancy girls
- Pregnancy teenage
- Pregnancy teenager
- Pregnancy teens

Important Sites

New York Online Access to Health (NOAH): Ask NOAH about Pregnancy: Teenage Pregnancy: <http://www.noah-health.org/english/pregnancy/teenpreg.html>

Quality Life: Teenage Pregnancy Problems and Challenges: <http://www.qualitylife.org/teenage_problems.html>

Teen Pregnancy Information Center: Teen Pregnancy: <http://www.geocities.com/Wellesley/7746/teen pregnancy.htm>

WomensHealthChannel: Teen Pregnancy: <http://www.womenshealthchannel.com/teenpregnancy/index.shtml>

84. Pregnancy at Later Age

Recommended Search Terms

- "At-risk" age pregnancy
- "Older age" pregnancy
- "Older mothers"
- Childbearing later
- Delayed childbearing
- Older "primiparous women" pregnancy
- Pregnancy "after 35"
- Pregnancy "after 40"
- Pregnancy "later age"
- Pregnancy "older women"

Important Sites

BabyCenter: Pregnancy: Prenatal Health: Ask the Experts: What Are the Risks of Having a Baby after Age 35: <http://www.babycenter.com/expert/pregnancy/prenatalhealth/3127>

Estronaut: Pregnancy at a Later Age: <http://www.womens health.org/a/pregnant_older.htm>

March of Dimes: Pregnancy and Newborn Health Education Center: Pregnancy after 35: <http://www.marchof dimes.com/pnhec/173_812.asp>

Medem: Medical Library: American College of Obstetricians and Gynecologists: Later Childbearing: <http://www.medem.com/>

85. Multiple Births

Recommended Search Terms

- "Maternal complications" multiples
- "Maternal complications" triplets
- "Multiple gestation" complications
- "Multiple pregnancies" complications
- "Pregnancy complication" "multiple births"
- "Pregnancy complications" twins
- Pregnancy problems "multiple births"
- Pregnancy risks "multiples"
- Multiparous problems
- Multiparous complications

Important Sites

American Society for Reproductive Medicine: Patient's Fact Sheet: Complications of Multiple Gestation: <http://www.asrm.org/Patients/FactSheets/complications-multi.pdf>

Dartmouth-Hitchcock Medical Center: Departments: High Risk Obstetrics: Patient Education: Monochorionic Twins: <http://www.dhmc.org/>

MedlinePlus: Twins, Triplets, Multiple Births: <http://www.nlm.nih.gov/medlineplus/twinstripletsmultiple births.html>

Resolve: Pregnancy/Parenting: Pregnancy after Infertility: Pregnancy with Multiples: <http://www.resolve.org/pregparent/multiples/multiples1.shtml>

WomensHealthChannel: Multiple Pregnancies: Maternal Complications: <http://www.womenshealthchannel.com/multiplepregnancies/risks_maternal.shtml>

86. Diagnosis of Pregnancy Complications

[*See also* "Birth Defects," p.154.]

Recommended Search Terms

- "Pregnancy complications" diagnosis
- "Pregnancy problems" "obstetric ultrasound"
- "Pregnancy problems" testing
- Pregnancy "blood tests"
- Pregnancy "estradiol"
- Pregnancy "estrone tests"
- Pregnancy CBC
- Pregnancy urinalysis
- "Pregnancy complications" monitoring

Important Sites

Lab Tests Online: Estrogen Tests: <http://www.labtests online.org/understanding/analytes/estrogen/test.html>

March of Dimes: Pregnancy and Newborn Health Education Center: Ultrasound: <http://www.marchofdimes.com/pnhec/159_523.asp>

Oregon Health and Science University (OHSU): OHSU Doernbecher Children's Hospital: Child Health A-Z: High-Risk Pregnancy: Maternal and Fetal Testing: <http://www.ohsuhealth.com/dch/health/hrpregnant/fetal_index.asp>

87. Common Pregnancy Complications and Problems

[*See also* " Diabetes," p. 51, vol. 2; "Heart and Circulatory Diseases: Hypertension," p. 90, vol. 2; "Anemias," p. 7, vol. 2.]

Recommended Search Terms

- "Gestational diabetes"
- "RH incompatibility"
- "Pre-eclampsia"
- Preeclampsia
- Pregnancy "pre-existing diabetes"
- Pregnancy preexisting diabetes

- Pregnancy "high blood pressure"
- Pregnancy "incompetent cervix"
- Pregnancy "uterine fibroids"
- Pregnancy anemia
- Pregnancy asthma
- Pregnancy hypertension

Important Sites

American Academy of Periodontology: Oral Health Information for the Public: Preterm Low Birth Weight Births: <http://www.perio.org/consumer/mbc.baby.htm>

Dartmouth-Hitchcock Medical Center: Departments: High Risk Obstetrics: Patient Education: Incompetent Cervix: <http://www.dhmc.org/>

eMedicine: eMedicine Specialties: Emergency Medicine: Obstetrics and Gynecology: Pregnancy, Preeclampsia: <http://www.emedicine.com/emerg/topic480.htm>

KidsHealth: Parents: Pregnancy and Newborns: Pregnancy and Childbirth: What is Rh Incompatibility? <http://kidshealth.org/parent/pregnancy_newborn/pregnancy/rh.html>

Life Clinic: Blood Pressure: Hypertension and Pregnancy: <http://www.lifeclinic.com/focus/hypertension/default.asp>

March of Dimes: Professionals and Researchers: Quick Reference and Fact Sheets: Diabetes in Pregnancy: <http://www.marchofdimes.com/professionals/681_1197.asp>

Medical Center Online: Children's Health: High-Risk Pregnancy: Anemia in Pregnancy: <http://www.mccg.org/childrenshealth/hrpregnant/aip.asp>

MedlinePlus: Diabetes and Pregnancy: <http://www.nlm.nih.gov/medlineplus/diabetesandpregnancy.html>

MedlinePlus: Medical Encyclopedia: Uterine Fibroids: <http://www.nlm.nih.gov/medlineplus/ency/article/000914.htm>

National Heart, Lung, and Blood Institute (NHLBI): Information for Patients and the Public: Publications: High Blood Pressure in Pregnancy: <http://www.nhlbi.nih.gov/health/public/heart/hbp/hbp_preg.htm>

Pregnancy and Asthma: Frequently Asked Questions: <http://www.pregnancyandasthma.com/pregnancy/asthma-pregnancy-questions.asp>

88. Risks in Pregnancy

[*See also* "Alcoholism," p. 250, vol. 2.]

Recommended Search Terms

- Pregnancy "alcohol use"
- Pregnancy "drug use"
- Pregnancy alcohol
- Pregnancy drinking
- Pregnancy drugs
- Pregnancy smoke
- Pregnancy smoking

Important Sites

Centers for Disease Control and Prevention (CDC): *Morbidity and Mortality Weekly Report (MMWR)*: Alcohol Use among Women of Childbearing Age—United States, 1991–1999: <http://www.cdc.gov/mmwr/preview/mmwrhtml/mm5113a2.htm>

Medical University of South Carolina (MUSC): Children's Hospital: High-Risk Pregnancy: Smoking and Pregnancy: <http://www.musckids.com/health_library/hrpregnant/presmoke.htm>

National Institute on Alcohol Abuse and Alcoholism (NIAAA): Graphics Gallery: Fetal Alcohol Syndrome: <http://www.niaaa.nih.gov/gallery/fetal/fetal.htm>

National Institute on Alcohol Abuse and Alcoholism (NIAAA): Publications: Drinking and Your Pregnancy: <http://www.niaaa.nih.gov/publications/brochure.htm>

Substance Abuse and Mental Health Services Administration (SAMHSA): National Household Survey on Drug Abuse (NHSDA): The NHSDA Report: Pregnancy and Illicit Drug Use: <http://www.samhsa.gov/oas/2k2/pregDU/pregDU.htm>

89. Ectopic Pregnancy

Recommended Search Terms

- "Abdominal pregnancy"
- "Cervical pregnancy"
- "Ectopic pregnancy"
- "Tubal pregnancy"

Important Sites

Baby Center: Pregnancy: Pregnancy Complications: Ectopic Pregnancy: <http://www.babycenter.com/refcap/pregnancy/pregcomplications>

KidsHealth: Parents: Pregnancy and Newborns: Pregnancy and Childbirth: Ectopic Pregnancy: <http://kidshealth.org/parent/pregnancy_newborn/pregnancy/ectopic.html>

MedlinePlus: Medical Encyclopedia: Ectopic Pregnancy: <http://www.nlm.nih.gov/medlineplus/ency/article/000895.htm>

Northwestern Memorial Hospital: Health Library: Illnesses and Conditions: Ectopic Pregnancy: <http://health_info.nmh.org/Library/HealthGuide/IllnessConditions/topic.asp?hwid=hw144921>

90. INFECTIONS IN PREGNANCY

Recommended Search Terms

- Cytomegalovirus
- Pregnancy "childhood illnesses"
- Pregnancy "fifth disease"
- Pregnancy "German measles"
- Pregnancy "Group B strep"
- Pregnancy "parvovirus B19"
- Pregnancy chickenpox
- Pregnancy CMV
- Pregnancy rubella
- Pregnancy toxoplasmosis

Important Sites

American Academy of Family Physicians (AAFP): Family Doctor: Women: Pregnancy and Childbirth: Group B Strep Infection in Pregnancy: <http://familydoctor.org/handouts/281.html>

Centers for Disease Control and Prevention (CDC): Division of Bacterial and Mycotic Diseases: Disease Information: Group B Streptococcal Disease (GBS): <http://www.cdc.gov/ncidod/dbmd/diseaseinfo/groupbstrep_g.htm>

Centers for Disease Control and Prevention (CDC): National Center for Infectious Diseases: Parvovirus B19 Infection (Fifth Disease) Infection and Pregnancy: <http://www.cdc.gov/ncidod/diseases/parvovirus/B19andpreg.htm>

March of Dimes: Pregnancy and Newborn Health Education Center: Complications: Cytomegalovirus: <http://www.marchofdimes.com/pnhec/188_671.asp>

March of Dimes: Pregnancy and Newborn Health Education Center: Complications: Toxoplasmosis: <http://www.marchofdimes.com/pnhec/188_667.asp>

March of Dimes: Professional and Researchers: Quick Reference and Fact Sheets: Childhood Illnesses in Pregnancy: Chickenpox and Fifth Disease: <http://www.marchofdimes.com/professionals/681_1185.asp>

March of Dimes: Professionals and Researchers: Quick Reference and Fact Sheet: Rubella: <http://www.marchofdimes.com/professionals/681_1225.asp>

91. SEXUALLY TRANSMITTED DISEASES IN PREGNANCY

[*See also* "AIDS and HIV," p. 3, vol. 2; "Sexual Health Issues," p. 178.]

Recommended Search Terms

- Pregnancy "genital herpes"
- Pregnancy "genital warts"
- Pregnancy "hepatitis B"
- Pregnancy "human papillomavirus"
- Pregnancy "sexually transmitted diseases"
- Pregnancy AIDS
- Pregnancy chlamydia
- Pregnancy gonorrhea
- Pregnancy HIV
- Pregnancy HPV
- Pregnancy STD
- Pregnancy syphilis
- Pregnancy trichomoniasis

Important Sites

Centers for Disease Control and Prevention (CDC): National Center for HIV, STD and TB Prevention: Division of Sexually Transmitted Diseases: STDs and Pregnancy: <http://www.cdc.gov/nchstp/dstd/Fact_Sheets/facts_stds_and_pregnancy.htm>

Dartmouth-Hitchcock Medical Center: Departments: High Risk Obstetrics: Patient Education: Sexually Transmitted Diseases: <http://www.dartmouth.edu/>

Health on the Net (HON) Foundation: HON Dossier: Mother and Child Glossary: Reproduction: Gynaecologic Problems: Syphilis: <http://www.hon.ch/Dossier/MotherChild/gynae_problems/std_syphilis.html>

iVillage: iVillageHealth: Experts: Infectious Diseases: Chlamydia and Pregnancy: <http://www.ivillagehealth.com/experts/infectious/qas/0,11816,531912_175406,00.html>

March of Dimes: Professionals and Researchers: Quick Reference and Fact Sheets: Genital Herpes: <http://www.marchofdimes.com/professionals/681_1201.asp>

March of Dimes: Professionals and Researchers: Quick Reference: Infections and Diseases: HIV and AIDS in Pregnancy: <http://www.marchofdimes.com/printableArticles/681_1223.asp>

MedlinePlus: AIDS and Pregnancy: <http://www.nlm.nih.gov/medlineplus/aidsandpregnancy.html>

National Institute of Allergy and Infectious Diseases (NIAID): Health Matters: Human Papillomavirus and Genital Warts: <http://www.niaid.nih.gov/factsheets/stdhpv.htm>

March of Dimes: Pregnancy and Newborn Health Education Center: Complications: Trichomoniasis: <http://www.marchofdimes.com/pnhec/188_734.asp>

New York Online Access to Health (NOAH): Ask NOAH About: Pregnancy and Sexually Transmitted Diseases: <http://www.noah-health.org/english/illness/stds/stds.html#Pregnancy>

TheBody: Hepatitis B Prevention and Pregnancy: <http://www.thebody.com/cdc/hepbprevent.html>

WebMD: Health: Gonorrhea and Pregnancy: <http://my.webmd.com/content/article/1680.51323>

92. BEDREST

Recommended Search Term

- Pregnancy "bedrest"

Important Sites

Dartmouth-Hitchcock Medical Center: Departments: High Risk Obstetrics: Patient Education: Bedrest in Pregnancy: <http://www.dhmc.org/>

Pregnancy Bedrest.com: <http://www.pregnancybedrest .com/>

93. COMPLICATIONS IN LABOR AND DELIVERY

Recommended Search Terms

- "Abruptio placentae"
- "Amniotic fluid problems"
- "Breech births"
- "Excessive bleeding" labor
- "Placenta accreta"
- "Placenta previa"
- "Placental abruption"
- "Placental complication"
- "Postpartum hemorrhage"
- "Post-term labor" complications
- "Postterm labor" complications
- "Premature labor"
- "Premature rupture" membranes
- "Preterm labor" complications
- "Prolapsed umbilical cord"
- "Shoulder dystocia"
- "Uterine rupture"
- Birth complications
- Childbirth complications
- Delivery problems
- Labor complications

Important Sites

About: Health and Fitness: Pregnancy/Birth: Amniotic Fluid: Articles: Disorders of Amniotic Fluid: <http:// pregnancy.about.com/library/weekly/aa010499.htm>

American Academy of Family Physicians (AAFP): Family Doctor: Women: Pregnancy and Childbirth: Pregnancy: What to Expect When Your Due Date Has Passed: <http://familydoctor.org/handouts/143.html>

Baby Center: Pregnancy: Labor and Delivery: Labor Complications: <http://www.babycenter.com/pregnancy/ childbirth/index>

Baby Center: Baby: Postpartum Recovery: Labor Complication: Postpartum Hemorrhage: <http://www.baby center.com/refcap/baby/physrecovery/1152328.html>

Childbirth.org: Complications: Labor and Birth: Difficult Births: <http://www.childbirth.org/articles/labor/ difficultbirth.html>

Dartmouth-Hitchcock Medical Center: Departments: High Risk Obstetrics: Patient Education: Placental Abruption: <http://www.dhmc.org/>

Health on the Net (HON) Foundation: HON Dossier: Mother and Child Glossary: Birth: Prolapsed Umbilical Cord: <http://www.hon.ch/Dossier/MotherChild/ labor_complications/birth_cordprolapse.html>

Health on the Net (HON) Foundation: HON Dossier: Mother and Child Glossary: During Pregnancy: Abruptio Placentae: <http://www.hon.ch/Dossier/ MotherChild/complications/placenta_abruptio.html>

Health on the Net (HON) Foundation: HON Dossier: Mother and Child Glossary: During Pregnancy: Placenta and Amniotic Fluid Problems: <http://www.hon .ch/Dossier/MotherChild/complications/complicate _placenta.html>

iVillage: Pregnancy/Babies: Pregnancy: Labor, Birth: Labor Complications: <http://www.ivillage.com/topics/preg baby/0,10707,166369,00.html>

March of Dimes: Pregnancy and Newborn Health Education Center: Complications: Placenta Accreta, Increta and Percreta: <http://www.marchofdimes.com/pnhec/ 188_1128.asp>

National Institutes of Health (NIH): National Institute of Nursing Research: NIH News Release: Risk of Uterine Rupture During Labor Higher for Women with a Prior Cesarean Delivery: <http://www.nih.gov/news/ pr/jul2001/ninr-04.htm>

Pregnancy, Birth and Beyond: Breech Babies: Breech Births: <http://www.pregnancy.com.au/breech_babies .htm>

94. PREGNANCY LOSS

Recommended Search Terms

- "Incomplete miscarriage"
- "Neonatal death"
- "Pregnancy loss"
- "Spontaneous abortion"
- Miscarriage
- Stillbirth

Important Sites

Discovery Health Channel: Diseases and Conditions: Encyclopedia: Incomplete Miscarriage: <http://health .discovery.com/diseasesandcond/encyclopedia/1961 .html>

GrowthHouse: Infant Death and Pregnancy Loss: <http:// www.growthhouse.org/natal.html>

March of Dimes: Professionals and Researchers: Quick Reference and Fact Sheets: Stillbirth: <http://www.marchofdimes.com/professionals/681_1198.asp>

MedlinePlus: Medical Encyclopedia: Abortion-Spontaneous: <http://www.nlm.nih.gov/medlineplus/ency/article/001488.htm>

Fertility Place: Miscarriage: Miscarriage Support and Information Resources: <http://www.fertilityplus.org/faq/miscarriage/resources.html>

MedlinePlus: Pregnancy Loss: <http://www.nlm.nih.gov/medlineplus/pregnancyloss.html>

New York Online Access to Health (NOAH): Pregnancy and Childbirth Problems and Risks: Problems after Pregnancy: Miscarriage, Stillbirth: <http://www.noah-health.org/english/pregnancy/pregproblems.html#MISCARRIAGE>

95. Postpartum Depression

Recommended Search Terms

- "Post partum" depression
- "Baby blues"
- Postpartum depression
- Postpartum blues

Important Sites

American Academy of Family Physicians (AAFP): Family Doctor: Women: Pregnancy and Childbirth: Postpartum Depression and the "Baby Blues": <http://familydoctor.org/handouts/379.html>

KidsHealth: Parents: Pregnancy and Newborns: Pregnancy and Childbirth: Postpartum Depression and Caring for Your Baby: <http://kidshealth.org/parent/pregnancy_newborn/pregnancy/ppd_baby.html>

StorkNet: Pregnancy and Birth: Postpartum Depression: <http://www.storknet.com/cubbies/pregnancy/ppd.htm>

Hotlines

America's Pregnancy Helpline:
1-800-672-2296

Sidelines National Support Network: High-Risk Pregnancy Support:
1-888-447-4754

FAQs

BabyCenter: Pregnancy: Pregnancy Complications: <http://www.babycenter.com/pregnancy/pregcomplications/index>

National Women's Health Information Center: 4woman.gov: Frequently Asked Questions about Women's Health: Pregnancy and Reproductive Health: <http://www.4woman.gov/faq/index.htm#16>

Sidelines National Support Network: Frequently Asked Questions: <http://www.sidelines.org/faq1.htm>

StorkNet: Pregnancy Complications: Carolyn M. Salafia, MD's FAQ (Frequently Asked Questions): <http://www.storknet.com/complications/salafia>

Pregnancy Complication-Related Publications on the Internet

Merck Manual of Medical Information, 2nd home ed.: Section 22: Women's Health Issues: Chapter 258. High-Risk Pregnancy (2003): <http://www.merck.com/mrkshared/mmanual_home2/sec22/ch258/ch258a.jsp>

Medical Specialties

Family physicians; Midwifery; Obstetrics; Gynecology

Professional Organizations

NOTE: There are some Web sites specifically for physicians and medical personnel working with obstetrics and pregnancy. Web sites from the individual medical specialties associated with pregnancy or obstetrics sometimes, but not always, have separate pages on the various pregnancy complications for the general public.

American Academy of Family Physicians: <http://www.aafp.org/>

American College of Obstetricians and Gynecologist (ACOG): <http://www.acog.org/>

American College of Physicians: Internal Medicine/Doctors for Adults: <http://www.acponline.org/>

Patient Support Organizations/ Discussion Groups

BabyCenter: Pregnancy Complications: <http://www.babycenter.com/pregnancy/pregcomplications/index>

iVillage: Parents Place.com: OB/GYN Pregnancy Complications: "Find a Board" or "Family Health Resources": <http://www.parentsplace.com/expert/obgyn/archive/0,10693,240200,00.html>

March of Dimes: Pregnancy and Newborn Health Education Center: Ask Us Now: <http://www.marchofdimes.com/pnhec/188.asp>

Sidelines National Support Network: High-Risk Pregnancy Support: <http://www.sidelines.org/>

Storknet: Pregnancy Complications: <http://www.storknet.com/complications/>

BEST ONE-STOP SHOPS

Dartmouth-Hitchcock Medical Center: Departments: Obstetrics and Prenatal Diagnosis Gynecology: High Risk Obstetrics: Division of Maternal Fetal Medicine: <http://www.dhmc.org/>

Health on the Net (HON) Foundation: HON Dossier: Mother and Child Glossary: During Pregnancy: Pregnancy Problems and Complications: <http://www.hon.ch/Dossier/MotherChild/complications/problems.html>

MedlinePlus: Health Topics: High Risk Pregnancy: <http://www.nlm.nih.gov/medlineplus/highrisk pregnancy.html>

New York Online Access to Health (NOAH): Ask NOAH About: Pregnancy and Childbirth Problems and Risks: <http://www.noah-health.org/english/pregnancy/preg problems.html>

OBCyberbook: <http://www.obfocus.com/resources/ob cyberbook.htm>

Sidelines National Support Network: <http://www.side lines.org/>

Part X: Prostate Disorders

Robert Young

SPECIAL SEARCHING ISSUES FOR THIS TOPIC

It may seem like an unfair generality but, unlike women, most men are not familiar with their internal sexual/urinary system. Until there is a medical problem, men tend to be ignorant of the prostate gland, from its location to its function. It is also part of the sexual and urinary systems, so men are hesitant to discuss it, and using the Web for information can turn up a multitude of sex and pornography sites as well as sites that play on ignorance and fear.

TOPIC PROFILE

Who

Any mature male with a prostate gland can develop a prostate disorder. Although it is not known why, African-American men develop prostate disorders earlier than Caucasian men. Men with a familial history of prostatic disorders are also more prone to prostate problems.

What

Urinary problems ranging from difficulty in urinating (including pain) to blood in the urine or the semen. There are basically three prostatic disorders: benign prostatic hyperplasia (BPH), prostate cancer, and prostatitis. Each can produce an enlargement of the prostate gland (and similar symptoms) and a man can have any or all of them at the same time.

Where

Penis and bladder. In advanced conditions, there may be pain in the pelvis and lower back.

When

The possibility of a prostatic disorder increases with age, especially at 45 or older, but younger ages should not be discounted.

ABBREVIATIONS USED IN THIS SECTION

ACS = American Cancer Society

AFUD = American Foundation for Urologic Disease

CBP = Chronic bacterial prostatitis

CaP = Cancer of the prostate, when cancer originates in the prostate gland. Also abbreviated PCa.

DRE = Digital rectal examination. This is when a physician inserts a lubricated, gloved finger into the rectum and feels for irregularities. Because the prostate gland sits against the rectal wall, the physician can determine if the gland is swollen or has any irregular features.

FDA = Food and Drug Administration

NBP = Nonbacterial prostatitis

NCI = National Cancer Institute

NIDDK = National Institute of Diabetes and Digestive and Kidney Diseases

NLM = National Library of Medicine

OCCAM = Office of Cancer Complementary and Alternative Medicine (NCI)

PCa = Prostate cancer, when cancer originates in the prostate gland. Also abbreviated CaP.

PDy = Postatodynia

PSA = Prostate-specific antigen. Every prostate gland, including in healthy males, produces PSA. It facilitates the seminal fluid. The level of PSA is found with a blood test. A rise in PSA is one of the primary markers of a prostatic disorder and, along with a DRE, may prompt additional tests, including a biopsy.

UC = University of California

YANA = You Are Not Alone (Prostate cancer support group message board)

PROCEDURES AND SPECIAL TOPICS

96. GENERAL

Because of the anatomy of the prostate gland, prostate disorders can all produce the same symptoms and diagnostic markers. For example, all prostate disorders can produce urinary difficulties and elevated PSA levels. On the other hand, some symptoms, such as blood in the urine or urinary pain, may not be caused by the prostate but by another condition— kidney stones can cause blood in the urine and an infection in the penis can cause pain. Only a full medical diagnosis can determine the cause.

Diagnosis will come from a medical examination and laboratory tests. If the diagnosis is severe such as, prostate cancer, the patient may not know to ask for details, but he, his companion, or both should ask for the exact findings that prompted the diagnosis. It may very well be in a language that is completely foreign (for prostate cancer there will be a PSA and a Gleason score, for example), but he should get the figures for each so that later he can understand what they mean.

Once the patient has the exact diagnostic information, he can then start his education, for he may have to approve the recommended treatment or select a treatment option. Diagnostic information is critical for determining what treatment options are available. Some treatments have side effects that may last a lifetime, so the patient needs to learn the side effect of each treatment and use that information in his selection or approval of a treatment. A variety of resources can be used and are listed below.

Using a search engine can be overwhelming. At press time, a search of Google <http://www.google.com> produced the following:

- Prostate disorders – 581,000 pages/hits
- Prostate gland – 222,000 pages/hits
- Prostatitis – 155,000 pages/hits
- Prostate cancer – 1,710,000 pages/hits

As with any disease, these include some dangerous treatments as well as con games that play on the frightened, so it is highly recommended that the newly diagnosed learn their basics from established organizations before wandering into the Internet. In other words, know before you go. Generic searches (such as "prostate gland," "prostate problem/disorder" or "urinary problem") are of little value to most because they are too vague. Questions such as "What is the prostate?" and "What does the prostate do?" produce better results.

Other important issues to keep in mind while searching are that all treatments can carry side effects, and that searching for information on any disorder of the genitals or on anything that affects sexual function may retrieve unwanted material. To avoid sexually explicit or pornographic sites, you may wish to add the following searching string to your Internet searches on this topic:

- -xxx -porn
- ".gov"
- ".org"
- ".edu"

Recommended Search Terms

- Prostate health ".gov"
- "Prostate disorders"
- "Prostate gland" ".edu"
- Prostatitis ".org"
- "Prostate cancer"
- "Urologic diseases" prostate
- Urological prostate
- Urology prostate

Important Sites

Commonwealth Department of Veterans' Affairs (Australia): You and Your Prostate: <http://www.dva.gov.au/media/publicat/2001/prostate/index.htm>

John Hopkins Medical Institutions: Brady Urological Institute <http://urology.jhu.edu/diseases/index.html>

National Cancer Institute (NCI): cancer.gov: Prostate Cancer Home Page: <http://www.cancer.gov/cancerinfo/types/prostate>

National Health Service (NHS) Direct (UK): Self-Help Guide: Prostate Problems: <http://www.nhsdirect.nhs.uk/SelfHelp/conditions/prostrateproblems/prostrateproblems.asp>

National Institute of Diabetes and Digestive and Kidney Diseases (NIDDK): National Kidney and Urologic Diseases Information Clearinghouse: Kidney and Urologic Diseases Topics List: <http://www.niddk.nih.gov/kudiseases/pubs/prostate_ez/index.htm>

National Institute of Diabetes and Digestive and Kidney Diseases (NIDDK): National Kidney and Urologic Diseases Information Clearinghouse: Kidney and Urologic Diseases Topics List: Medical Tests for Prostate Problems: <http://www.niddk.nih.gov/kudiseases/pubs/prostatetests/index.htm>

Phoenix5: The Prostate Cancer InfoLink Archive: Where Is Your Prostate and What Does It Do? <http://www.phoenix5.org/Infolink/Physiology.html>

Prostate Health Directory: Prostate Health Articles: What Is the Prostate Gland and What Does It Do? <http://www.prostatehealthdirectory.com/articles/what_prostate.html>

University of Maryland Medicine: Prostate Health Guide: Benign Prostate Problems: <http://www.umm.edu/prostate/problems.htm>

University of Michigan Health System: Comprehensive Cancer Center: Urologic Oncology Program: <http://www.cancer.med.umich.edu/prostcan/prostcan.html>

Urological Associates, S.C.: Health Information: Prostate—A Review: <http://www.urological.com/health/prostate.html>

97. BENIGN PROSTATIC HYPERPLASIA (BPH)

This non-cancerous (benign) enlargement of the prostate may occur in one of two ways. Either the number of prostate cells increase (hyperplasia), or the size of the existing cells increase (hypertrophy). Either way, the prostate gland enlarges, thus constricting the urinary flow or forcing more frequent urination. It is a common condition in older men and not itself life-threatening. BPH cannot be transmitted. A number of treatment options exist.

Recommended Search Terms

- "Benign prostate hyperplasia"
- "Benign prostate hypertrophy"
- "Benign prostatic hyperplasia"
- "Benign prostatic hypertrophy"
- BPH prostate
- BPH prostatic
- Hyperplasia prostate
- Hypertrophy prostatic
- "Large prostate"
- "Swollen prostate"
- "Prostate enlargement"
- "Prostate inflammation" "differential diagnosis"

Important Sites

About: Health and Fitness: Senior Health: Benign Prostatic Hypertrophy (BPH): <http://seniorhealth.about.com/library/men/blbph.htm>

American Academy of Family Physicians (AAFP): Family Doctor: Men's Health: Benign Prostatic Hyperplasia (BPH): <http://www.familydoctor.org/handouts/148.html>

Bandolier: Benign Prostatic Hyperplasia: Diagnosis and Treatment: <http://www.jr2.ox.ac.uk/bandolier/band11/b11-3.html>

British United Provident Association (BUPN): Health Information: ABC of Health: Enlarged Prostate (BPH): <http://hcd2.bupa.co.uk/fact_sheets/Mosby_factsheets/BPH.html>

Cleveland Clinic: Health Information: Learning the Facts about BPH (Benign Prostatic Hyperplasia): <http://www.clevelandclinic.org/health/health-info/docs/2100/2129.asp?index=8985>

Google Directory: Health: Conditions and Diseases: Urological Disorders: <http://directory.google.com/Top/Health/Conditions_and_Diseases/Urological_Disorders/>

Kidney and Urology Foundation of America: Patient Resources: Library: Prostatic Problems: What You Should Know about Common Prostate Problems: Prostatitis and Benign Prostatic Hyperplasia (BPH): <http://www.kidneyurology.org/Patient_Resources/PaR_Lib_ProstateProblems.htm>

National Institute of Diabetes and Digestive and Kidney Diseases (NIDDK): National Kidney and Urologic Diseases Information Clearinghouse: Kidney and Urologic Diseases: Prostate: <http://kidney.niddk.nih.gov/kudiseases/topics/prostate.asp/>

National Institute of Diabetes and Digestive and Kidney Diseases (NIDDK): National Kidney and Urologic Diseases Information Clearinghouse: Kidney and Urologic Diseases Topics List: Prostate Enlargement: Benign Prostatic Hyperplasia: <http://kidney.niddk.nih.gov/kudiseases/pubs/prostateenlargement/index.htm>

Oregon Health and Science University (OHSU) Health: Health Topics: Urology: Benign Prostatic Hyperplastia: <http://www.ohsuhealth.com/urology/bph.asp?sub=1>

Prostate.com: Understanding Benign Prostatic Hyperplasia: <http://www.prostate.com/understandingbph_c.htm>

University of Pittsburgh Medical Center: Benign Prostatic Hyperplasia (BPH): <http://prostate.upmc.com/>

Urology Channel: Prostate BPH (Benign Prostatic Hyperplasia): Diagnosis: <http://www.urologychannel.com/prostate/bph/diagnosis.shtml>

Urology Channel: Prostate BPH (Benign Prostatic Hyperplasia): Overview: <http://www.urologychannel.com/prostate/bph/index.shtml>

Yahoo (UK and Ireland) Directory: Health: Diseases and Conditions: Benign Prostatic Hyperplasia: <http://uk.dir.yahoo.com/health/diseases_and_conditions/benign_prostatic_hyperplasia__bph_/>

98. PROSTATE CANCER

The most feared of prostatic disorders, prostate cancer (PCa, CaP) is a cancer that originates in the prostate gland. Although there are various markers or tests (for example, PSA blood test or digital rectal exam) to help determine the possibility of PCa, *the only valid diagnostic method is a biopsy of the prostate gland.* This is because other non-cancerous, prostate disorders can cause similar symptoms. The markers and symptoms direct the physician to what tests should be done next to determine the actual problem.

Recommended Search Terms

- "Prostate cancer"
- "Cancer of the prostate"
- "Prostate adenocarcinoma"

Important Sites

American Cancer Society (ACS): Learn about Cancer: All about Prostate Cancer: <http://www.cancer.org/>

CancerLinks: Welcome to Prostate Cancer Links: <http://www.cancerlinks.org/prostate.html>

Prostate Cancer Foundation: Prostate Cancer: <http://www.prostatecancerfoundation.org/site/pp.asp?c=biJTJ8OTF&b=9066>

Centers for Disease Control and Prevention (CDC): National Center for Chronic Disease Prevention and Health Promotion (NCCDPHP): Cancer Prevention and Control: Prostate Cancer: The Public Health Perspective: <http://www.cdc.gov/cancer/prostate/prostate.htm>

Johns Hopkins Prostate Bulletin: <http://hopkinsprostate.com/>

University of Texas: MD Anderson Cancer Center: Prostate Cancer: <http://www.mdanderson.org/diseases/prostate/>

MedlinePlus: Prostate Cancer: <http://www.nlm.nih.gov/medlineplus/prostatecancer.html>

National Cancer Institute (NCI): cancer.gov: Cancer Information: Prostate Cancer (PDQ): Treatment: <http://www.cancer.gov/cancerinfo/pdq/treatment/prostate/patient/>

National Prostate Cancer Coalition: <http://www.4npcc.org/>

Oncolink: Types of Cancer: Prostate Cancer: Overview: <http://www.oncolink.com/types/index.cfm>

Open Directory Project (DMOZ): Health: Conditions and Diseases: Cancer: Genitourinary: Prostate: <http://dmoz.org/Health/Conditions_and_Diseases/Cancer/Genitourinary/Prostate/>

Phoenix5: <http://www.phoenix5.org/>

Phoenix5: Prostate Cancer InfoLink <http://www.phoenix5.org/Infolink/index.html>

Prostate-Help: <http://www.prostate-help.org/>

Prostate Pointers: <http://www.prostatepointers.org/prostate/>

PSA (Prostate Cancer Survivor) Rising Magazine: <http://psa-rising.com/>

University of Michigan Health System: Comprehensive Cancer Center: Urologic Oncology Program: <http://www.cancer.med.umich.edu/prostcan/prostcan.html>

WebMD Health: Diseases and Conditions: Prostate Cancer Health Center: <http://my.webmd.com/medical_information/condition_centers/prostate_cancer/default.htm>

YANA (You Are Not Alone Now): <http://www.yananow.net/>

99. PROSTATITIS

Prostatitis is an inflammation usually caused by bacteria and, thus, treatable with antibiotics. However, it can also be caused by a virus, or even stones in the prostate, as one might get in the kidney. Prostatitis is *not* a sexually transmitted disease.

Recommended Search Terms

- Prostate inflammation infection -".com" -".co.uk" -".biz"
- Prostatitis
- Prostatitis "differential diagnosis"
- "Chronic prostatitis"
- Prostatodynia
- "Nonbacterial prostatitis"
- "Chronic bacterial prostatitis"
- "Acute prostatitis"
- CBP prostate
- NBP prostate
- PDy prostate
- "painful prostate"

Important Sites

American Foundation for Urologic Disease (AFUD): Diseases and Conditions: Prostatitis: <http://www.afud.org/conditions/ps.html>

Columbia University Medical Center: Departments: Urology: Prostatitis at the Prostate Center: <http://cpmcnet.columbia.edu/dept/urology/prostatitis.html>

National Institute of Diabetes and Digestive and Kidney Diseases (NIDDK): National Kidney and Urologic Disease Information Clearinghouse: Kidney and Urologic Diseases Topics List: Prostatitis: Disorders of the Prostate: <http://kidney.niddk.nih.gov/kudiseases/pubs/prostatitis/index.htm>

Prostate Pointers: Prostatitis: <http://www.prostatepointers.org/prostate/>

Prostatitis Foundation: <http://www.prostatitis.org/>

Urology Channel: Prostatitis: <http://www.urologychannel.com/prostate/prostatitis/index.shtml>

100. Incontinence

Recommended Search Terms

- "Difficuly urinating"
- "Incontinence"
- "Urinating/urinary problem"
- "Frequent urination"
- "Trouble urinating"
- Urinating difficulty
- Urinary problem

Important Sites

About: Men's Health: <http://menshealth.about.com/>

American Foundation of Urologic Disease: Bladder Health Council: Incontinence.org: <http://www.incontinence.org/>

Johns Hopkins Medical Institutions: Department of Urology: Brady Urological Institute: <http://urology.jhu.edu//diseases/bladder/incontinence.html>

National Association for Continence (NAFC) <http://www.nafc.org/site2/index.html>

Urology Channel: Incontinence: <http://www.urologychannel.com/incontinence/index.shtml>

101. Erectile and Sexual Dysfunction

Recommended Search Terms

NOTE: This is one of the most difficult topics to search because common sexual words will produce hits to sites that are sexually explicit, including pornography, or that sell drugs or products that guarantee a sex life and are seldom relevant to sexual side effects of prostate disorders. It is vital the search be kept narrow, cautious (avoiding explicit terms), and relevant to the prostate disorder, if possible.

- "Erectile dysfunction" +prostate
- "Erectile dysfunction" -xxx -porn
- "Sexual dysfunction" -xxx -porn
- Sexuality +prostatitis
- Sex +"prostate cancer"
- Intimacy +"prostate surgery"
- Sex +"prostate surgery"

Important Sites

About: Health and Fitness: Men's Health: Man Matters: Articles: Understanding Impotence: <http://menshealth.about.com/cs/menonly/a/impotence.htm>

Alt.Support.Impotence on the Web: Frequently Asked Questions (FAQ): <http://www.alt-support-impotence.org/faq.htm>

American Foundation for Urologic Disease (AFUD): Diseases and Conditions: Impotence: <http://www.afud.org/education/sexualfunction/impotence.asp>

American Foundation for Urologic Disease (AFUD): Sexual Function Health Council: Impotence.org: <http://www.impotence.org/>

Bandolier: Bandolier Journal: Erectile Dysfunction Treatments: <http://www.jr2.ox.ac.uk/bandolier/band43/b43-3.html>

MedlinePlus: Impotence: <http://www.nlm.nih.gov/medlineplus/impotence.html>

National Institute of Diabetes and Digestive and Kidney Diseases (NIDDK): National Kidney and Urologic Diseases Information Clearinghouse: Kidney and Urologic Diseases Topics List: Erectile Dysfunction: <http://kidney.niddk.nih.gov/kudiseases/topics/erectile.asp>

Phoenix5: Sexuality and Intimacy: <http://www.phoenix5.org/sexaids.html>

Prostate Cancer UK: Erectile Dysfunction: <http://www.prostatecanceruk.org/erictile-sysfunction.html>

Prostatitis Foundation: Prostatitis—Pointers to Other Sites: <http://www.prostatitis.org/pointers.html>

University of Pittsburgh Medical Center (UPMC) Cancer Centers: Cancer Information: Prostate Cancer: Erectile Dysfunction: <http://www.upmccancercenters.com/cancer/prostate/erectiledysfunction.html>

Urology Channel: Erectile Dysfunction: <http://www.urologychannel.com/erectiledysfunction/index.shtml>

Viagra (Pfizer): <http://www.viagra.com/>

Wayne State University: Department of Urology: Urological Conditions: Individual Urological Conditions: Impotence and Sexual Function: <http://www.med.wayne.edu/urology/DISEASES/impotence.html>

WebMD Health: Medical News Archive: Men Eager to Renew Activities After Prostate Surgery: <http://my.webmd.com/content/article/32/1728_60522?>

102. Drugs and Medications

Recommended Search Terms

NOTE: Because there are hundreds of drugs and medications for prostate disorder treatments, search by the name or the disorder. Inserting a reputable resource will help.

- BPH drug treatment ACS
- BPH drug treatment NCI
- BPH drug treatment NIDDK
- BPH medication ACS
- Hyperplasia drugs prostate NCI
- Hyperplasia medication prostate NIDDK

Important Sites

About: Health and Fitness: Senior Health: (Benign Prostatic Hyperplasia) Treatment: <http://seniorhealth.about.com/library/men/blbph6.htm>

DrugDigest: Health Conditions: Benign Prostatic Hyperplasia (BPH): How Is It Treated? <http://www.drugdigest.org/DD/HC/Treatment/0,4047,550246,00.html>

Food and Drug Administration (FDA): FDA Consumer Magazine: Prostate Cancer: No One Answer for Testing or Treatment: <http://www.fda.gov/fdac/features/1998/598_pros.html>

HealthWise: Medications: Alpha-Blockers for Benign Prostatic Hyperplasia (BPH): <http://www.information-therapy.org/kbase/topic/detail/drug/hw59707/detail.htm>

National Cancer Institute (NCI): cancer.gov: Cancer Information: Know Your Options: Understanding Treatment Choices for Prostate Cancer: The Decision Is Yours: <http://www.cancer.gov/CancerInformation/understanding-prostate-cancer-treatment/page9>

National Cancer Institute (NCI): cancer.gov: Cancer Information: Prostate Cancer (PDQ): Treatment: <http://www.nci.nih.gov/cancer_information/doc_pdq.aspx?viewid=f4c08184-f6a9-49d5-8521-7540e59224ac>

National Institute of Diabetes and Digestive and Kidney Diseases (NIDDK): National Kidney and Urologic Diseases Information Clearinghouse: Kidney and Urologic Diseases Topics List: What I Need to Know about Prostate Problems: <http://kidney.niddk.nih.gov/kudiseases/pubs/prostate_ez/index.htm>

Physician's Desk Reference (PDR): <http://www.pdr.net>

University of California–Davis Health System: Health and Wellness: Benign Prostatic Hyperplasia: What Drugs Are Used for Benign Prostatic Hyperplasia? <http://www.ucdmc.ucdavis.edu/health/a-z/71BenignProstaticHyperplasia/doc71drugs.html>

University of Pennsylvania Health System: Institute on Aging: Health Center: Benign Prostatic Hypertrophy: Treatment: <http://www.uphs.upenn.edu/aging/turtle_springs/hc_files/bph/bph_medication.html>

103. Clinical Trials

Recommended Search Terms

NOTE: The condition or the gland must be included. You can also include the drug. Including your city/state may restrict the search too much.

- "Clinical trial" prostatitis
- "Clinical trial" BPH
- "Clinical trial" "benign prostatic hyperplasia"
- "Clinical trial" "benign prostatic hypertrophy"
- "Clinical trial" "prostate cancer
- "Clinical trial" "erectile dysfunction"
- "Clinical trial" "prostate zometa"

Important Sites

CenterWatch:<http://www.centerwatch.com/>

CenterWatch: Patient Resources: Clinical Trials: Benign Prostatic Hyperplasia (Enlarged Prostate) <http://www.centerwatch.com/patient/studies/cat276.html>

CenterWatch: Patient Resources: Clinical Trials: Erectile Dysfunction: <http://www.centerwatch.com/patient/studies/cat371.html>

CenterWatch: Patient Resources: Clinical Trials: Prostate Cancer: <http://www.centerwatch.com/patient/studies/cat36.html>

ClinicalTrials.com (from Pharmaceutical Research Plus): <http://www.clinicaltrials.com/>

ClinicalTrials.gov (from the U.S. National Institutes of Health): <http://www.clinicaltrials.gov/>

National Cancer Institute (NCI): cancer.gov: Clinical Trials: <http://www.nci.nih.gov/clinical_trials/>

National Cancer Institute (NCI): Office of Cancer Complementary and Alternative Medicine (OCCAM): Clinical Trials: <http://www3.cancer.gov/occam/trials.html>

National Institute of Diabetes and Digestive and Kidney Diseases (NIDDK): Clinical Research: <http://www.niddk.nih.gov/patient/patient.htm>

Search the Studies: <http://clinicalstudies.info.nih.gov/>

University of California – Los Angeles (UCLA): Oncology: UCLA Medical Oncology and Southern California Prostate Cancer Study Group Program in Prostate Cancer: <http://www.medonc.med.ucla.edu/Prostate_Cancer_Trials.htm>

University of California–San Francisco (UCSF): Department of Urology: Clinical Trials: <http://urology.ucsf.edu/clinicalTrials.html>

Veritas Medicine: <http://www.veritasmedicine.com>

Yahoo! Health: Clinical Trials: Urology/Nephrology: <http://health.yahoo.com/health/clinical_trials/uro.html>

104. Diet

There are countless diet and health fads touted as cures to the newly diagnosed and the frightened. At press time, a search for "diet + prostate" gave nearly 865,000 hits, "prostate + health" gave 1,580,000 and "diet + cancer" produced over 2,800,000 hits. It is strongly recommended that you rely on fundamental nutrition information from authoritative and reliable sources.

Important Sites

U.S. National Institutes of Health (NIH): Office of Dietary Supplements: <http://dietary-supplements.info.nih.gov/>

National Cancer Institute (NCI): Office of Cancer Complementary and Alternative Medicine (OCCAM): <http://www3.cancer.gov/occam/about.html>

105. Diagnosis

Recommended Search Terms

- "Prostate gland" diagnosis
- "Prostate screening"
- "Prostate test"
- "Prostatitis testing"
- "BPH test"
- "Prostate cancer tests"
- "Prostate cancer" "differential diagnosis"
- "BPH symptoms"
- "Prostatitis symptoms"
- "Prostate cancer symptoms"

Important Sites

American Cancer Society (ACS): Cancer Reference Information: Detailed Guide: Prostate Cancer: Can Prostate Cancer Be Found Early? <http://www.cancer.org/docroot/cri/content/cri_2_4_3x_can_prostate_cancer_be_found_early_36.asp?sitearea=cri>

BPH (Benign Prostatic Hyperplasia) Partners: BPH Symptoms: <http://www.bphpartners.com/symptoms.htm>

Cancer Treatment Centers of America: Prostate Cancer Symptoms: <http://www.cancercenter.com/prostate-cancer-symptoms-a.htm>

CancerBackUp (UK): About Cancer: Screening and Prevention: The Prostate Gland: <http://www.cancerbacup.org.uk/info/psatest/psatest-1.htm>

Cornell University: Department of Urology: BPH: Signs and Symptoms: <http://www.cornellurology.com/uro/cornell/bph/symptoms/>

Discovery Health Channel: Health Centers: Sexual Health: PSA (Prostate Specific Antigen): <http://health.discovery.com/centers/sex/sexpedia/psa.html>

Food and Drug Administration (FDA): FDA Consumer Magazine: Prostate Cancer: No One Answer for Testing or Treatment: <http://www.fda.gov/fdac/features/1998/598_pros.html>

Medical College of Wisconsin: HealthLink: Medical Opinions Differ on Testing for Prostate Cancer: <http://healthlink.mcw.edu/article/962132605.html>

MedlinePlus: Prostate Cancer: <http://www.nlm.nih.gov/medlineplus/prostatecancer.html>

Memorial Sloan-Kettering Cancer Center: Cancer Information: Cancer and Treatment: Types of Cancer: Prostate Cancer: Diagnsosis: <http://www.mskcc.org/mskcc/html/1819.cfm>

Methodist Health Care System: Prostate Cancer: Diagnostic and Evaluation Procedures: <http://www.methodisthealth.com/Urology/MthTopics/prced.htm>

National Cancer Institute (NCI): cancer.gov: Cancer Information: Prostate Cancer Home Page: <http://www.cancer.gov/cancerinfo/types/prostate>

Oncology Channel: Prostate Cancer: Diagnosis: <http://www.oncologychannel.com/prostatecancer/diagnosis.shtml>

Penn State University: Milton S. Hershey Medical Center: College of Medicine: Health and Disease Information A to Z Topics: Prostate-Specific Antigen (PSA) Testing: <http://www.hmc.psu.edu/healthinfo/pq/psa.htm>

ProstateDisease.org: Prostatitis: <http://www.prostatedisease.org/prostatitis/index.asp>

Prostatitis Foundation: Prostatitis: Diagnosing and Treating Chronic Prostatitis: Do Urologists Use the Glass Test? <http://www.prostatitis.org/stameymeares.html>

PSA (Prostate Cancer Survivor) Rising Magazine: Finding Prostate Cancer: <http://psa-rising.com/caplinks/medical_psa.htm>

Seven Hills Urology Center: Prostate Symptom Score: <http://www.sevenhillsurology.com/bphtest.html>

University of Maryland Medicine: Health Information: Prostate Health Guide: Diagnosis and Evaluation: <http://www.umm.edu/prostate/prced.htm>

University of Pennsylvania Health System: Benign Prostatic Hyperplasia (BPH): Symptoms: <http://www.uphs.upenn.edu/aging/turtle_springs/hc_files/bph/bph_symptoms.html>

Urology Channel: Prostatitis: Signs and Symptoms: <http://www.urologychannel.com/prostate/prostatitis/symptoms.shtml>

106. Glossaries and Dictionaries

Cambridge Dictionaries Online: <http://dictionary.cambridge.org/>

Department Veterans Affairs (Australia): You and Your Prostate: Glossary of Medical Terms: <http://www.dva.gov.au/media/publicat/2001/prostate/glossary.htm>

Merriam-Webster Online: <http://www.m-w.com/dictionary.htm>

National Cancer Institute (NCI): cancer.gov: Dictionary: <http://www.nci.nih.gov/dictionary/>

OneLook: Dictionary Search: <http://www.onelook.com/>

Phoenix5: Phoenix5 Illustrated: Prostate Cancer Glossary: <http://www.phoenix5.org/glossary/glossary.html>

Prostate Cancer Research Institute: Glossary of PCa (Prostate Cancer) Related Terms: <http://www.prostate-cancer.org/resource/glossary.html>

Prostate Pointers: Glossary of PCa Related Terms: <http://www.prostatepointers.org/prostate/ed-pip/glossary.html>

University of California—Davis: Cancer Center: Prostate Cancer Information: <http://cancer.ucdmc.ucdavis.edu/info/publications/prostate_cancer_info/glossary.html>

WebMD: Health: A Basic Prostate Glossary: <http://my.webmd.com/content/article/4/1680_50808?>

Hotlines

American Cancer Institute:
1-800-4-CANCER/1-800-422-6237
American Cancer Society:
1-800-227-2345
American Institute for Cancer Research:
1-800-843-8114
Prostate Wellness Hotline:
1-800-394-7546

FAQs

Memorial Sloan-Kettering Cancer Center: Cancer Information: Cancer and Treatment: Types of Cancer: Prostate Cancer: Questions and Answers about Prostate Cancer: <http://www.mskcc.org/mskcc/html/410.cfm>

Prostate.com: BPH (Benign Prostatic Hyperplastia): <http://www.prostate.com/BPH/BPH.asp>

Prostate.com: Prostate Cancer FAQs (Frequently Asked Questions): <http://www.prostate.com/pcfaq_g.htm>

Prostatitis Foundation: Prostatitis Frequently Asked Questions: <http://www.prostatitis.org/prosfaq.html>

Professional Organizations

American Cancer Society (ACS): <http://www.cancer.org/>

American Foundation for Urologic Disease (AFUD) <http://www.afud.org>

Prostate Cancer Foundation: <http://www.prostatecancerfoundation.org/site/pp.asp?c=biJTJ8OTFandb=6477>

Prostate Cancer Research Institute: <http://www.prostate-cancer.org/>

Patient Support Organizations/ Discussion Groups

American Cancer Society (ACS): Support for Survivors and Patients: Support Programs and Services: ACS Man to Man Support Groups: <http://www.cancer.org/docroot/SHR/SHR_2.asp>

Open Directory Project (DMOZ): Health: Conditions and Diseases: Cancer: Genitourinary: Prostate: Support Groups: <http://dmoz.org/Health/Conditions_and_Diseases/Cancer/Genitourinary/Prostate/Support/>

Phoenix5: Prostate Cancer Support Groups: <http://www.phoenix5.org/supportgroups.html>

Association of Cancer Online Resources (ACOR): <http://www.acor.org/index.html>

Prostate-Help: <http://www.prostate-help.com/>

US TOO: Prostate Cancer Education and Support: <http://www.ustoo.com/>

YANA (You Are Not Alone) Prostate Cancer Support Group Message Board: <http://pub1.bravenet.com>

Best One-Stop Shops

MedlinePlus: [A service of the US National Library of Medicine, it is the largest medical library in the world and has illustrations. Use it to find health and drug information.] <http://medlineplus.gov>

National Cancer Institute (NCI): [The NCI has considerable information on prostate disorders other than cancer, with free booklets and an extensive glossary plus a toll-free number for telephone information.]: <http://www.cancer.gov>

National Institute of Diabetes and Digestive and Kidney Diseases (NIDDK): [NIDDK is part of the US National Institutes of Health. Although "prostate" is not in their name, it is in their research and so the NIDDK site has some excellent information]: <http://www.niddk.nih.gov/>

Open Directory Project (DMOZ): Health: Conditions and Diseases: Cancer: Genitourinary: Prostate: <http://dmoz.org/Health/Conditions_and_Diseases/Cancer/Genitourinary/Prostate/>

Part XI: Sexual Health Issues

Kristine Alpi

[*See also* relevant parts of "Life Stages," vol. 3; "Sexual Safety;" p. 23; "Pregnancy and Childbirth," p. 144; "AIDS/HIV," p. 3, vol. 2; Infectious Diseases," p. 98, vol. 2.]

Special Searching Issues for this Topic

Sexual health comprises sexual development, sexual identity, sex education, reproductive health (including birth control), sexually transmitted infections, sexuality across the life span, and sexual assault recovery. The synonyms for sexual activities are endless. Because of this, try to use medical terminology when searching. When slang terms are used, take extra care in reviewing the quality of search results since those terms may lead to sites with poor quality information. For example, searching with common euphemisms such as the "facts of life" or the "birds and the bees" will retrieve many nonrelated sites. This is also true when searching on slang words for sexually transmitted diseases (STDs). A Google search for the slang term "the clap" brings up sites about a British band; searching on the medical term "gonorrhea" brings up information from the Centers for Disease Control and Prevention (CDC). A final example of the problems with searching with slang terminology comes from the topic of emergency contraception, which is often called the "morning-after" pill, even though it may be used up to 72 hours after unprotected intercourse. You will also find that some clinicians and consumers mistakenly refer to the "morning-after" pill as the "abortion-pill" confusing it with RU-486.

In addition to the choice of search terms, there are also several other issues to be aware of when searching for information on sexual health issues. First, some low-quality sexuality Web sites also link to sexual commerce (pornography) sites. Second, schools, libraries, and homes using Internet filtering software may not be able to access many sexual health resources. Finally, images on these sites, especially pictures to assist in the diagnosis of sexually transmitted diseases, may be disturbing. If you run into problems with too many inappropriate sites, you can use a search engine that can limit results to those from ".edu" and ".org" Web site addresses. This will eliminate many commercial sites; unfortunately, some good ones along with the bad ones.

What to Ask

It is a good idea to spend some time thinking about what you want before you start searching. In this preparation phase, you may want to take the following questions into consideration. What am I looking for? Do I want images? Do I need materials geared toward a certain age level or cultural group? How comfortable am I with the possibility of accidentally finding links to pornographic Web sites? To avoid pornographic sites, but still be able to find good material on sexuality or sexual health issues, please refer to the chapter "Strategic Searching with Search Engines" (p. 49) in Volume 1.

Where to Start

Since sexual health is such a broad topic, searching may be difficult. It would be valuable to start by finding the best pages from respected organizations and building

from their links, or building keywords based on topics of interest. This will help define a search strategy appropriate to the topic.

Topic Profile

Who

People at almost every age, gender, and life stage have the possibility of needing information on sexual well-being, including abstinence or celibacy.

What

Sexuality is part of every day existence. We are bombarded with messages about our sexuality daily, whether we realize it or not. Knowing where to find straight talk about sexual health concerns can relieve a lot of the stress that people may feel when confronted by questions about their development, reproductive health decisions, and preventing sexually transmitted diseases.

Where

Sexual health is not just about erogenous zones. The major participating organ in sexual health is the brain. These sites address both the physical and mental issues involved in healthy sexuality.

When

Since sexual health is important at all stages of life, it's never too early to start learning.

Abbreviations Used In This Section

CDC = Centers for Disease Control and Prevention
HPV = Human papillomavirus
IUD = Intrauterine devices
LGBT = Lesbian, gay, bisexual, transgender
STD = Sexually transmitted diseases
STI = Sexually transmitted infections
TB = Tuberculosis

Procedures and Special Topics

107. General

Recommended Search Terms

- "Reproductive health"
- "Sexual health"
- Sexuality
- "Sexuality and health"

Important Sites

Aetna InteliHealth: Diseases and Conditions: Sexual and Reproductive Health: <http://www.intelihealth.com/>

Alan Guttmacher Institute: <http://www.agi-usa.org/>

EngenderHealth: <http://www.engenderhealth.org/>

Family Health International (FHI): <http://www.fhi.org/>

healthfinder: Health Library: Prevention and Wellness: Sexuality: <http://www.healthfinder.gov/>

Johns Hopkins University: Reproductive Health Online: Reproline: <http://www.reproline.jhu.edu/>

Kaiser Family Foundation: Women's Health Policy: Reproductive Health: <http://www.kff.org/womenshealth/repro.cfm>

MedlinePlus: Reproductive Health: <http://www.nlm.nih.gov/medlineplus/reproductivehealth.html>

MedlinePlus: Sexual Health Issues: <http://www.nlm.nih.gov/medlineplus/sexualhealthissues.html>

New York Online Access to Health (NOAH): Ask NOAH About: Sexuality: <http://www.noah-health.org/english/sexuality/sexuality.html>

Planned Parenthood Federation of America (PPFA): <http://www.plannedparenthood.org/>

Sexual Health Network: <http://www.sexualhealth.com/>

108. Sexual Development and Sex Education

Recommended Search Terms

- Intimacy
- Masturbation health -xxx -porn
- "Oral sex" -xxx -porn
- Puberty
- "Sex behavior"
- "Sexual activity"
- "Sexual development"
- "Sex education" (or "sex eEd")
- "Sexual education"
- "Sexual maturation"

Important Sites

American Social Health Association (ASHA): iwanna know.com: <http://www.iwannaknow.org/>

Coalition for Positive Sexuality (CPS): <http://www.positive.org/>

Go Ask Alice! <http://www.goaskalice.columbia.edu/>

MedlinePlus: Teen Sexual Health: <http://www.nlm.nih.gov/medlineplus/teensexualhealth.html>

Sexuality Information and Education Council of the United States (SIECUS): <http://www.siecus.org/>

Talking with Kids about Tough Issues: Talking with Kids about Sex and Relationships: <http://www.talkingwithkids.org/sex.html>

Planned Parenthood Federation of America: teenwire: <http://www.teenwire.com/>

109. Sexual Identity

When searching on sexual identity, you will find many opinion pieces, often with strong religious points of view. Assessing the results from a search on homosexuality, for example, will require you to evaluate the Web page author's bias.

Recommended Search Terms

NOTES: (1) Add identity or health or some other terms to further narrow the search. (2) Intersexuality means a person is born with sex chromosomes, external genitalia, and/or an internal reproductive system that are discordant.

- Bisexual
- Bisexuality
- Gay lifestyle
- Gay sexuality
- "Gender Dysphoria"
- "Gender identity"
- "Gender reassignment"
- Heterosexual
- Heterosexuality
- Homosexual
- Homosexuality
- Intersexuality
- Lesbian
- LGBT
- Lesbian gay bisexual transgender
- "Sex change"
- "Sex reassignment"
- "Sexual identity"
- "Sexual orientation"
- "Sexual preference"
- Transgender
- Transgenderism
- Transsexual
- Transsexualism
- Transsexuality
- Transvestite
- Transvestism

Important Sites

American Psychological Association: Public Topics: What You Need to Know about Lesbian/Gay/Bisexual Health Issues: <http://www.apa.org/psychnet/lgbc.html>

Bisexual Resource Center: <http://www.biresource.org/>

Document for Lesbian, Gay, Bisexual and Transgender (LGBT) Health: <http://www.glma.org/policy/hp2010/PDF/HP2010CDLGBTHealth.pdf>

Gay and Lesbian Medical Association (GLMA): Public Policy: Healthy People 2010 Companion Harry Benjamin International Gender Dysphoria Association (HBIGDA): <http://www.hbigda.org/>

Intersex Society of North America (ISNA): <http://www.isna.org/>

Seattle and King County Public Health: Gay Lesbian Bisexual and Transgender (GLBT) Health Webpages: <http://www.metrokc.gov/health/glbt/>

110. Birth Control and Contraception

Recommended Search Terms

- Abstinence
- "Birth control"
- "Birth control patch"
- Celibacy
- Cervical cap
- Condoms
- Contraception
- "Contraceptive sponges"
- Contraceptives
- Diaphragm
- Emergency contraception"
- Family planning
- Female condoms
- Intrauterine devices
- IUDs
- Norplant
- "Safe Sex"
- Spermicides
- Sterilization
- "Tubal ligation"
- Vasectomy

Important Sites

MedlinePlus: Birth Control/Contraception: <http://www.nlm.nih.gov/medlineplus/birthcontrolcontraception.html>

NOT-2-LATE.com: The Emergency Contraception Website: <http://ec.princeton.edu/>

Resource Center for Adolescent Pregnancy Prevention: <http://www.etr.org/recapp/>

111. Sexual Health and Fertility

Recommended Search Terms

- "Assisted reproduction techniques"
- "Erectile dysfunction"

- Fertility sexuality
- Impotence
- Infertility
- Menopause sexuality
- Sexuality disability
- Sexuality disabilities
- "Sexual dysfunction"
- "Sexual performance anxiety"
- Sexuality aging

Important Sites

Centers for Disease Control and Prevention (CDC): CDC's Reproductive Health Information Source: Assisted Reproductive Technology Reports: <http://www.cdc.gov/nccdphp/drh/art.htm>

MedlinePlus: Infertility: <http://www.nlm.nih.gov/medlineplus/infertility.html>

MedlinePlus: Impotence: <http://www.nlm.nih.gov/medlineplus/impotence.html>

National Women's Health Information Center: 4woman.gov: Women with Disabilities: Sexuality and Disability: <http://www.4woman.gov/>

New York Online Access to Health (NOAH): Ask NOAH About Pregnancy: Fertility, Infertility and Surrogacy: <http://www.noah-health.org/english/pregnancy/fertility.html>

SeniorSex: Older Adult Sexuality Reference: <http://instruct1.cit.cornell.edu/courses/psych431/student2000/dp51/>

Sexual Function Health Council of the American Foundation for Urologic Disease: International Impotence Education Month: <http://www.iiem.org/>

Sexual Health and Fertility after Brain and Spinal Cord Impairment: <http://www.scisexualhealth.com/>

112. Sexual Violence

[*See also* "Personal Safety and Domestic Violence," p. 20.]

Recommended Search Terms

- Child sexual abuse
- "Date rape"
- "Domestic violence"
- Incest
- Molestation
- "Partner abuse"
- Rape
- "Sexual abuse"
- "Sexual assault"
- Sexual "child abuse"
- "Sexual violence"

Important Sites

Gay Partner Abuse Project (Canada): <http://www.gay partnerabuseproject.org/>

MedlinePlus: Rape: <http://www.nlm.nih.gov/medlineplus/rape.html>

New York Online Access to Health (NOAH): Ask NOAH About: Family Violence and Sexual Assault: <http://www.noah-health.org/english/illness/mental health/domestic.html>

Rape, Abuse and Incest National Network (RAINN): <http://www.rainn.org/>

Sexual Assault Nurse Examination (SANE)-Sexual Assault Resource Team (SART): <http://www.sane-sart.com/>

113. LIFE CHOICES: ABORTION AND ADOPTION

Recommended Search Terms

- Abortion
- Adoption
- "Elective abortion"
- Mifepristone
- Pregnancy choices
- "Pregnancy termination"
- RU-486

Important Sites

Administration for Children and Families: National Adoption Information Clearinghouse (NAIC): Resources for Expectant Patients Considering Adoption: <http://naic.acf.hhs.gov/brelativ/expect.cfm>

Medem: Medical Library: American College of Obstetricians and Gynecologists: Pregnancy Choices: Raising the Baby, Adoption and Abortion: <http://www.medem.com/>

MedlinePlus: Adoption: <http://www.nlm.nih.gov/medlineplus/adoption.html>

MedlinePlus: Abortion: <http://www.nlm.nih.gov/medlineplus/abortion.html>

Planned Parenthood:Choosing Abortion: Questions and Answers: <http://www.plannedparenthood.org/abortion/abortquestions.html>

114. SEXUALLY TRANSMITTED DISEASES/INFECTIONS

Recommended Search Terms

- "Sexually transmitted diseases"
- STDs
- "Sexually transmitted infections"
- STIs

NOTE: You may wish to use the names of specific infections or organisms. such as chancroid, Chlamydia, pubic lice (crabs), gonorrhea, herpes, human papillomavirus (HPV), genital warts, molluscum contagiosum, syphilis, trichomoniasis, and so on, combined with prevention, diagnosis, or treatment.

- "Genital warts" treatment
- HPV prevention
- Gonorrhea diagnosis

Important Sites

American Social Health Association (ASHA): <http://www.ashastd.org/>

Centers for Disease Control and Prevention (CDC): National Center for HIV, STD and TB Prevention: Division of Sexually Transmitted Diseases: STD Prevention: <http://www.cdc.gov/nchstp/dstd/dstdp.html>

healthfinder: Health Library: Prevention and Wellness: Sexually Transmitted Diseases: <http://www.healthfinder.gov/>

MedlinePlus: Sexually Transmitted Diseases: <http://www.nlm.nih.gov/medlineplus/sexuallytransmitteddiseases.html>

New York Online Access to Health (NOAH): Ask NOAH About: Sexually Transmitted Diseases: <http://www.noah-health.org/english/illness/stds/stds.html>

HOTLINES

Emergency Contraception Hotline:
1-888-NOT-2-LATE
National Sexual Assault Hotline:
1-800-656-HOPE
National STD and AIDS Hotline:
1-800-277-8922 or 1-800-342-AIDS (2437)
National Women's Health Information Center:
1-800-994-WOMAN

FAQS

National Women's Health Information Center: 4woman.gov: Frequently Asked Questions about Women's Health: <http://www.4woman.gov/faq>

Planned Parenthood Federation of America (PPFA): Research and Media: Frequently Asked Questions: <http://www.plannedparenthood.org/library/FAQs.html>

SEXUAL HEALTH PUBLICATIONS ON THE INTERNET

Electronic Journal of Human Sexuality: <http://www.ejhs.org/>

Family Health International (FHI): Reproductive Health: Frequently Asked Questions: <http://www.fhi.org/en/RH/FAQs/index.htm>

Alan Guttmacher Institute: Publications: *Perspectives on Sexual and Reproductive Health*: <http://www.agi-usa.org/journals/fpp_archive.html>

Sexuality Information and Education Council of the United States (SIECUS): *SIECUS Report*: <http://www.siecus.org/pubs/pubs0004.html#REPORT>

MEDICAL SPECIALTIES

Gynecology; Urology; Reproductive medicine; Infectious disease; Psychiatry; Public health

PROFESSIONAL ORGANIZATIONS

American Association of Sex Educators, Counselors, and Therapists (AASECT): <http://www.aasect.org/>

American College of Obstetricians and Gynecologists (ACOG): <http://www.acog.org/>

Association of Reproductive Health Professionals (ARHP): <http://www.arhp.org/>

PATIENT SUPPORT ORGANIZATIONS/ DISCUSSIONS GROUPS

Coalition for Positive Sexuality: Let's Talk: <http://www.positive.org/LetsTalk/welcome.html>

OBGYN.net: Online Discussion Forums: <http://www.obgyn.net/english/forums/forums.asp>

BEST ONE-STOP SHOPS

Johns Hopkins University: Reproductive Health Online: Reproline: <http://www.reproline.jhu.edu/>

New York Online Access to Health (NOAH): Ask NOAH About: Sexuality: <http://www.noah-health.org/english/sexuality/sexuality.html>

Planned Parenthood Federation of America (PPFA): <http://www.plannedparenthood.org/>

Sexuality Information and Education Council of the United States (SIECUS): <http://www.siecus.org/>

List of Contributors

Kristine Alpi, M.L.S., M.P.H., AHIP
Library Manager
Public Health Library
New York City Department of Health and Mental Hygiene
New York, NY

Lecturer in Public Health
Weill Medical College of Cornell University
New York, NY

Theresa Arndt, M.L.S.
Head of Outreach Services
Taubman Medical Library
University of Michigan
Ann Arbor, MI

Sheila J. Bryant, M.L.I.S., AHIP
Health Sciences/Veterinary Medicine Librarian
Michigan State University
East Lansing, MI

Gary L. Cheatham, M.Div., M.S.L.S.
Assistant Professor of Library Services
Northeastern State University
Tahlequah, Oklahoma

Erinn Faiks, M.S.I.
University Library Associate
Public Health Informatics Services and Access (PHISA)
University of Michigan
Ann Arbor, MI

NLM Associate Fellow
National Library of Medicine
Bethesda, MD

Gillian Goldsmith Mayman, M.L.S.
Reference and Instruction Librarian
Public Health Informatics Services and Access (PHISA)
University of Michigan
Ann Arbor, MI

Susan K. Kendall, Ph.D., M.S.L.I.S.
Health Sciences Librarian
Michigan State University
East Lansing, MI

Martin L. Knott, M.S.I.
Cataloger, University Library
University of Michigan
Ann Arbor, MI

Deborah L. Lauseng, A.M.L.S.
   Administrative Associate
   Public Health Informatics Services and Access (PHISA)
   University of Michigan
   Ann Arbor, MI

   Information Services Librarian
   Taubman Medical Library
   University of Michigan
   Ann Arbor, MI

Helen Look, M.S.I.
   Collection Management Coordinator
   Public Health Informatics Services and Access (PHISA)
   University of Michigan
   Ann Arbor, MI

Alana O'Neal, B.A.
   Information Resource Specialist
   Public Health Informatics Services and Access (PHISA)
   University of Michigan
   Ann Arbor, MI

Katherine Ott, M.L.S.
   Instructor of Library services
   Northeastern State University
   Tahlequah, OK

Karyn L. Pomerantz, M.L.S., M.P.H.
   PI, Partners for Health Information
   School of Public Health and Health Services
   George Washington University
   Washington, DC

Nancy Pulsipher, M.S.I.
   Reference and Instruction Librarian
   Public Health Informatics Services and Access (PHISA)
   University of Michigan
   Ann Arbor, MI

   NLM Associate Fellow
   National Library of Medicine
   Bethesda, MD

Anna Ercoli Schnitzer, A.M.L.S.
   Information Services Librarian
   Taubman Medical Library
   University of Michigan
   Ann Arbor, MI

Christopher J. Shaffer, M.S.
   Assistant Director, Public Services
   Hardin Library for the Health Sciences
   University of Iowa
   Iowa City, IA

Shelley Barker Shea, M.L.S.
    Library Administrator
    Professional Library and Archives
    Jefferson County Public Schools
    Golden, CO

Bryan S. Vogh, M.L.S.
    Technology Coordinator
    National Network of Libraries of Medicine
    Southeastern/Atlantic Region (NN/LM-SE/A)

Brian D. Westra, M.S.I.
    Head Librarian
    Hazardous Waste Management Program
    Seattle, WA

Robert Young, M.A.
    Webmaster, Founder and President Phoenix5
    <http://www.phoenix5.org/>

About the Editors

P. F. ANDERSON

Patricia Anderson has been the Head Librarian for the University of Michigan (Ann Arbor) Dentistry Library since 1998. In this role, she consulted with the National Institutes of Health (NIH) as an expert searcher for the NIH Consensus Development Conference on Diagnosis and Management of Dental Caries, and is currently serving on the Program Planning Committee for the forthcoming NIH-sponsored working conference "Dental Informatics and Dental Research: Making the Connection." Patricia regularly serves as a member of an international instructional team on evidence-based dentistry, systematic reviews, and meta-analytic methodologies. She applies a similar searching conceptual approach to her instructional, consulting, and research activities related to Internet searching.

Prior to her work with the University of Michigan, Patricia served as the Head of the Galter Health Sciences Library, Barnes Learning Resource Center, Chicago. During her tenure there, Patricia was the first chair of the HealthWeb Design Working Group, coordinating interface and design resources for the HealthWeb multi-institution project and serving on their Board of Directors for five years. She uses conceptual models much like those in these books in her instructional, consulting, and research activities.

NANCY J. ALLEE

Nancy J. Allee is Director of Public Health Informatics Services and Access (PHISA) at the University of Michigan. In this position she oversees the library, instructional technology, online learning, outreach, and Web services for the School of Public Health. She holds a B.A. in English literature from DePauw University (Greencastle, IN), an M.L.S. from Indiana University, and an M.P.H. from the University of Oklahoma. She is a fellow in the National Library of Medicine (NLM)/Association of Academic Health Sciences Libraries leadership program, chair of the Public Health Training Subcommittee of the Partners in Information Access for the Public Health Workforce, a past chair of the Public Health/Health Administration Section of the Medical Library Association, a distinguished member of the Academy of Health Information Professionals (AHIP), and a recipient of the Agent for Cooperative Efforts (ACE) Award from the University of Michigan Library.

About the Medical Library Association

The Medical Library Association, founded in 1898, is an educational organization of more than 1,100 institutions and 3,600 individual members in the health sciences information field, committed to educating health information professionals, supporting health information research, promoting access to the world's health sciences information, and working to ensure that the best health information is available to all.

Cumulative Index

For lists of topics included on a specific disease, such as varieties of cancers discussed, readers should use the table of contents. Use the index for exact terminology, such as retinopathy or sigmoidoscopy or ibuprofen, with cross references and suggested alternate terms on the referenced pages and at the chapter level. See the Searching Instructions at the beginning of each volume for more detail.

N